To my mother, with love, gratitude & mostly joy

Praise for CONSCIOUS HEALING: BOOK ONE ON THE REGENETICS METHOD ...

"CONSCIOUS HEALING is one of the most important books I have ever read ... From Mr. Luckman's own personal, debilitating illness to discovery and transformation, we are brought to extraordinary levels of understanding."

—Andrea Garvey, Publisher, CREATIONS MAGAZINE

"In this paradigm-reworking book, author Sol Luckman develops the concept of 'Ener-genetics,' a synthesis of age-old and new-age wisdom with a sound- and light-based technology that has huge potential for human evolution and self-enlightenment ... This is revolutionary healing science that's expanding the boundaries of being."

—NEXUS NEW TIMES

"A welcome addition to personal, professional, and academic library Alternative Medicine reference collections, CONSCIOUS HEALING is to be given high praise for its remarkable coverage of the many intricacies of Regenetics and its progressive discovery, and is very highly recommended to all seeking an education on alternative self-healing procedures."

—Midwest Book Review

CONSCIOUS HEALING might "be the key that unlocks a new way of being."

—ODYSSEY MAGAZINE, Editor's Choice Book

ALSO BY SOL LUCKMAN

NONFICTION

Conscious Healing: Book One on the Regenetics Method

FICTION

Snooze: A Story of Awakening

HUMOR

The Angel's Dictionary: A Spirited Glossary for the Little Devil in You

POTENTIATE YOUR DNA

A PRACTICAL GUIDE TO HEALING & TRANSFORMATION WITH THE REGENETICS METHOD

Sol Luckman

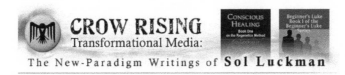

CROW RISING
Transformational Media:
The New-Paradigm Writings of **Sol Luckman**

POTENTIATE YOUR DNA: A PRACTICAL GUIDE TO HEALING &
TRANSFORMATION WITH THE REGENETICS METHOD

First Edition printed in 2010 by Crow Rising Transformational Media through Lulu Enterprises, Inc., 3101 Hillsborough Street, Raleigh, North Carolina USA 27607

http://stores.lulu.com/solluckman

ISBN: 978-0-9825983-1-3

Library of Congress Control Number: 2010936142

Library of Congress Cataloging in Publication Division, 101 Independence Avenue, SE, Washington, DC 20540-4320

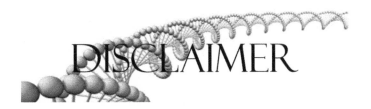

DISCLAIMER

Performing your own, or another's, in-person or distance Potentiation implies your tacit acknowledgement that you have read, understood and agreed to the terms contained in the Potentiation Consent Form found in Appendix B.

The reader understands that the author of *Potentiate Your DNA* and the developers of the Regenetics Method are not engaged herein in making medical claims or providing advice, recommendations, protocols, techniques or services designed to diagnose, prevent or treat illness of any kind.

Where the term *medicine* is used in relation to Potentiation or Regenetics, as in "Era III medicine," it is intended merely philosophically, not as implying the actual practice of medicine on the part of the author or developers.

The author and developers offer the information in *Potentiate Your DNA*, and the reader accepts it, with the understanding that people act on it at their own risk and with full knowledge that they should consult with medical professionals for any medical assistance they need.

The author and developers shall have neither liability nor responsibility to any person or entity with respect to any loss, damage or injury caused, or alleged to be caused, directly or indirectly, by the information provided in this book.

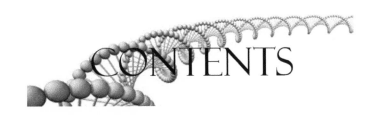

CONTENTS

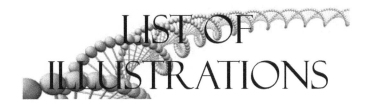

LIST OF ILLUSTRATIONS

IMPORTANT NOTE

All DNA activations in the Regenetics Method employ one or more notes from the ancient Solfeggio scale.

Potentiation Electromagnetic Repatterning, the focus of this book, uses the note "Mi," a frequency (528 Hz.) that has been employed by pioneering researchers to repair genetic defects.

Although some readers will be attracted solely to the leading-edge theoretical and scientific material presented herein, those desirous to "potentiate" themselves will need the Mi tuning fork.

You can order either the single Mi tuning fork or the six-fork original Solfeggio scale from the Phoenix Center for Regenetics at www.phoenixregenetics.org or www.potentiation.net. Our competitively priced tuning forks are of the very highest quality.

If you think that at some point you might pursue Facilitator certification in subsequent levels of the Regenetics Method, which progressively introduce the full Solfeggio, or if you simply desire to experiment with this extraordinary scale, it may be worth considering the whole set of six tuning forks.

Virtually anyone who commits to learning the Potentiation technique can perform this work effectively for him or herself, as well as for others.

If for any reason you are uncomfortable performing your own Potentiation, but still wish to experience this life-changing DNA activation, there are certified Regenetics Method Facilitators throughout the world who would be happy to do it for you— remotely or in person.

A complete and regularly updated list of certified Facilitators grouped by country is available at www.phoenixregenetics.org and www.potentiation.net.

Finally, while Potentiate Your DNA *is designed for individuals with no knowledge of the Regenetics Method, those with prior experience of Potentiation or other Regenetics activations stand to benefit greatly from reading this book.*

"The heart of the discipline
of the personality is
threefold. One, know your
self. Two, accept your self.
Three, become the Creator."
— The Law of One

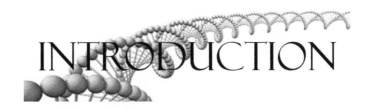

INTRODUCTION

Illness as a Teacher

It has been said by many people in many ways that illness—whether physical, mental, emotional, or spiritual—can be a valuable teacher. In my case, this observation proved absolutely true.

My nearly decade-long chronic autoimmune illness was a stern and sobering mentor, matriculating me through a veritable shamanic initiation of (near) death and rebirth, from which I emerged both a wiser and humbler man.

Wiser, in that the "crash course" I enrolled in during my self-healing tutorial that began in earnest in 2002—involving liberal doses of new science and metaphysics—led to such a novel understanding of human nature that during this terrifying and exhilarating period when I thought I was dying, I often felt like a different person each morning when I awoke.

Humbler, in that having been athletic to the point of cockiness my whole life, as well as something of a know-it-all in my chosen field of study (literature), I was reminded consistently of how dead wrong I had been about so many things.

Specifically, I was forced to admit how little I actually knew about reality and the way *the universe is only material as an afterthought, being fundamentally structured on and operating through consciousness.*

Thus in all ways, as I elaborate in Book One on the Regenetics Method, my initiatory education through and beyond disease was one of *Conscious Healing.*

Today, nearly five years after the initial publication of that bestselling book that has been translated into multiple languages, having personally facilitated the Regenetics Method for thousands of clients worldwide and taught it to many students, it is time to share the first phase of this uniquely empowering work, Potentiation, with you.

May learning, performing and perhaps offering Potentiation to your family, friends and even pets be as filled with daily miracles as was my own healing and transformational experience of this powerful "ener-genetic" activation.

What Is Potentiation?

Potentiation Electromagnetic Repatterning is the first of four integrated DNA activations, performed on a specific minimum Timeline explained in Part III, that make up the Regenetics Method. Additional information on the second, third and fourth phases of this work also is provided in Part III.

As detailed hereafter, Potentiation employs specific sound and light codes—produced vocally and mentally—to stimulate a self-healing and transformational potential in DNA.

The Potentiation session initiates a progressive repatterning designed to "reset" your bioenergy fields, which serve as the blueprint for your body-mind-spirit and, as such, when distorted by trauma or toxicity (or both), can induce dysfunctions of various kinds.

By "resetting" the bioenergy blueprint, Potentiation facilitates an integrated, manageable release of often deeply held traumas and toxins while establishing a higher harmonic resonance with life-enhancing "torsion" energy.

Just as crucially, Potentiation also transforms the bioenergetic disruption known as the *Fragmentary Body* through a process called *sealing*.

Central to true healing, or "wholing," sealing the Fragmentary Body enhances one's sense of unity consciousness and, by itself, can lead to tangible and lasting improvement. The critically important notion of the Fragmentary Body is discussed at various points throughout this text.

Initiated by a single thirty-minute session, which can be performed in person but often is done remotely, as explained, the entire Potentiation process takes just over nine months (forty-two weeks, or a "gestation cycle") to unfold.

To the best of my knowledge, such a remarkable "rebirth," set in motion by one short session that requires neither repeating nor reenergizing, is unique in the world of energy healing.

In addition, this process of recalibration charts a highly specific pattern through the bioenergy blueprint. We will explore the nature and experience of this profound bio-spiritual metamorphosis in much greater detail as we go along.

Benefits of Potentiation

Since my partner Leigh and I first began to offer Potentiation to clients back in 2003, we have received reports of a variety of benefits spanning the body-mind-spirit continuum. Some of these benefits have been subtle, while others have been quite dramatic.

The most common reported benefits include:

Allergy Elimination

Enhanced Energy

Parasite Cleansing

Pain Relief

Physical Strengthening

Improved Respiration

Better Digestion

Sharper Thinking

Deeper Sleep

Straighter Posture

Healthier Urination

Regular Stools

Stronger Immunity

Clearer Skin

Thicker Hair

Fewer Migraines

Clearer Boundaries

Healthier Relationships

Increased Serendipity

Heightened Manifestation

Greater Abundance

I share some of my own remarkable benefits from Potentiation toward the end of Part I. Also, a selection of categorized Testimonials from clients who have experienced Potentiation concludes Part II.

What This Book Is & Is Not

Divided into three sections, this book is designed to assist you, step by step, in understanding (Part I), performing (Part II) and integrating (Part III) an apparently simple, but potentially reality-altering DNA activation for yourself—and maybe others.

Throughout, I expand on the perhaps foreign (for some) concept of DNA activation. I trust you will find this material, if not essential to experiencing and benefiting from Potentiation, content-rich and thought-provoking.

I wish to clarify from the outset that *this is not a book primarily concerned with science.* You do not have to be a scientist or student of science to grasp and implement the self-empowering tools I have to share.

Rather, *Potentiate Your DNA* is about a singularly potent type of energy healing—one that I contend operates simultaneously at the genetic and energetic levels. Thus my regular use of the term *ener-genetic* to describe many aspects of Regenetics.

In Part I, I provide a clear and concise conceptual framework for how DNA activation functions. But as they say, "the proof is in the pudding."

We can discuss Potentiation forever—but the only meaningful way to "prove" that Potentiation works is to experience it yourself. Insisting on wrapping your "left brain" around every detail is, in the final analysis, like anything over-intellectualized, counterproductive.

If you are the type of person who feels intimidated by the mere mention of DNA, know this: I used to be, too.

In the interest of accessibility, I have stripped the intellectual material contained herein down to the bare bones while making sure to include enough personal narrative to move the story along.

I recommend that you get all you can out of Part I; then put it behind you as you focus on mastering your Potentiation technique in Part II; before turning your attention to integrating and maximizing the energies of Potentiation with the help of Part III.

This is also not a book about music or musicology. You do not have to be a musician or have studied music to master Potentiation. While you will be learning a form of sound healing, you do not have to be able to read music or be blessed with perfect pitch to perform and benefit from this work.

If you are a sound healer or have prior experience with sound healing, I encourage you to release any preconceptions as to what Potentiation "should" sound like while engaging this deceptively simple work with an ongoing attitude of openness and experimentation.

In addition, *this is not a book that advocates a predetermined lifestyle change*. You do not need to devote any more time to this work than the amount it takes to read this material, thoroughly and thoughtfully, and "potentiate" yourself.

Nor do you need to meditate regularly, repeat mantras, use affirmations, do yoga or adopt a special diet to heal and transform your life with Potentiation. You do not even have to believe in this "kind of stuff" for it to unfold in extraordinary ways.

On the other hand, you do need to:

1. Be open to your own healing;

2. Listen to your heart's wisdom; and

3. Allow your life to transform naturally as your everyday existence becomes more and more a living meditation.

This process typically occurs as "potentiators" find themselves increasingly present in the Now and releasing those things which do not contribute to the embodiment and manifestation of their potential.

Also, for those concerned with such things, *this is not a book about 2012, the Mayan calendar, or related topics*. I write in detail on these subjects in *Conscious Healing*—where I propose that humanity is undergoing a massive and positive Shift in consciousness, a metamorphosis into a more enlightened way of being that can be promoted by Potentiation and the Regenetics Method.

But Potentiation's ability to activate you to higher levels of consciousness and wellbeing really has nothing to do with whether anything "out of the ordinary" happens around the end of 2012, whether you suddenly wake up to find yourself in a completely new reality, or wake up in your old bed.

As many recipients of Potentiation have attested, for those open to healing and transformation without drugs or therapies, DNA activation truly is "strong medicine."

Indeed, because they can be so effective in addressing a range of issues that traditional "materialistic" approaches cannot begin to unravel, ener-genetic modalities—especially those focused on the revolutionary potential of consciousness—are fast becoming the medicine of the future in the here and now.

Finally, to be perfectly clear, *you do not have to have read Book One on the Regenetics Method to potentiate yourself,* although you may find it helpful to read it before, during or after your Potentiation process.

What Is Conscious Healing?

Here, I am calling attention to the concept, not the book. One of the foundational ideas behind Potentiation and the Regenetics Method can be summarized:

Consciousness not only is primary to matter; it also gives rise to and modifies matter, including human genetics and physiology, through a process that is energetic in nature.

The hyperdimensional, generative energy to which I refer—dubbed *torsion* energy in literally thousands of scientific studies conducted mainly in Russia—can be understood as *universal creative consciousness.*

The two principal manifestations of this consciousness, both of which are capable of operating instantaneously at a distance, or "nonlocally," are *sound* and *light* (Figures 1 and 4). These closely related types of torsion energy are employed synergistically in all Regenetics activations.

Whether you realize it or not, you have heard of torsion energy before. When the Book of John opens with the statement "In the beginning was the Word," the Word referenced is torsion energy.

In this instance, the Creator employs the Word, which is pure torsion energy in the form of sound waves, to create (and subsequently develop) the light-based material world—human biology included.

The biblical story of Genesis (read: genetic origin) according to John, which finds parallels in virtually all religions and wisdom traditions throughout the world, specifies that:

1. The universe literally was *spoken* into being; and

2. Language, embodied in sound and light, not only *affects*, but *effects* the genesis of life.

The related new sciences of genetic linguistics and wave-genetics have established beyond any reasonable doubt that universal creative consciousness, or torsion energy, gives rise to and evolves DNA through an inherently linguistic interface.

This revolutionary research, which proves that the basic storyline of creation in the Bible and many other ancient cosmologies is far more than myth, further implies that *we ourselves can employ linguistically energized torsion consciousness to activate DNA and promote healing and transformation.*

In the case of Potentiation, as explained in Part I and taught in Part II, this ener-genetic activation is prompted by specific combinations of vowel-based "words."

To Your Potential!

I will conclude this brief Introduction by returning to you, the reader, because *Potentiate Your DNA* is nothing if not about teaching you to promote your own conscious healing and personal evolution.

We can talk theory ad infinitum, but this book is really about *practice*—the practice of activating your potential to become and live your true and authentic self.

On this subject, allow me to offer a bit of friendly advice from one who has walked this path and assisted many others in walking it.

Read this book thoroughly, enjoying the story of the development of Potentiation in Part I—but paying particular attention to Part II so that you perform your Potentiation correctly, and Part III so that you get the most out of this work.

Then, go live your passion(s) with all the joy, gratitude, laughter and love you can muster!

This is not merely superficial advice and, appearances notwithstanding, does not have its roots in "new age" philosophy, the Law of Attraction, the Power of Now, or anything of the sort.

Instead, this advice is based on scientific experiments by cell biologist Glen Rein proving that positive emotions benefit DNA, making DNA stronger, healthier and—it stands to reason—more available to activation through linguistically expressed consciousness.

On the other hand, feelings such as fear and anger can do considerable harm to DNA so that it is less available for activation through consciousness.

Let me emphasize that I am far from judging so-called negative emotions, as we all experience them from time to time. It does nobody, least of all ourselves, any good pointing the proverbial finger at the mirror during our moments of inadequacy—and may even do us considerable harm.

The best we can do, when we inevitably slip up, is to follow the time-honored wisdom of "forgive and forget," allowing ourselves to reengage life-affirming attitudes that, based on hard science, ener-genetically promote our healing and the realization of our innate potential.

To yours!

—Sol Luckman

July 2010

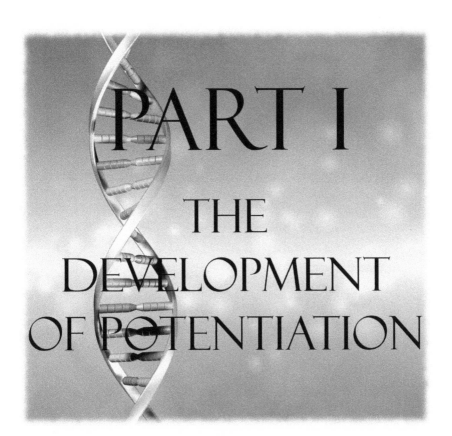

PART I

THE
DEVELOPMENT
OF POTENTIATION

CHAPTER 1
The Fires of Initiation

Since 2003, when Leigh and I performed the first memorable Potentiation on ourselves while living in Brazil and soon thereafter began offering it to clients, we have fielded literally thousands of questions on all aspects of the Regenetics Method.

Many of these questions have been of an intellectual nature, asked with a desire for greater understanding of the philosophical and scientific principles behind this unique DNA activation technique.

Other questions have sought greater clarity relative to how Regenetics sessions are performed, the Timeline for Regenetics activations (Figure 19), or how to interpret the many possible unfoldments occasioned by Potentiation or other phases of the Regenetics Method.

As a service to readers with similar questions, I have endeavored to address as many aspects of this work as possible in these pages. A number of remaining questions that did not fit into the main text are answered in the FAQ in Appendix A.

In addition, recipients of Potentiation, including "self-potentiators" who have learned and performed this DNA activation for themselves using this book, are encouraged to join the Regenetics Method Forum online.

Rather than via individual correspondence with the Phoenix Center for Regenetics, the Regenetics Method Forum is the place to ask any outstanding questions about Potentiation you might have after reading *Potentiate Your DNA*.

On the Forum, many far-ranging subjects relative to this work are discussed. Membership guidelines and registration instructions are available at **www.phoenixregenetics.org** and **www.potentiation.net**.

Over the years, perhaps the single most common question Leigh and I have fielded—one having little to do with mental understanding—has stemmed mostly from plain curiosity and goes something like this:

How in the world did you guys come up with Potentiation in the first place?

This question, which I never have answered fully in writing, requires more than a brief summary. Now, in Part I it is my pleasure and honor to share the extraordinary story of the development of Potentiation with you.

In this chapter, I elaborate on my personal initiation involving a mysterious and potentially life-threatening autoimmune disease that ultimately was resolved by Potentiation.

Over the course of the following chapters, I flesh out my personal story with an account of the steps leading up to Potentiation and how this DNA activation helped me regain my physical strength and stamina; rid myself of debilitating nutritional and environmental allergies; and begin a new life as a healing innovator.

The Golden Boy Syndrome

To grasp the level of desperation that was necessary for Potentiation to be born, how it was only by finding myself at the bottom that I was able to surrender and get out of my own way enough to let this radical work flow through, it is necessary to paint a picture of the Olympian height from which I so suddenly and unexpectedly had fallen.

I used to be perfect. I mean that in a tongue-in-cheek way. To an outside observer, I appeared to have my act completely together.

Ever since high school, when I played first-team quarterback for the varsity, graduated first in my class and was the first ever from my rural Southern county to be awarded arguably the nation's most prestigious undergraduate scholarship, I had been destined, it seemed, for worldly success.

Nothing about my collegiate career, in which I majored in literature and graduated at the top of my scholarship class, appeared to contradict this Hollywood script for my glorious destiny.

Nor did what happened next as I won a Fulbright award, received an Ivy League doctoral-student fellowship, and was selected for two coveted national research grants in the humanities.

Meanwhile, I was the picture of health. Having declined a chance to play Division I football to pursue my academic path, in order to stay fit I had devoted myself to basketball, often playing three hours a day—to the point that I more than held my own against the varsity players at the university where I was working on my doctorate.

Little did I suspect, as I went about my ostensibly perfect existence, powered by no small ego, largely oblivious to the world of spirit and often ignoring my heart's wisdom in favor of a predominantly mental approach to life, that *true health is more than a material state of being.*

But to paraphrase Jim Morrison, our pale reason often hides our infinite potential from us. Certainly, I had no consciousness of the fact that my Golden Boy Syndrome was just that: an unhealthy façade that needed to be broken through if ever I was to access the real me and fulfill my true calling.

Breakdown & Breakthrough

In stating that my fake veneer of wellbeing needed to be broken through for genuine healing to take place, I mean that as literally as you possibly can imagine.

Initially, however, my nightmarish experience of emotional trauma and genetic collapse that initiated—and initiated me, spiritually speaking—in 1995 resembled anything but a teaching tool, guided by my Higher Self, designed to wake me up from what Ken Carey calls the "spell of matter" to a knowledge of my authentic nature as a bio-spiritual being with a divine purpose.

Since that time, through working with so many clients who came to Regenetics with a similar sense of desperation, and watching so many utilize Potentiation and subsequent levels of this Method to better their lives beyond anything recognizable from the perspective of their starting point, I have been blessed repeatedly to witness a profound truth in action:

Breakdown is often a precondition for breakthrough.

In Chinese, in fact, the same word for "crisis," *wei-chi*, also can be understood to mean "dangerous opportunity."

That breakthrough often requires breakdown does not mean, necessarily, that something of a physical nature (such as an illness) must occur as we wake up to the fact that, to paraphrase a famous quote by Pierre Teilhard de Chardin, *we are not human beings on a spiritual journey, but spiritual beings on a human journey.*

Just as there are many types of people, there are many varieties of wake-up calls to our greater life in spirit.

The growing literature on this subject, exemplified in the writings of Carl Jung and often told from a first-person perspective, reveals an astonishing creative methodology on the part of the Higher Self when endeavoring to remind us of our authentic nature and purpose—the "why we came here in the first place" aspect of our existence.

For some the initiatory fires come in the form of financial distress. For others initiation involves divorce or loss of a loved one. Still others experience mental illness, emotional wounding or spiritual crisis as spurs to conscious evolution.

But lest the reader think that only tragedy can foster spiritual development, let me be clear that, for many, "breakdown" takes the far more benign (if for that reason, more ambiguous) form of an inner knowing that something is missing ... that life must be more ... that there has to be a *reason* why we are here.

At the risk of sounding like a party pooper to those who might be influenced by certain proponents of the Law of Attraction who at times appear to offer quick fixes with less than pure motivations, it must be stated that *manifestation of a higher spiritual and material reality is usually neither easy nor immediately forthcoming when we embark on our initiatory path.*

There are also numerous energetic modalities that make similar promises of instantaneous healing. While this may be theoretically possible, and even appropriate for some, many clients of Regenetics have "been there, done that," with less than satisfying results.

The real Secret so many people do not arrive at their destination by steering down such supposedly straightforward avenues is that the intention of their Higher Self is not to experience a "miracle healing" in the blink of an eye, without explanation and engendering little understanding.

Instead, the intention is to utilize initiation as a catalyst for an inward journey that teaches love—for self and others—and imparts compassion and wisdom as prerequisites for healing and enlightenment.

The foregoing sentence contains the essence of what I call *conscious personal mastery*, which the Regenetics Method was created to encourage as explained in Part III.

If true healing were otherwise, if healing were simply a synonym for *curing*, alleviating symptoms, and had nothing to do with increasing consciousness, you would not be reading this book because it would not have been written.

But healing, as I define it based on experience and observation, is much more than curing. When engaged consciously, *healing often pushes us through the fires of initiation so that we might be transformed and become purer vessels for spirit to flow through in service.*

While we are on this subject, there is absolutely no guarantee that our desired manifestation of healing and transformation will occur, in this lifetime anyway, as despite embracing the initiatory experience in good faith, some people simply do not survive it.

There are also some individuals who achieve transformation without visible healing, as my mother did during her own inspiring experience of conscious dying. During the last month of her life, many of those who knew her best felt that everything about her was transformed—with the exception of her body.

Faced with such unpleasant—and certainly, inconvenient—truths, we would do well to ask ourselves:

If there is any validity to the notion that life is a classroom where our core curriculum centers on learning the lessons of love (for ourselves as well as others), how could such conscious personal mastery be fostered if we never really had to study because our teacher always assured us of a passing grade in our tests?

This analogy encapsulates our student-teacher relationship with our Higher Self, including the "tough love" and "kicks to the backside" we often receive as spurs to our spiritual evolution.

Fortunately, many people, myself included, "live to tell about it," having passed their initiatory tests and—despite a variety of challenges—graduated into personal realities that are much more in alignment with their soul's purpose.

In criticizing the lure of instant gratification of many contemporary spirituality and healing philosophies, I am far from suggesting that miracles do not happen. They most certainly do, all the time.

Many children, thanks to living so much in their imagination, understand that everyday miracles are the norm. The problem is that *as we grow older, we can become so caught up in our personal—and sometimes collective— dramas that we fail to recognize miracles when they occur.*

This phenomenon, which Leigh and I observe on a regular basis with clients, can be rather humorous.

While a majority of our clients have felt and often taken time to express gratitude for the many breakthroughs this work has helped them achieve, and a small minority have perceived little benefit from Regenetics, with a third group we tend to dialogue to this effect:

Client: "I had my Potentiation six months ago, and I just don't know if it's working."

Us: "That's understandable. Sometimes the effects can be subtle. How's your insomnia that you mentioned in a previous email?"

Client: "Well, it's a lot better, come to think of it."

Us: "Great. How are you getting along with your husband these days? We recall things weren't going too smoothly when you first started this process."

Client: "You know, we went through a rocky period just after my session. But things are much better now. Thanks for asking."

Us: "Fantastic. You're welcome. How are those terrible allergies to wheat and dairy these days?"

Client: "You know, they were pretty bad for a while. But now they're gone. I'm eating whatever I like. Do you think maybe this has something to do with Potentiation?"

Breakdown and breakthrough. This is a central dynamic of initiation in general, and often a prominent feature before and during the sequence of Regenetics activations.

The better we understand this dynamic, and the more we engage our personal evolution consciously, the faster manifestation of our potential can occur.

As we powerfully activate our DNA and embark on our evolutionary journey, which is bound to have its ups and downs, it is vital that we grasp the cyclical aspect of true healing.

I like to call healing *wholing*. And I regularly remind people that this process typically has a way of ushering us through darkness on our way to the light.

From a spiritual viewpoint, *this journey can be envisioned as one from stagnation to transformation.* And it always helps to keep our eyes peeled for signs that we are on the right path—whether these manifest as a seemingly insignificant serendipity or an unmistakable miracle.

Dark Night of the Soul: Part One

The phrase "dark night of the soul" stems from the writings of Saint John of the Cross, a Spanish Catholic priest in the 16th Century, being the name of one of his poems and its commentary on mystical development and the stages one passes through on the way to reunion with the Creator.

In popular parlance, *dark night of the soul* has come to signify the aftermath of any serious breakdown—whether physical, mental, emotional, or spiritual.

My own dark night of the soul took the form of a body-mind-spirit initiation of the most deadly serious kind that, in retrospect, I should have seen coming as early as the summer of 1995—when I took a leave of absence from graduate school and first traveled to Rio de Janeiro for dissertation research.

I was tremendously excited at the prospect of spending five months in Brazil practicing Portuguese and studying Brazilian fiction, but also entertained mixed feelings since my girlfriend of four years had elected to remain behind.

We had decided to maintain a long-distance relationship; and being something of a romantic at heart, I was naïve enough to think this was a good idea.

I immediately fell in love—not with another woman, but with Rio, a city unlike any other which later, looking back on its sun-splashed, samba-filled backdrop out of the unspeakable bleakness of illness, I wrote about nostalgically in my seriocomic novel series, *Beginner's Luke*.

In the meantime, back in the United States my girlfriend also was falling in love—not with a city, but with another man. This emotionally devastating fact I learned hardly a month into my first visit to the Cidade Maravilhosa.

Another strange thing happened right about this time that helped set the stage for my dark night of the soul. On a visit to a remote Atlantic island, I apparently managed to contract the parasite that causes a theoretically incurable type of sleeping sickness known as Chagas' disease, which according to some killed Charles Darwin.

The odds of this happening to a twentieth-century tourist like myself staying in well-maintained lodgings were slim at best. In hindsight, I interpret this weird twist as yet another log thrown on the fires of my initiation by my Higher Self.

In the final book of *Beginner's Luke, Morphametosis,* I offer a fictional account of the intense recurring fevers I experienced after contracting *mal de Chagas,* which some say kills over a hundred thousand people a year in South America alone.

Thankfully, after Potentiation and the Regenetics Method, three different forms of energy-based diagnostics have failed to detect even a trace of this parasite in my system.

While I can make no medical claims as to a causal relationship, "sealing" the Fragmentary Body, which occurs at around the five-month mark following the Potentiation session, often appears to "squeeze out" all types of parasites—without recourse to pharmaceuticals, supplements, special diets, or energy devices.

Clients of Potentiation have been known to contact Leigh and myself along these lines:

Client: "I just went to my naturopath for a routine checkup, and she said I was full of parasites!"

Us: "Interesting. How far are you into your Potentiation?"

Client: "About seven months. How can I be full of parasites? I thought Potentiation was supposed to raise my personal frequency so that this kind of thing wouldn't happen!"

Us: "We believe it does. If you don't mind our asking, what are your stools like these days?"

Client: "Oh, they're copious. I go two or three times a day."

Us: "Do they look at all ... strange?"

Client: "Yes, now that you mention it. They're really ... shaggy."

Us: "How do they smell?"

Client: "Awful. Just terrible. Like nothing I've ever smelled. Do you think maybe I'm starting to release old parasites?"

Our theory is that the Fragmentary Body, which is associated with the second bioenergy field from the bottom and related sex *chakra* (Figures 3, 5, and 10a), constitutes an ener-genetic disruption that allows us to take on parasites—physical ones, etheric "entities," and even "parasitic" people—in the first place.

By sealing the Fragmentary Body, which occurs roughly five months into Potentiation, we repattern our bioenergy blueprint so that parasites (of all types) encountering us find it difficult to gain a foothold in our systems. Thus external parasites might be repelled, while internal ones can be weakened and gradually expelled.

The observable phenomenon of detoxification that regularly occurs over the weeks and months following Potentiation applies not just to parasites, but to other nasty pathogens, such as those introduced under the radar of the immune system through "immunizations."

In addition, detoxification can—and often does—include heavy metals, pesticides, solvents and even residue from old hormones, histamines and neurotransmitters that team up with pathogens to compromise health and wellbeing.

The bad news is that while not everyone experiences detoxification following Potentiation, a significant percentage of people attracted to this work are more compromised by toxicity than they ever would have suspected.

In my own admittedly extreme case, to indulge in a moment of embarrassingly honest indelicacy, I spent the first few months following my Potentiation releasing insanely fluorescent green stools I called the Swamp Thing.

The good news is that through DNA activation, we *can* release these highly toxic elements that typically end up killing other people, sooner or later.

On this note, the suggestion by some new age writers that toxins simply "go dormant" or are "transmuted" entirely during our conscious evolution makes little sense, either experientially or philosophically.

From the perspective of conscious personal mastery, *toxins are teachers designed to be felt coming out, to some degree, so that we might learn from our own dysfunctional creations in the past.*

The detoxification process is not always easy, and rarely pretty, but it usually is manageable. And when it passes, people often notice fewer allergies, the disappearance of a chronic rash, healthier hair, greater energy, or some other undeniable sign that something positive has transpired.

And even when there is no external indication immediately forthcoming, releasing pathogens and toxins leaves most people feeling cleaner, clearer, and happier.

Dark Night of the Soul: Part Two

Certainly, my inevitable breakup with my girlfriend, involving cutting my stay in Rio short and returning to my hometown to regroup, combined with contracting a serious parasite that attacks—of all things—the heart, were important ingredients in my personal recipe for disaster. But they were not the key ingredient.

The proverbial straw that broke the camel's back already was at work in my system before I ever traveled to Brazil, although at the time I did not know it.

In my mind's eye, I often visualize my feet in basketball sneakers strolling along the sidewalk to the university health clinic. This was where in the spring of 1995 I received the hepatitis and yellow fever vaccines that, starting in 1996, wrecked my health and sent me spiraling into the lightless abyss of my dark night of the soul.

Almost overnight, during my second year of leave of absence during which I was attempting to pull myself together again, my life exploded into a thousand pieces like a wine glass hitting the floor.

Inexplicably, at the time anyway, I developed devastating food and environmental allergies, extreme chronic fatigue, bizarre muscle twitching, facial neuralgia, awful bloating, terrible insomnia, horrific migraines, and twenty-odd other mysterious symptoms that baffled every doctor and therapist I visited—and I visited many.

The only straightforward medical diagnosis I received was as unhelpful as it was meaningless: "depression." Naturally, I was depressed. But I knew perfectly well that was not what had *initiated* my undeniable physical deterioration.

The main reason Regenetics avoids the negative diagnostic model, the centerpiece of allopathic medicine, is that diagnosis played absolutely no role in my own healing or that of many recipients of Potentiation and the Regenetics Method who have shared their inspiring stories.

In fact, more often than not diagnosis is the "kiss of death," bestowed by a so-called medical authority, that negates our justified belief in our natural ability to heal ourselves.

According to some statistics, *medical diagnosis is off the mark more than ninety percent of the time*—in many thousands of cases resulting in unnecessary, doctor-induced fatalities.

That said, of course there are instances when allopathic medicine is entirely appropriate. We would not want carpenters setting broken bones or electricians performing emergency brain surgery.

But with many, even most conditions, *diagnosis is useless mental baggage of a negatively oriented nature that, if our interest truly is in healing, we would do well to jettison in favor of a medical model that focuses positively on the ever-present possibility of sustained wellbeing.*

I relate the story of my rapid decline and panicked attempts at saving myself through hundreds of mostly ineffective therapies, "miracle cures" and the like in *Conscious Healing,* where I also cite a wealth of research proving that *vaccines potentially cause genetic damage resulting in a variety of autoimmune conditions running the gamut from lupus to AIDS.*

There is no doubt in my mind that, while I never tested positive for HIV, my illness, which involved disturbing fluctuations in my white blood cell count and a number of immunological problems such as systemic Candidiasis like that often observed in AIDS patients, had many similarities to AIDS—starting with the fact that it was induced by vaccines.

I often have asked myself why I chose to get vaccinated before my trip to Brazil, other than the fact that my travel guidebook recommended it, when there was already so much literature warning of the risks of vaccines that far outweigh the potential rewards.

But like many people, having swallowed the dubious logic of contemporary medical dogma hook, line and sinker, I simply neglected to do my homework.

I encourage skeptics to do their own homework on the subject of vaccines before subjecting themselves or their loved ones to this type of antiquated barbarism.

Autism has been regularly linked, unlinked and linked again (depending on which authors you read and whether they have ties to pharmaceutical companies) to vaccinations for years.

Throughout 2009 there was tremendous global opposition—from individuals as well as whole unions of medical workers—to the swine flu vaccine.

This vaccine, which the World Health Organization pushed to be included in regular seasonal flu vaccines, has been associated with a killer nerve disease called Guillain-Barre Syndrome (GBS).

Yet although this is undeniably the case, and swine flu before predictably petering out proved to be no more dangerous than normal flu, a fact even the Centers for Disease Control and Prevention admitted publicly, the medical-pharmaceutical establishment ratcheted up the fear for a year in an attempt to scare the population into being vaccinated.

What was really going on here? David Wilcock summed up at least part of the underlying rationale wittily in the title to one of his blogs: "Swine Flu + Mainstream Media = $$$."

Sure enough, the *Washington Post* later accused the WHO of 1) greatly exaggerating the H1N1 threat and, even more alarmingly, 2) having financial ties to two manufacturers of antiviral medications used against the swine flu virus.

In the words of the creators of one of dozens of websites devoted to telling the ugly truth about vaccines, "The most effective marketing strategy on the planet is to convince the consumer that if he doesn't buy the product, he'll die!"

This same website, which unfortunately went down shortly before publication of this book, contained a wonderful graphic showing how epidemic statistics traditionally have been made to lie.

If you just read the bottom of the graph, it appeared that vaccines were responsible for stopping particular deadly diseases. This interpretation is taught in our medical schools. But the whole picture suggested that the diseases went into decline all by themselves—prior to introduction of vaccines!

Moreover, many reputable studies have offered convincing evidence based on historical data that in all probability, *vaccinations actually trigger a rise in infections and death.*

After the polio vaccine became compulsory in the United States in 1959, the four states (Connecticut, North Carolina, Ohio, and Tennessee) and one city (Los Angeles) that kept records showed a marked increase in the incidence of polio in the year *after* mandatory vaccination.

In 1977, according to a number of sources, Dr. Jonas Salk, developer of the first polio vaccine, testified with a panel of other scientists that mass polio inoculation was really the cause of the majority of polio cases in the United States dating back to its introduction.

Make no mistake: we are not talking about just polio vaccine. In the words of former United States Secretary of War Henry Stimson, in one half-year period at an American boot camp, sixty-three deaths and over 25,000 cases of hepatitis occurred as "a direct result of the yellow fever vaccine."

Even as this book was being completed, according to well-known "health ranger" Mike Adams, a mumps outbreak spread among people in New York and New Jersey who recently had been vaccinated against mumps.

While there is no hard scientific data that definitively proves vaccines protect people from anything, there is an overwhelming abundance of information indicating that vaccines cause many diseases.

This is an assertion with which many in the allopathic community would disagree. Yet a growing number of physicians, researchers and epidemiologists—among them, the outspoken medical doctor Joseph Mercola—have reached similar conclusions.

The simple, irrefutable fact is that just because vaccines create an increase in specific antibodies *under a microscope* does not prove, in a *scientific* way, that this translates into effective immunity *in a live human being.*

Many people get positively furious and claim that you are putting them and their children at risk by not vaccinating. Never mind that this is an untenable position, since these same people also believe themselves to be protected by vaccines!

I also understand that, for parents and others, it can be difficult (although by no means, impossible) to navigate in today's world without vaccinating.

But regardless of whether vaccines damage our genetics through insertion of pathogenic genetic (or "pathogenetic") material into our DNA, as suggested by a great deal of research, they remain a highly toxic cocktail—full of mercury (Thimerosol), formaldehyde, squalene and other potent toxins that damage nerves and decrease our natural immunity.

Now, while it is true, and maybe a little scary for some readers, that vaccines nearly killed me, it is also true that over time Potentiation and the Regenetics Method successfully undid the vast majority of my vaccine damage.

It also is worth pointing out that, as explained in Chapter Thirteen, *not all people are damaged equally by vaccines.* If you do not need to take on vaccination fallout as a potential catalyst for spiritual growth, it is highly unlikely that you will.

To Be or Not To Be

Hamlet's famous existential query pretty much sums up the question I asked myself repeatedly starting in 1996, after my Brazil vaccines had had time to wreck my immunity and, so it seemed, destroy everything I had to live for.

Thankfully, in 1997 after researching the detrimental role dental mercury plays in many autoimmune conditions, I experienced a brief respite after I made the decision to have my mercury-containing amalgam ("silver") fillings replaced with benign materials.

Based on my extensive research, considerable personal experience and long-term professional observation, it appears that *for those genetically damaged by vaccines, the body has a greater tendency than normal to retain powerful environmental toxins, such as mercury, in order to slow down the growth of vaccine-induced pathogens at the cellular level.*

This helps explain why some people tend to develop pronounced immunological sensitivities to their toxic dental work—whereas others appear to tolerate whatever experimental materials the dental establishment deems appropriate to affix permanently in human heads.

The genetically modified individual's tendency to hoard externally introduced toxins also sheds light on why such people nearly always develop problems with systemic yeast overgrowth in the form of Candidiasis.

In their case, *Candida albicans*, a toxin-scavenging organism essential to healthy biological function, is trying to clean up the pathogenetic mess that results from the body's self-preserving response to genetic damage. A similar observation relative to Candida's affinity for heavy metals has been made by Dr. Dietrich Klinghardt.

Nevertheless, a popular misconception even in the alternative health community is that Candida is "bad." This is a gross misunderstanding. *When Candida proliferates, it actually is trying to cleanse, not harm, the body.*

This is why restrictive diets (which may be necessary for a period) and even antifungal medications rarely get rid of systemic Candida, which always returns *because it must.*

Fortunately, for those genetically compromised enough to have to put up with them, Candida overgrowth problems are often reported to lessen and even disappear eventually as the body detoxifies during Potentiation and the Regenetics Method.

Not that this was any comfort to me at the nadir of my illness prior to the development of Potentiation, after my brief respite following my new dental work, when whatever ground I had gained in terms of energy and allergies suddenly dissolved as I tumbled like a boulder from the heights of my Golden Boy existence to the very bottom of a mountain of despair.

Before long, owing to crippling allergic reactions involving severe Candidiasis, I lost my ability to eat anything other than meat and vegetables. Drinking wine or beer was totally out of the question.

Additionally, I was forced to stop playing basketball, an activity I loved, because of lack of energy accompanied by musculoskeletal pain and stiffness. I also had to give up swimming (another form of exercise I enjoyed) due to fatigue and sensitivity to chlorine.

As my bizarre symptoms multiplied over the course of 1998 and I became someone I never thought I would be, a "sick person," I found myself losing still other things that mattered to me.

Socially, most of my friends disappeared as it became obvious I was no longer the life of the party. Romantically, I could not keep a steady girlfriend under any circumstances.

Mentally, I started having difficulty thinking clearly for prolonged periods owing to intense "brain fog." After managing to complete my master's degree, I was forced to drop out of graduate school before finishing my dissertation.

At the time, this last loss, that of my envisioned career as a tenured literature professor, felt like the one that might tip the scales of my existential questioning in the direction of opting *not* to be.

But luckily, it had exactly the opposite effect—provoking me, in the middle of my dark night of the soul, to challenge many of my long-held assumptions about reality and embrace extraordinary new possibilities for thinking and being.

I experienced the truth that "the most important thing," to quote Charles Dubois, is "to be able at any moment to sacrifice what we are for what we could become."

In hindsight, leaving the constricting world of mainstream academics was precisely the moment during my initiation when I set myself free to begin pursuing my own path of thought and deed that, step by step, led me back up the mountainside toward a state of genuine wellness.

This state I eventually came to realize not just physically—but also, for the very first time, mentally, emotionally, and spiritually.

CHAPTER 2
Up from the Ashes

In many cultures throughout the world, initiation of young people involves elaborate rites of passage that are typically frightening, sometimes painful, and occasionally dangerous.

Some initiatory paths force initiates to submit to deprivation, abuse, or even bodily mutilation. In certain shamanic traditions, initiates literally are buried alive before being permitted to be "reborn" into their new identities.

Whatever form initiation takes, the basic concept is that you are not the same person afterward, but have transformed into one who is stronger, wiser, and qualified to play a new role—often that of healer—in your community.

Ever since becoming ill in the mid-1990s, I have read a great deal on the subject of initiation, ranging from anthropological studies to the more fanciful (although still insightful) writings of Carlos Castaneda.

The overwhelming impression I have maintained for nearly a decade is that my experience of a serious health crisis, followed by my dark night of the soul, which gave way to inspiration, healing and transformation, meets all the criteria for a genuine spiritual initiation—one perhaps best symbolized by the mythical creature known as the phoenix.

Circa A.D. 170, the phoenix was mentioned by Flavius Philostratus as a bird from India that occasionally migrated to Egypt. Since that time, the legend of the phoenix has grown and changed, but usually the phoenix is described as a large mythical bird.

Near the end of its days, according to legend, the phoenix constructs a nest for itself that spontaneously combusts. Both bird and nest burn to ashes—from which arises a fresh, young bird, reborn and set to embark on a new life cycle.

After Leigh and I performed the first Potentiation on ourselves and my health improved dramatically, we began offering this potent DNA activation to others while evolving our methodology into what eventually became the four-part Regenetics Method.

When it came time to create an online presence in order to share this work with a wider audience, we were drawn naturally to the phoenix, a symbol that perfectly captured my own initiatory "ascension" out of the ashes of my former life. Thus the Phoenix Center for Regenetics was born.

In this chapter, I relate four important, sometimes overlapping stages of my bio-spiritual rebirth that prepared the way for the development of Potentiation. All four of these preparatory experiences played two key roles.

First, each fostered greater awareness on my part of the fundamentally energetic and consciousness-based nature of so-called physical reality.

Second and even more crucially, from my perspective, each of these experiences sustained me energetically through critical phases of my illness when, without them, I believe I would have lacked the vital force to remain alive.

Vision Quest

No sooner had I left graduate school at the end of May, 1998, than I was on my way to a brand-new variety of education that tremendously broadened my horizons—while also imparting much life energy, or *chi* (sometimes spelled *qi*), to my depleted and struggling systems.

Qigong is an ancient technique of energy healing related to tai chi. Through one of my remaining friends, I had been put in contact with a gifted qigong teacher, an American also in his early thirties who, several years previously, had traveled to China to study this venerable art to cure his extreme chronic fatigue syndrome (CFS or CFIDS).

I did not travel to China. But after the yard sale of yard sales, I crammed my scant belongings into my car and spent two days driving nearly twenty-four hours from the East Coast to New Mexico, where my qigong teacher taught a popular class attended by as many as a hundred students three times a week at dawn.

I think of this transitional, challenging and magical period of my life as my own personal "vision quest" that, for the first time, opened my eyes to the often misunderstood and underestimated worlds of spirit and energy.

In many indigenous cultures, the vision quest is the form initiation takes and constitutes the transition from adolescence to adulthood. When the initiate is old enough for vision questing, he (or she) typically spends several days or weeks alone in nature, often while fasting.

Eventually, a particular animal, sometimes called the "totem animal" or "animal medicine," visits the initiate in a dream, vision, or (more rarely) waking state.

The appearance of the totem animal embodying a specific spiritual power indicates the individual's innate calling—which after returning to the tribe, the newly initiated young person pursues following a time of apprenticeship.

Curiously, I did not realize (at least consciously) that I was on any kind of vision quest. To be honest, I did not even know what a vision quest was.

I simply was living like a hermit in the windy, sage-covered high desert; eating the few foods my ravaged immune and digestive systems could tolerate; and practicing qigong often half the day because I intuitively felt I had to in order to survive.

Certainly, I had no awareness of being a shaman in training!

Now, anyone who has ever regularly spent half an hour "hugging the tree," the primary practice in medical qigong, knows two things.

For starters, an enormous amount of bioenergy (chi) is pooled by maintaining this oddly difficult position between standing and squatting, arms loosely draped around an invisible trunk, eyes remaining calmly unfocused on nothing in particular.

The first time I experienced this powerful energy, it literally knocked me on my rear. I lay on the ground outside my rental panting for thirty minutes as waves of electric heat like cosmic hot flashes shook my body again and again.

This was the energy I ultimately used to strengthen myself enough to go on with my life. But I needed an entire summer of practice just to be able to accommodate it gracefully.

The second observation made by serious "tree huggers" is that in that meditative state where you are supposed to think about nothing, sometimes you successfully empty your head. But more often, you think about anything and everything.

Such was my case at first, but then an odd thing started to happen: every time I hugged the tree and aligned myself with the flow of spiritual energy, I thought of crows.

Ever since I was a kid, strangely, I had felt a strong affinity for crows, learning to imitate their caws and always appreciating their presence. But now, whenever I did qigong, crows were all I could think about. Not just that—crows started to appear *everywhere* in my life.

They circled raucously around me as I hugged the tree under the autumnal sky and perched beside me on my porch as I sipped herbal tea and wrote in my journal. Crow statues seemed to appear like weeds, suddenly and uncontrollably, all over my quaint little New Mexican town.

Almost every night, I dreamed of crows. I realized I was into the music of the Counting Crows. And when I started dabbling with watercolors, for the longest time crows were all I wanted to paint.

A fellow student in my qigong class, overhearing me describe my weird fascination with crows, was kind enough to loan me a copy of *Medicine Cards: The Discovery of Power through the Ways of Animals.*

Turning to the section on Crow Medicine, I learned that in many native wisdom traditions, Crow is the totem animal, or "medicine," that "knows the unknowable mysteries of creation," guards holy texts, and upholds the sacred laws of being.

As keeper of the Creator's linguistically based knowledge of creation, as recorded in sacred texts, Crow is gifted with the special ability to modify universal rules and "shape-shift," both personally and collectively.

In other words, Crow's innate talent involves knowing how to manifest new ways of living and being.

When shortly thereafter I was prompted intuitively to read a magazine article (featuring a crow graphic) on vision questing, I realized in an epiphany that for months I had been receiving visits from my totem animal!

Apparently, Crow was trying to tell me through its repeated cawing that my calling involved recalling that I knew something important about creation, holy texts, and sacred law.

Humorously, I visualized myself as a phoenix-crow hybrid, a jet-black bird engulfed in indigo flames, hugging the tree with my wings alight as I stood pooling chi in the middle of my ashes. I actually painted a little watercolor close to this description.

The only problem was, while the phoenix imagery was crystal clear, it was years before I was able to grasp the meaning of the crow part of the picture.

But eventually, as I came to fathom the true nature of DNA—which you will not find in biology textbooks, but will learn more about shortly—while developing Potentiation, I understood why Crow had come to me so insistently.

DNA is the language-based holy text, the sacred law of creation that Crow guards and shape-shifts by calling out its inherent potential through linguistic means.

In fact, as I explain in detail in *Conscious Healing*, the Regenetics Method very well may be an example of a type of ancient healing speech applied to genetics referred to in the Koran as the "Language of the Birds."

The Art of Allowing

Meanwhile, in the lonely and starkly beautiful high desert of northern New Mexico, my apprenticeship in the ways of spirit continued in earnest as winter approached.

It is my belief that the appearance of Crow Medicine during my unwitting vision quest by itself provided me with a much-needed boost of healing energy.

Be that as it may, for the first time I glimpsed—if briefly and inchoately—a foundational truth that would go on to inform every aspect of the Regenetics Method:

Spirit is not just energy, as it currently is understood by most Westerners, but a form of consciousness that underwrites all being.

True healing, which I have called wholing but which also might be described as *transformation*, being fundamentally spiritual in nature, cannot be achieved without activation of higher consciousness through energetic means of one kind or another.

Since everything is a form of conscious energy, including our bodies, activating ourselves ener-getically to raise our consciousness often, if not always, results in physical improvement.

Integrating this higher consciousness, the subject of Part III, requires knowledge and acceptance of the fact that *from the limited perspective of our egos, we really do not control much of anything in our lives.*

To get at this important truth, I often say that "life lives us"—by which I mean something rather different from the old hippy adage to just "go with the flow."

Going with the flow implies a lack of guiding purpose behind our existence, a disposition to let things happen as they may and accept whatever occurs with a detached expression and shrug of the shoulders.

When we acknowledge that *life lives us*, on the other hand, we still are riding the currents of our individual destiny. But if I may reason oxymoronically, by embracing our true purpose and potential as beings embodying particular aspects of Great Spirit, which expresses itself through us, we embrace a decidedly more active role in our personal surrender and service to divine will.

Here, it is important to emphasize that unlike much Eastern spirituality, in no way do I advocate that we suppress, repress or attempt to destroy our egos.

Achieving healing and transformation does not mean that we instantly dissolve back into the primordial soup of Source where we completely lose all sense of individuality.

Rather, genuine wholing involves a willingness to evolve our perception of identity away from a self mired in separation and fragmentation, to an identity rooted in the Self from which all things of a seemingly individual nature flow.

Ken Carey eloquently describes the relationship between spirit and ego: "*For if your ego is a reflection of spirit, then even at its core, your ego is spirit.*" In a healthy state, "both spirit and ego perform their respective roles equally centered in God."

During the healing process, as consciousness increases, Carey explains that

> your sense of self blossoms into an accurate awareness of who you are. This transformed awareness includes your former sense of being one among many, but it also includes an awareness ... rooted in the singularity of Eternal Being from which all individuality unfolds.

Lacking such awareness, you remain "a latent possibility, a programmed product of human culture. You are not truly yourself."

The awakening process, the Shift in consciousness that is fundamental to genuine healing and transformation, can be envisioned as an evolutionary movement from "victim consciousness," in which we see ourselves as separate from the world, to "unity consciousness," in which we realize not just that we are part of the world—but that we *are* the world.

Surrender at the level of our ego to this thoroughgoing personal metamorphosis, which is guided in all instances by our Higher Self, is not optional.

Rather, *surrender is the first, all-important step in our ongoing journey toward realization of our inherent potential.*

To be absolutely clear, as I am using the term, surrender does not mean that we must maintain a lukewarm attitude relative to the occasionally frustrating and sometimes bewildering unfoldment of our lives.

To the contrary, as we evolve our perspective and raise our consciousness, we begin to appreciate surrender to the spiritual guidance of our Higher Self as a viable means to an end, the only workable strategy for healing, wholing and becoming the complete individuals we were meant to be.

The reason Leigh and I counsel clients of the Regenetics Method to listen to their intuition and engage their imagination when making decisions is that *spirit always speaks to us through the heart. Anything coming from the head is likely unchecked ego and usually serves to sidetrack us.*

Not that we ever fully surrender the ego. As we move forward on our path of conscious personal mastery, the ego continues to play a valuable role by, most importantly, helping us protect and care for our physical body so that we may fulfill our spiritual purpose.

But having awakened to our true divine nature through stepping into unity consciousness, the ego no longer is leading the way. Instead of being our guide, the ego is now a follower—and this is as it should be.

Qigong, which is associated with Taoism, was a wonderful teacher in what I like to call the *Art of Allowing,* for which the Taoist term in Chinese, *Wu Wei,* can be translated as "doing by not doing."

As opposed to mentally directed action, considered artificial, the philosophy of Wu Wei, which is at the heart of both Taoism and qigong, encourages intuitive, or natural, action.

As a practical example, the *doing nothing* of remaining motionless hugging the tree results in *doing something* obviously life-affirming by pooling huge amounts of bioenergy that can be used for healing, creativity, sex, and many other activities.

From a more philosophical perspective, the practice of Wu Wei can be thought of as your ego—"you"—learning to get out of your spirit's "way" so that "thy will be done" and miracles of personal healing and transformation can occur.

As an American with a background in mainstream academics, the idea that there was any art to allowing initially was every bit as foreign to me as the words "Wu Wei."

Although I considered myself a "free thinker," I quickly discovered that I was far more culturally conditioned in the ways of ego, individualism, materialism and having to "make things happen" than I was comfortable admitting.

Shockingly, for something whose chief requirement was doing nothing, Wu Wei was the hardest thing I had ever (not) done. I came very close to throwing in the towel, cutting down the tree instead of hugging it every day.

Having facilitated the Regenetics Method for years now and worked with many westernized clients, I know I am far from alone in my culturally ingrained tendency to doubt the power of spiritual energy and resist allowing things to manifest naturally.

Not infrequently, Leigh and I receive emails from clients following their Potentiation like this:

Client: "I just can't tell if I'm making any progress. I'm trying so hard."

Us: "We're sorry to hear that. How in particular do you feel that you're not making progress?"

Client: "Well, I just feel rough all the time. I know I'm detoxing. Our last conversation really helped me understand that part of the process. But it's just so uncomfortable."

Us: "It certainly can be difficult. If you don't mind our asking, are you doing any other things besides Regenetics to get well?"

Client: "Oh, yeah. Lots of things."

Us: "Like what?"

Client: "Well, I'm doing ionized footbaths to draw out toxins—three times a week. I'm also getting regular lymphatic drainage and using a zapper several hours a day for parasites. I take a lot of homeopathics and supplements. And I just started a round of colonics and a colon cleansing diet—"

Us: "Hold on. You're doing all of that, in addition to having just received Potentiation a few months ago?"

Client: *"Yeah. What's the matter?"*

Us: *"Didn't you read in our materials to proceed gently with other modalities, since Potentiation can be a powerful activation?"*

Client: *"Of course. I just thought that, you know, since Regenetics only involves energy, I had to make something happen here. Do you think maybe I'm pushing myself too hard?"*

Fortunately, I had an excellent qigong teacher who helped me integrate the Art of Allowing into my life because he was a living example of its power to strengthen the body.

From a chronically fatigued and emaciated young man on his deathbed, he had transformed through his own practice of qigong and Wu Wei into a robust, physically imposing martial artist who appeared the epitome of radiant physical health.

I am forever grateful to my teacher, a generous and gifted person whom I credit with helping me get back on my feet at one of the lowest points of my dark night of the soul.

But as one suffering acutely from chronic fatigue myself, I observed two subtle behaviors on his part that made me question whether he really had cured his illness—or simply had put it into remission by building up vast chi reserves through continuous qigong practice.

My teacher's dependence on qigong was itself a possible sign that all was not entirely well in him. By his own admission, if he skipped hugging the tree more than a day or two, he started to feel "lousy."

But even more indicative that his health probably remained compromised at a deep level was that he felt compelled to maintain a very strict diet, one nearly as severe as my own that almost completely avoided sugars and starches, which he admitted he still did not tolerate well.

In retrospect, my teacher's unrelenting food sensitivities were a "red flag" that, despite years of qigong practice and an ascetic lifestyle, suggested he remained damaged genetically—most likely by vaccines.

Later, as I became aware of the role vaccines play in inducing autoimmunity, and thus many allergies, by negatively programming DNA, I started to wonder if it might be possible to "reprogram" damaged DNA to a state of healthy functioning.

I asked myself if this kind of reset might be capable of undoing sensitivities and other symptoms experienced by individuals suffering from autoimmune conditions such as chronic fatigue syndrome, fibromyalgia, multiple chemical sensitivity (MCS), and other essentially empty diagnoses.

Although I enjoyed qigong and never had been opposed to hard work, I wondered if there might be an even purer form of Wu Wei, an even more effective method of engaging the Art of Allowing that would empower me—and maybe others—to heal at a more profound level and leave behind meditation and daily practice in favor of being fully present in the world of daily activity.

It was this line of "passively purposeful" questioning, made possible by Wu Wei in the first place, that steered me unerringly downstream during the development of Potentiation.

Allowing My Art

But I still had years ahead of me and much to learn before Potentiation came through and I felt healthy enough to let go of qigong and devote my renewed energy to activities that were aligned more directly with my calling.

Meanwhile, that winter in the high desert, as snow blanketed the Sangre de Cristo Mountains and I spent more and more time indoors and inwardly focused, a third preparatory stage in my bio-spiritual rebirth commenced.

Having undergone my own Vision Quest accompanied by a solitary intensive in the Art of Allowing, one day, for the first time in my career as a fiction writer, a character who seemed every bit as real as I was introduced himself to me.

While this should make perfect sense to fellow writers and artists, the phenomenon of meeting a fully developed character in the imagination in much the same way you might encounter an interesting character at a bar may strike some readers as strange.

Perhaps by recalling some of the unforgettable figures who have appeared in your dreams, you can understand how this might occur in waking life.

His name was Luke Soloman. He was about six feet tall and Hollywood handsome but for a slightly overlarge nose, with sandy blond hair and mischievous eyes that seemed to alternate between shades of green and blue.

He wore a red T-shirt, faded jeans and tennis shoes, and carried a buffalo leather duffel bag slung nonchalantly over one shoulder. His first act, even before introducing himself, after walking into the room where I sat at my computer desk gazing out at the snow, was to ask, "Got a smoke?"

I did not have a smoke because I did not—could not—smoke. The question, which seemed insensitive, annoyed me. In fact, *he* annoyed me.

Here I was trying to overcome a life-threatening illness, for God's sake, and into my allergen-free sanctuary walks this brash, sarcastic character wanting to light up. But more than that—the guy wants me to write down, word for word, the story of *his* imaginary life!

"What are you waiting for?" he asked, plopping down on the beanbag in the corner. "Start typing. This is important."

Maybe it was because my life ever since moving to the Southwest already bordered on surrealism, or maybe I was bored, but I started taking dictation from a character I had just met.

Thus began *Beginner's Luke* in the only way it could have—illogically and improbably—with these two philosophically loaded paragraphs:

It all began with a mysterious fire in my belly, a burning desire to go everywhere, meet everyone, see and do everything. It began with a life-or-death decision to remove the Needle of False Security from my arm, turn away from the Medusa of Routine, part the Veil of Bogus Guarantees and pass on into that vital place where, regardless of the question, all you have to say is *yes*.

It began with the Wisdom of Foolishness, a commitment to remain fluid, receptive, in process, part of the Membrane of Things as I struck out on that spiritual Route 66, the Experience Trail, determined to follow it to the end. It began with yours truly spontaneously ceasing to be myself and becoming someone else, assuming in the blink of an "I" the role of a drifter, a rolling stone, a wayward mariner lone and visionary on the High Seas of Chance and Possibility.

Having shared this literary anecdote, allow me to clarify that I was not "channeling" anything other than a previously submerged aspect of my own consciousness.

This should be obvious from the playful similarity of the names Sol Luckman and Luke Soloman, who are indeed mirror images, twisting helices of my own complex psyche—simultaneously serious and ludicrous, respectful and irreverent, profound and absurd.

Channeling is an overused term and concept, particularly among new agers, for many of whom if a message is not "channeled" from Archangel This or Galactic That, it is not valid.

But the question must be asked, especially of those who espouse a cosmology (as do I) where everything is seen as ultimately One Being, a Creator seeking to experience itself through the illusion of multiplicity:

How is it possible to channel anything other than parts of ourselves?

To think and act otherwise is, at best, not to be in unity consciousness; and at worst, to adopt an irresponsible attitude that allows us to say anything we like while attributing it to the "higher authority" of some outside source.

But there is no outside. As award-winning musician and longtime student of *A Course in Miracles* Larry Seyer likes to say, "There is only one of us here."

By far, the healthiest attitude toward so-called channeled transmissions embraces the fact that, ultimately, we always are speaking to ourselves. Even our Higher Self can be understood as part of our so-called individual identity—and an integral one at that.

I am far from implying that no interesting or useful information can come through channeling. To the contrary, much of the inspired and inspiring material in the Bible and other holy texts could be considered channeled.

As I elaborate in Chapter Seven, in the final analysis, my extensive background research notwithstanding, the actual sound and light codes used in Potentiation were derived intuitively through nonrational processes that might best be described as mystical.

In the case of Luke Soloman, his "transmissions," which eventually ran to 1,100 pages and six volumes, constitute a major portion of Sol Luckman's life's work. This may not be immediately apparent to readers who interpret Luke's imaginary Adventure as merely an absurd lark.

While it is that, most assuredly, Luke is also a profound teacher in the role consciousness (specifically, the imagination) plays in creating and re-creating our reality.

All joking aside, Luke's message is that it is crucial that we learn to live consciously in our imagination—for only in this manner can we reinvent ourselves and our world.

In order to come to life in our imagination, and thereby awaken to our greater spiritual identity and purpose, Luke taught me in no uncertain terms that *we must be willing to leave the old reality and its historical limitations behind.*

In his own words, our awakening to the possibility of radical healing and transformation begins "with a life-or-death decision to remove the Needle of False Security from [our arms], turn away from the Medusa of Routine, part the Veil of Bogus Guarantees and pass on into that vital place where, regardless of the question, all [we] have to say is *yes.*"

Often willingly but sometimes grudgingly, over the next five years I listened more and more to what Luke had to tell me as I recorded his laugh-and-cry-out-loud narrative in a mode that usually felt, bizarrely enough, less like composition than transcription.

Thus well before Potentiation, yet in a fictional manner that was preparatory to it, I immersed myself in the philosophy that I could begin a new life in and through consciousness—one where sickness was merely a memory and I was healthy enough to imagine and live my own inspiring Adventure. And lo and behold, I did.

Allowing my art to flow through me in as unadulterated a form as possible was facilitated greatly by the Art of Allowing. Without some mastery of the latter, I would have been incapable of staying out of my own way long enough to let Luke utter his typically trenchant wit and wisdom.

And like the Art of Allowing, allowing my art, which despite my debilitated physical condition often sent me into spasms of giggling at the shocking sentences I found myself typing, provided its own palpable influx of healing energy.

Clearing the Way

By the following May, having accepted a teaching job at a boarding school, I said goodbye to the high desert now abloom with countless yellow and lavender asters and headed back East to get ready for the fall semester.

Amazingly, after a year of vision questing, hugging the tree and writing almost daily, my body was strong enough to take on a demanding position where I would do much more than just teach English.

I also would spend considerable time and energy guiding groups of high school students through the woods and mountains of Appalachia carrying a heavy backpack.

Deep down, however, I knew that my health remained problematic. In addition to residual fatigue and annoying symptoms such as headaches and muscle spasms, I still suffered from disturbing food allergies and chemical sensitivities.

While continuing my qigong regimen, I started seeing a therapist who used an electrodermal screening device to determine and treat allergies—to little effect. In addition, I began regular intravenous chelation to draw heavy metals out of my system—also money poorly spent.

The next year, my health relatively unchanged, I accepted another teaching position at an international school. Out of the blue, midway through the school year I developed back-to-back abscessed teeth that required antibiotics followed by root canals.

The shock to my already shaky system was swift and severe. Within a matter of weeks, my old problems with Candida were back with a vengeance, as was my debilitating fatigue.

At the same time, my allergies, which had been manageable, became so intense I could no longer season my meat and vegetables because of crippling reactions to simple spices.

My existential agony at having rolled back down to the bottom of the mountain like Sisyphus's boulder was almost too much to bear. To have been so close to reaching the summit and taking flight, and now to be wallowing in my own ashes again, very nearly led me to despair.

Not even daily qigong could tip the scales at this stage when, more clearly than ever before, I came face to face with my own mortality.

Thankfully, my nightmarish relapse was short-lived and, as before, breakdown soon gave way to breakthrough. I managed to survive— literally—the remaining two months of the school year, at the end of which I resigned for medical reasons and returned home with little direction and less hope like a soldier wounded in battle.

And yet, it was at this exact juncture that I discovered the remarkable world of allergy clearing through Devi Nambudripad's Allergy Elimination Technique.

NAET employs a form of muscle testing called kinesiology to determine and (in tandem with a type of acupressure) treat various kinds of allergies that often are associated with chronic conditions.

For all its promise, NAET left something to be desired. Still, I noticed a slight improvement in my allergic responses that led me to try a similar therapy called BioSET, developed by one of Dr. Nambudripad's students.

BioSET expanded on NAET by clearing not just for allergens, but simultaneously for underlying toxic factors such as heavy metals. While initially providing some additional symptom relief, BioSET also failed to undo the Gordian knot of my mysterious chronic illness.

Nevertheless, allergy elimination technique, an energy-based methodology described in the next chapter, fostered the most substantial health improvements in me since learning qigong. Indeed, in terms of reducing (if not actually eliminating) my sensitivities, allergy elimination was even more effective than qigong.

I became so enthusiastic about the possibilities of allergy clearing that I hounded my BioSET practitioner to train me in her own variety of allergy elimination technique she was in the process of developing—after which I spent a year working with her.

Thus a powerful new period of apprenticeship in understanding and utilizing spiritual energy began for me—clearing the way for Potentiation and the Regenetics Method both energetically and through a series of life-changing insights into the true nature of healing and transformation.

CHAPTER 3
Spirits in the Material World

The tendency to view the human body as a machine, composed of matter and regulated biochemically, has become increasingly widespread since the dawn of Cartesian thinking in the 17th Century.

This materialistic view flies in the face of so-called primitive ways of understanding our physical bodies, and the material realms in general, as merely bio-spiritual epiphenomena created and sustained by spiritual energy.

Fortunately, over the last several decades more and more thinkers have become disillusioned with the limitations and dangers of materialistic thought.

Guided by an inner knowing that such a restrictive mentality, divorced from meaning or purpose, only serves to obscure the important truth that humans are, to quote Sting, "Spirits in the Material World," many individuals and groups have contributed to a veritable renaissance in how we envision ourselves and our environment.

This renaissance has impacted (and in many cases, revolutionized) numerous fields of study—often foregrounding through the work of pioneers the ancient wisdom that *behind everything we perceive exists a blueprint of conscious energy.*

Such a revelation is the basis for psychology's focus on unity consciousness; physics' longtime obsession with a unified theory; and biology's realization that DNA constitutes a "morphogenetic" information field that unites the human species much like the Internet.

The fascinating new science of quantum bioholography accepts as its core premise that human beings are, in essence, holograms composed of intersecting frequencies of energy transduced and directed by DNA.

This line of thinking, supported by compelling theory and evidence, has led physician Richard Gerber, author of *Vibrational Medicine*, to state bluntly that humans are "crystallized or precipitated light."

Quantum bioholography is related to the emerging field of wave-genetics, a leading-edge science—of which the Regenetics Method is a human-potential-based application—that employs what has been called torsion energy generated by sound and light to stimulate a self-healing potential in DNA.

This science, like the Regenetics model, recognizes that our bioenergy blueprint—which we can access by stimulating DNA through linguistic means and which I describe in the next chapter—holds the key to permanent healing and radical transformation.

But before examining the bioenergy blueprint, first we must gain some insight into the nature of bioenergy.

Going Deeper

Allergy elimination technique, of which Nambudripad's version, NAET, was the first and remains the most famous, derives from the homeopathic discovery that bioenergy signatures can be imprinted in tiny glass vials with an electro-acupuncture device.

For instance, the frequency for an allergen such as sugar can be held permanently in a vial containing pure water and a drop of alcohol. The immune system's response to the vial is practically indistinguishable from its reaction to the actual allergen.

Although their cause remains unexplained, allergies are defined in NAET as chemical, environmental or nutritional sensitivities that derange the immune system, contributing to a variety of chronic ailments.

Given the role such factors as vaccines play in creating many sensitivities, however, a more accurate definition of allergies sees them as potentially *resulting from* genetically induced autoimmune conditions—not the other way around.

Another fuzzy area in the theory behind the majority of allergy elimination techniques concerns the nature of bioenergy, which comes across as a nebulous concept. I hope to shed more light on bioenergy momentarily.

In NAET, whose ability to produce tangible results is attested to by the fact that it is used by thousands of alternative doctors, the patient holds the vial containing the allergen's energy signature while the practitioner performs acupressure along the spine in order to initiate a "clearing" by way of the nervous and Eastern meridian systems.

The basic idea, similar to that of acupuncture, is to eliminate "blockages" that keep bioenergy (however defined) from flowing freely through the body. In theory, clearings reprogram the immune system to accept substances formerly rejected as allergens.

BioSET improved on the rather simplistic methodology of NAET by recognizing that if it is possible to "clear" a person using one vial at a time, it should be possible to clear with multiple vials.

One can clear sugar allergies alongside *Candida albicans*, which can feed on sugar, and also add vials that represent the pancreatic system, since insulin and sugar are interrelated. Hypothetically, one can clear even for heavy metals, viruses and other pathogens that might be hindering pancreatic function.

In order to avoid having to work with dozens of pesky little vials that are difficult for the patient to hold, as well as prone to being misplaced, computer software and equipment have been developed to perform various offshoots of allergy elimination technique.

I was greatly encouraged by this approach—especially after some of my allergies began to wane. I enthusiastically underwent allergy elimination treatments from my mentor for approximately a year.

In total, I received in the neighborhood of seventy treatments from her. Doing the math, 70 x $75 at the going rate, I received over $5,000 of treatments. In today's economic terms, I spent closer to $10,000 on allergy elimination technique.

Unfortunately, after a short-lived plateau I found myself sliding downhill again. My chronic fatigue was inching its way back; I was losing many of the foods I partially had recovered; and most frustrating of all, I was experiencing a variety of new symptoms.

My professional observation as a former practitioner of allergy elimination technique led me to believe that my experience of improvement followed by losing ground was not altogether uncommon.

While NAET and its derivatives at times can work wonders, for seriously immuno-compromised individuals long-term exposure to allergy clearing sometimes appears to weaken the immune, irritate the nervous and overstimulate the adrenal systems. Without a doubt, this was my personal experience.

The reason for such shortcomings is straightforward. As previously mentioned, traditional allergy clearings work through the nervous and meridian systems.

But in order to reset our bioenergy blueprint, where allergy-producing distortions are imprinted, and establish a "clean slate" for permanent healing and transformation, we must go deeper.

Indeed, we must go all the way to the regulator of the ener-genetic patterns—both dysfunctional and healthy—that manifest in our bioenergy blueprint: DNA.

Only by properly activating DNA, I realized, is it possible to reestablish the systemic harmony and coherence necessary for sustained wellbeing.

I concluded that in order to stimulate the self-repair mechanism in the supposedly inactive portion of DNA, it is necessary to employ sound and light waves of torsion energy, which can be generated linguistically.

I zero in on this central subject in Chapters Six and Seven, before teaching you how to do it yourself in Part II.

Field Testing

Soon after I began working with a version of allergy elimination technique, four critical factors converged to lay the theoretical foundation for a clearer comprehension of bioenergy—as well as the development of Potentiation.

For starters and most crucially, I met my life partner Leigh, who provided me with tremendous support in both my ongoing healing journey and intensive ener-genetic research that began around this time. With wonderful serendipity, I met her in the Health & Body Care section of our local health food store.

Later, as our relationship grew, Leigh came to work as an assistant in my mentor's office. Her extensive background in herbology, nutrition, homeopathy, flower essences and energy medicine came into play early and often as we began "field testing" our ideas about the bioenergy blueprint and DNA.

A second factor associated with my stint with allergy elimination technique that played a role in shaping Regenetics was simply an observation.

The very fact that Leigh and I were using bioenergy to perform clearings that by themselves were capable of reducing allergies and providing other palpable benefits was proof positive that bioenergy can have a measurable impact on the body-mind-spirit complex and its functioning.

To medical "experts" who categorically dismiss the hundreds of thousands of success stories associated with energetic therapies as merely examples of the "placebo effect," it has been countered that the same can be said of the curative effects of many pharmaceuticals and even surgical procedures.

This point has been made eloquently and emphatically by a number of medical doctors and researchers, including respected cardiologist and author Larry Dossey.

In fact, rather than an aberration to be belittled and ignored, the placebo effect remains an open invitation to explore the extraordinary ability of consciousness to change physical reality—in many cases, replacing a medical "death sentence" with a state of glowing health.

Never was it more obvious that bioenergy profoundly affects the body than when an allergy elimination session instantly set off a major detoxification, or "healing crisis," in recipients.

This sometimes startling phenomenon, which Leigh and I observed and experienced personally on a frequent basis, fueled our desire to find a more integrated way to address distortions in the bioenergy blueprint and facilitate purification and healing.

Thirdly, it is worth emphasizing that we were employing a type of muscle testing known as kinesiology, or applied kinesiology, to determine allergies, sensitivities, underlying toxic factors, pathogenic elements, and emotional traumas.

These so-called blockages then were cleared energetically—at times quite successfully, and other times less so—through allergy elimination technique.

Over the decades since 1964, when American chiropractor George Goodheart first observed that a weak muscle could be treated using nonphysical methods and its strength significantly improved, kinesiology has constituted the predominant form of energetic assessment used by chiropractors and other healthcare professionals worldwide.

There are literally hundreds of spins on kinesiology. Leigh and I experimented with a lot of them as we conducted over a year's worth of exhaustive "field tests" with each other and our clients in order to "map" the human bioenergy blueprint.

Our methodology involved a huge number of checks and cross-checks, as well as experiential and intuitive ways of gathering knowledge, and would exceed the parameters of this book to outline adequately.

While muscle testing was critical to establishing a conceptual framework out of which the Regenetics Method emerged, *learning and performing this work now requires absolutely no prior knowledge of or experience with kinesiology.*

Within the context of Potentiation, the only use for kinesiology comes *after* the actual session, when muscle testing can be used to:

1. Verify that the session was successful; and

2. Determine the recipient's Electromagnetic Group, or bioenergy family, and corresponding Electromagnetic Schematic (Figures 15, 16, and 17).

Both of these applications are covered in Part III, where I share a simple but effective muscle testing technique that can be mastered in less than five minutes (Figure 14).

Fourth and finally, many of the ideas Leigh and I field tested were suggested by my extensive reading. My reading selections often were prompted by my intuitive faculties that had been honed during my initiation in the high desert, while my ability to synthesize so much information had been developed in graduate school.

I felt like a student all over again as I found myself devouring a book nearly every other day. But instead of literature and literary theory, now I was tackling texts on molecular biology, biochemistry, genetic science, quantum physics, energy healing, and metaphysics.

Out of this mountain of material, many pieces of which made their way into *Conscious Healing,* came numerous questions that seemed to me then, as they do now, essential to understanding true health and wellness.

The six primary questions Leigh and I sought answers to through kinesiology and other ways of knowing were:

1. What is the nature of bioenergy?

2. What would a map of our bioenergy blueprint look like?

3. What is DNA?

4. Is there a relationship between the bioenergy blueprint and DNA?

5. What role, if any, does DNA play in mediating between our bioenergy blueprint and our biology?

6. How might it be possible to activate DNA so as to correct distortions in the bioenergy blueprint and thus facilitate healing and transformation?

In what is left of this chapter and the remainder of Part I, I endeavor to provide helpful perspectives on these far-reaching questions in ways that readers with little or no scientific background can grasp easily.

Bioenergy = Torsion Energy = Consciousness

In 1913 Dr. Eli Cartan, observing an apparently novel form of energy with a spiraling motion through the fabric of space and time, coined the term *torsion* to characterize it.

I first encountered this word in 2002 and, initially having dismissed it, soon began seeing it regularly in relation to consciousness and DNA. Needless to say, given the nature of the field testing Leigh and I were conducting, my interest was piqued.

I learned that torsion energy was distinguishable from both gravity and electromagnetic energy, as well as strong and weak atomic forces. Translated: according to traditional Newtonian physics, torsion energy should not exist.

But clearly, it did, and a lot of people with fancy letters after their names had produced a lot of fancy names for it—including zero point energy and subspace energy. To which terms I was able to add several less scientific ones: bioenergy, life force, chi, *prana*, and *kundalini*.

Arguably, the best name for torsion energy was one of oldest: ether, or *aether* (from a root word meaning to burn or shine), the term the ancient Greeks used to describe this omnipresent field of background energy.

Aether might be the most appropriate term for torsion energy because, etymologically, it captures the important idea that the most obvious manifestation of the hyperdimensional energy we are discussing is light.

Unfortunately, although Albert Einstein admitted that it was essential to explaining the unified field, aether long has had a bad rap in the scientific community. At least partly, this is because its existence is hard to prove using scientific instrumentation designed to measure grosser forms of energy that fit neatly into Newtonian physics.

Nevertheless, Russian scientists, who in many ways are well ahead of their counterparts in the West, have measured aether and developed numerous practical applications—particularly in the healing field—for what they refer to as torsion energy.

To speak plainly about Western science's denial of aether, *it is hard to find something you categorically refuse to look for.*

For the past century, traditional science has maintained a tenacious and myopic belief in the primacy of the material over the spiritual—simply deleting the concept of aether from its lexicon despite many recurring, theory-deflating proofs of the existence of this important energy dating back at least to the 19th Century.

When I think about Western science's tendency to ignore reality in favor of theory, I am reminded of a poster my high school guidance counselor had on the wall in her office showing a person contorting to cover her eyes and stop up her ears whose caption read, "Don't confuse me with the facts!"

Comparing mainstream science to a "fetish," one that constrains many would-be open-minded scientists to worship foolish hobgoblins of concept and belief, Joachim-Ernst Berendt in *The World Is Sound* explains that since

> analysis is more important to the predominant sciences than synthesis, scientists tend to ... think narrowly and rigidly rather than widely and flexibly. Thus ... most scientists still cling stubbornly to Aristotelian logic and its linear causal chains. As a result of this rigidity, scientists accept findings that are a product of their own methodology within a few years or even months after they are published, but pass over all those findings that represent a danger to their traditional methods, even half a century after these findings are made.

Relative to the matter at hand, healing, Berendt notes that the "failure of the conventional methodology of science is especially apparent in the field of medicine."

Today's medicine "still looks at its 'object,' man, as if he were a 'machine' or a chemical plant" and "does not seem to be able to understand that it is still oriented toward a physical worldview that, in its basic conception, is outdated."

Berendt is far from alone in his assessment. According to physics pioneer Sir James Jeans, "The stream of knowledge is heading toward a nonmechanical reality; the universe begins to look more like a great thought than like a great machine. Mind no longer appears to be an accidental intruder into the realm of matter [but] the creator and governor of … matter."

Biologist and author Bruce Lipton describes the situation this way: "Although quantum mechanics was acknowledged eighty years ago as the best scientific description of the mechanisms creating our universe, most scientists rigidly cling to the prevailing matter-oriented worldview simply because it 'seems' to make better sense out of our existence."

"However," continues Dr. Lipton, "quantum laws must hold at every level of reality. We can no longer afford to ignore that fact. We must learn that our beliefs, perceptions and attitudes about the world create the world."

Recently, Lipton points out, physicist R. C. Henry of Johns Hopkins University "suggested that we 'get over it' and accept the inarguable conclusion: 'The universe is immaterial—mental and spiritual.'"

Similarly, in the words of world-renowned physicist John Hagelin, "If you scratch below the surface and get to the molecular, atomic and sub-atomic levels, you find that these worlds are not material worlds. They are worlds of intelligence and ultimately worlds of consciousness."

There is much more that could be written about this topic. But what I wish to stress is the simple observation that *traditional materialistic science, like the physically based medicine that grows out of it, represents merely a hypothetical description of reality that, at its core, is fundamentally in error.*

I realize this may be a hard pill to swallow for many scientists. But the fact is that mainstream science and medicine utterly fail to take into account the conscious spiritual energy that gives rise to the universe we inhabit.

Thus the logic behind our current scientific and medical models is critically flawed—being based on the false premise that matter is all that matters.

If we are to evolve beyond this distorted worldview in the direction of a more holistic perception, we must turn the tables on such faulty reasoning.

It would benefit all of us to realize that instead of inhabiting an essentially material universe that can be measured, weighed, dissected and placed in a box, we live in a malleable reality that forever transcends our boxes of concept and belief because *our very concepts and beliefs condition reality.*

Decades ago the Heisenberg Uncertainty Principle established that our perceptions of an event automatically affect the event's outcome. This theoretical assertion has been verified through numerous experiments proving that *human consciousness can, and does, alter physical reality.*

To be clear, I am far from stating that the material world does not exist. Rather, I propose that what we think of as the real world is a holographic consciousness construct that—in all ways at all times—is subject to modification by our consciousness (or unconsciousness) of it.

The original *Matrix* movie artfully charts this life-changing idea through Keanu Reeves' character. Faced with a variety of initiatory challenges, Neo steadily expands his perceptions from those of a heedless victim of the Matrix, to those of its purposeful master.

With the Matrix symbolizing our initial experience of reality as victims, Neo's development can be interpreted as a psychological evolution that embraces our greater reality and power as spiritual beings. Moreover, it is patently obvious that Neo's ability to change reality evolves in direct proportion to his consciousness.

While this way of looking at reality as a consciousness construct can make it seem as if there is no longer any firm ground to stand on, precisely this same truthful lens gives us wings to fly as soon as we accept reality's basic operating principle: *consciousness creates.*

Indeed, returning to the subject with which this section began, *another name for aether, bioenergy or torsion energy is simply consciousness.*

The purest form of torsion energy is that of the Creator and might be thought of as the Consciousness of Love (Figures 1 and 4). After all, the Bible states unequivocally that *God is love.*

Out of this universal creative consciousness, which constitutes the background spiritual energy on which what we think of as reality plays out in all its breathtaking diversity, emerges the Word (primal sound) that calls into being the galaxies by "let[ting] there be light" (Figures 1 and 4).

"In the beginning was the sound, the sound as logos," explains Berendt. "God's command 'Let there be ...' at the beginning of the biblical story of creation was first tone and sound. For the Sufis, the mystics of Islam, this is the core of things: God created the world from sound."

Figure 1 depicts how the Creator utters—consciously, energetically, and literally—the holographic construct of the world into existence. This illustration also shows how we ourselves can re-create our reality construct, starting at the ener-genetic level.

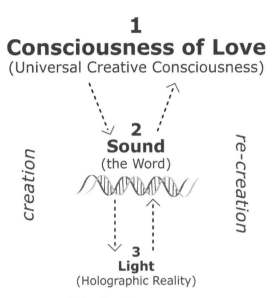

Figure 1: Three Forms of Torsion Energy

The above image illustrates the relational patterns of the three primary forms of torsion energy while also shedding light on how we are created and how we can re-create ourselves ener-genetically.

The Regenetics Method does not attempt to heal and transform the bioenergy blueprint through physical or biochemical manipulation, which would be to put the cart before the horse.

Instead, Regenetics respects the inherent order and nature of creation by employing the primary torsion energy produced by sound supported by torsion light waves emitted by thought—both of which are conveyed via special "words"—to activate DNA.

You can learn more about torsion energy by exploring the work of Russian scientist Nicolai Kozyrev, who in the 1950s proved the existence of this life-giving subspace energy.

Dr. Kozyrev demonstrated that, like time, torsion energy flows in a fractal spiral that has been referred to as *Phi*, the Golden Mean, and the Fibonacci sequence.

This spiraling energy mirrors the helical structure of DNA because, quite simply, as detailed in Chapter Six, it gives rise to the DNA molecule.

In addition, I regularly publish articles on torsion energy and related topics in my popular free ezine, *DNA Monthly*, current and back issues of which are available online at **www.potentiation.net**.

Last but not least, *Conscious Healing* provides a wealth of additional information and perspectives on DNA, torsion energy, and consciousness.

Space-time & Time-space

Happily, today a growing number of scientists and medical professionals are embracing the new paradigm that respects the profoundly spiritual, consciousness-based nature of the ostensibly material world.

As this crucial change in perspective gains momentum, more and more modalities designed to encourage permanent healing and radical transformation are being made available. Leigh and I are honored to play even a small part in this truly inspiring global movement.

So far we have determined that bioenergy is a form of consciousness. At the macrocosmic level, this conscious torsion energy, which David Wilcock refers to as the "consciousness field," constitutes the background spiritual energy out of which the physical universe "materializes" much in the way light projected through a holographic plate creates a lifelike three-dimensional image.

Microcosmically, *we ourselves emerge from the consciousness field, starting with our DNA, and ultimately are inseparable from it.* This realization, however it arrives and whatever form it takes, is a fundamental stepping stone to unity consciousness.

As explained in the next chapter, our very bioenergy blueprint is composed of torsion fields of consciousness within the greater consciousness field (Figure 3).

By far the most compelling conceptual model for understanding how the torsion energy of consciousness creates, sustains and modifies the material realms comes from American engineer and author Dewey Larson.

Larson's revolutionary Reciprocal System of physical theory was elaborated starting in 1959 through such seminal works as *The Structure of the Physical Universe* and *Basic Properties of Matter.*

By way of closing this chapter, in simple language I will describe the bare bones of Larson's thinking as viewed through the lens of contemporary torsion physics.

Going beyond Einstein's theoretical model, which assumed only five dimensions, Larson's Reciprocal System theory posited the existence of *six* dimensions: three of space and three of time.

Brilliantly insightful, Larson proposed that for a unified field to exist, in addition to a three-dimensional coordinate space (space-time), there also must be a three-dimensional coordinate time (time-space).

In practical terms, during our waking existence we live in space-time. But in our dreams and during the so-called afterlife, we find ourselves in time-space (Figure 2).

Larson grasped that these two realities are mirror images of one another—and even more importantly, that they are *connected.*

In essence, Reciprocal System theory posits a continuous flow of torsion energy from time-space, where our reality blueprints are stored, into space-time, where these blueprints are made manifest.

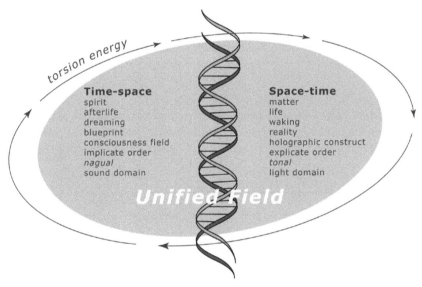

Figure 2: Space-time & Time-space

This chart lists various characteristics that distinguish time-space from space-time, while showing the unified field as a continuous torsion energy circuit between the sound and light domains.

The unified field is explained insofar as reality is thought to be a basically closed system in which the energy of consciousness originating in time-space travels into space-time and back again unceasingly (Figure 2).

Numerous small and large connection points exist between space-time and time-space. These include exactly twelve triangular areas on Earth's surface where planes and ships consistently disappear into and reemerge from time-space with names like the Dragon's Triangle and the Devil's Triangle.

For detailed information on the fascinating geophysical structure of our planet featuring twelve major connection points between space-time and time-space, I encourage you to explore biologist Ivan Sanderson's research on the twelve Devil's Graveyards.

In addition to the mysterious disappearance of planes and ships, the existence of time-space as a parallel reality where the energy templates for the observable world function explains a plethora of so-called paranormal phenomena that have baffled traditional science—from free energy technologies to Near Death Experiences (NDEs).

In a somewhat more mainstream manner, space-time and time-space find precise corollaries in physicist David Bohm's well-known explicate and implicate orders of existence (Figure 2).

Shamanically, for those familiar with this area of knowledge, space-time can be understood as the *tonal*, with time-space being the *nagual* (Figure 2).

In terms of human biology, as also shown in Figure 2, *DNA serves as the connection point between time-space and space-time*. But before we explore the profound implications of this observation, first we must understand our bioenergy blueprint in the context of time-space and space-time.

CHAPTER 4
Understanding Our Bioenergy Blueprint

To one such as myself who for years had wandered athirst seeking the waters of truth in the "desert of the real," to quote Morpheus in *The Matrix*, it was extremely gratifying to encounter a sound scientific theory that explains just how, in fact, we are spiritual beings on a human journey.

Dewey Larson's Reciprocal System of physical theory establishes that we are reciprocal creatures with one foot in the world of spirit, time-space, and the other foot in the world of matter, space-time (Figure 3).

Moreover, this model views the spiritual realm of time-space—being the repository of the consciousness templates from which our space-time reality is constructed—as primary.

In Larson's groundbreaking theory, the so-called physical world is seen as a secondary epiphenomenon that emerges directly from the consciousness field (Figure 3).

Stated otherwise, Reciprocal System theory provides an intellectual foundation for accepting the Primacy of Consciousness over the material (Figure 7).

Additionally, *this revolutionary model establishes a scientific rationale for addressing many issues related to physical reality—including the majority of health problems—using spiritual energy.*

If it is true that the blueprint for our existence, including that of our bodies and their dysfunctions, is held in the torsion field of time-space, a viable method for effecting permanent healing and fundamental transformation is to reset this blueprint when it is damaged.

In order to reset our blueprint, we can employ linguistic means to generate torsion waves that stimulate a self-repair capability intrinsic to DNA.

Activating this self-healing potential requires that we start at the genetic level, because in human biology DNA is the principal connection point between our space-time existence and time-space blueprint (Figures 1, 2, 3, and 4).

In this chapter, the nature and structure of the human bioenergy blueprint are examined. Particular attention is paid to the bioenergy fields, the chakras, and the energetic disruption known as the Fragmentary Body.

Sound & Light Domains

An early epiphany Leigh and I experienced while using kinesiology to field test ourselves and our clients was that the human bioenergy blueprint is divided into a series of interconnected fields, each having specific regulatory functions across the body-mind-spirit spectrum.

Esoteric science calls the composite of these linked levels the "aura," which is subdivided into a number of "auric fields" (Figures 3 and 10). Over the past several decades, numerous researchers have confirmed the existence of this critically important bioenergy structure surrounding the body.

In *Infinite Mind: Science of the Human Vibrations of Consciousness*, UCLA professor Valerie Hunt describes how she successfully used an encephalograph (EEG) machine to detect and better understand the multi-layered aura.

Dr. Hunt goes so far as to theorize that *the mind, instead of residing locally in the brain's neural network, actually exists nonlocally in the auric fields.*

Viewed from the perspective of Reciprocal System theory and torsion physics, Hunt's theory is right on the mark. Beyond any reasonable doubt, the bioenergy fields must be the mind (Figure 3).

In these torsion templates of consciousness functioning hyperdimensionally in time-space, we experience the core creative workings of inspiration, intuition, and imagination.

Only subsequently, passing into our space-time reality, are these subtle energy phenomena processed and actualized by the brain and central nervous system.

In the words of Bruce Lipton, "The switch from Newtonian to quantum mechanics changes the focus of psychology from physiochemical mechanisms to the role of energy fields."

Physicist and psychotherapist Arnold Mindell famously called our primary time-space manifestation the "Dreambody," whose secondary counterpart in space-time is the physical body.

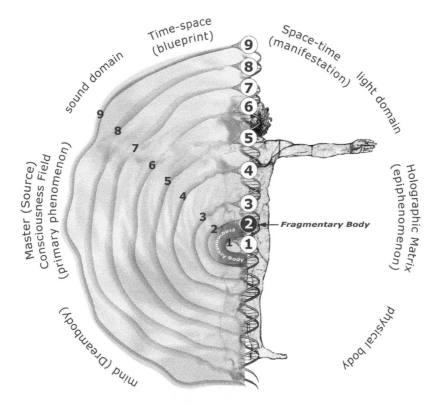

Figure 3: A Foot in Two Worlds

The above figure illustrates the interface between the sound domain of time-space and the light domain of space-time. Note the parallel existence of the bioenergy fields in the former and the chakras in the latter, including the placement of the Fragmentary Body.

Gifted psychic Sheradon Bryce sums up the situation straightforwardly: "Your mind is your electromagnetic field, your auric bands, or whatever you wish to call them. The thing in your head is your brain."

This statement brings up an important point in need of clarification: the term *electromagnetic* often has been employed erroneously to describe the bioenergy fields.

I have used it myself this way for years, as in Potentiation Electromagnetic Repatterning. Initially, I chose this term in order to emphasize the energetic quality of the bioenergy fields to a broad readership.

At the time, I felt that *auric* sounded too esoteric; *torsion* was too obscure; and *bioenergy*—lacking a fuller explanation such as the one I am providing now—seemed too vague. The problem with *electromagnetic* as a description of bioenergy is that this energy is not actually electromagnetic!

Rather, it is torsion energy, or consciousness. While it gives rise to such effects as electromagnetism, it is not measurable as such. Not surprisingly, many researchers using traditional techniques to look for the bioenergy fields have come up empty.

Nevertheless, the term electromagnetic is now a fixture in the Regenetics Method, where it is employed more descriptively than scientifically. Whenever you encounter it used in a way that seems to be a misnomer, I encourage you to substitute bioenergy or torsion, if this helps facilitate understanding of the Regenetics model.

Now, I mentioned in the previous chapter that torsion energy comes in three main varieties. All torsion energy ultimately stems from one Source, which I called the Consciousness of Love (Figures 1 and 4).

In *Conscious Healing*, elaborating on the three-phase cosmological model I am sketching here, I conceptualized this Source, our Creator, as Silent Stillness: the pure potential, or universal creative consciousness, associated with the center of our galaxy.

In the threefold process of creation, the Consciousness of Love differentiates first into torsion sound waves, then into torsion light waves. Biblically speaking, the Consciousness of Love is God, who speaks the Word (sound) in order to bring the World (light) into manifestation (Figures 1 and 4).

Such a framework for reality creation, in which a Supreme Consciousness literally speaks or sings a light-based (holographic) world into existence, is omnipresent in religions and mythologies. In the ancient *Vedas* of India, we read, "In the beginning was Brahman with whom was the Word."

The *Tao de Ching* introduces a cosmology wherein the "ten thousand things" constituting our holographic reality were brought into being through breath (sound).

In Mayan tradition, the *Popol Vuh* explains that the first humans were brought into being through speech. Similarly, the ancient Egyptians believed that life was created by language.

In terms of torsion physics and Reciprocal System theory as well, reality creation can be visualized as a three-step operation (Figure 4).

This process follows a specific order in which the Consciousness of Love employs linguistically generated blueprints of torsion energy in time-space in the form of hyperdimensional sound, which then transform into reality constructs in space-time that are light-generated, or holographic.

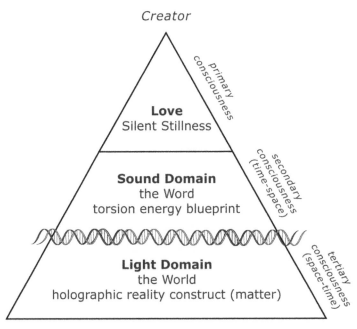

Figure 4: Threefold Process of Reality Creation

This diagram demonstrates how reality creation occurs in three phases, starting with the primary consciousness of the Creator, who employs sound to generate the light-based reality construct we inhabit—including biological life by way of DNA.

This tripartite model of reality creation highlights two points with particular relevance to DNA activation.

First, while it is true that we inhabit a light-based reality in space-time, *the primary energy that directly gives rise to our existence in space-time is sound*—just as so many ancient wisdom traditions have claimed.

For this reason, I often find it useful to refer to time-space as the "sound domain" and space-time as the "light domain" (Figures 2, 3, and 4).

Of course, both space-time and time-space contain sound as well as light energies. But while light is the operative principle here in space-time, the dreamlike domain of time-space appears to be governed by sound.

The reason clairvoyants insist that the aura is visible stems from the likelihood that by tapping into extrasensory perception (ESP), they can "see" this sonic energy as it filters through DNA into space-time via a genetic mechanism that translates sound into light (see Chapter Six).

Secondly, given that time-space is best understood as a function of sound energy, it should be obvious that *our bioenergy fields are sonic in nature.*

Keep in mind, however, that we are discussing hyperdimensional torsion sound waves, which means you cannot simply press a button and record the aura!

Since our consciousness blueprint in time-space is made of sound, and sound is the principal torsion energy for creating, supporting and evolving life, *using only light for healing, as the vast majority of energetic modalities do, often proves ineffectual.*

Hyperdimensional light is the form of torsion energy normally employed in energy medicine—whether we look at allergy elimination technique, acupuncture, reiki, radionics, meditation, or machines. But remember that *sound precedes and creates light.*

Compared to sound, light is superficial. Light is thought, form; sound is being, essence. Light diagnoses; sound restores. Light treats; sound heals.

Light is concerned with *information,* whereas sound is about *transformation.*

A tried and true way to pursue genuine wholing is to work with sound because *sound is capable of accessing and changing the sound domain,* where bioenergy distortions caused by trauma or toxicity, or both, are imprinted and states of illness are maintained.

Ener-genetically, *disharmony is disease.* Trauma- and toxicity-induced distortions in our bioenergy blueprint take the form of disharmonies that can be brought back into harmony using the right sounds.

Effective sound healing is a form of entrainment, or re-entrainment, of off-key tunes within the sound domain back to harmonious and healthy melodies. This approach encourages healing and transformation in a manner that exceeds the capabilities of light alone.

Here again, as illustrated in a number of Figures throughout this text, it is to be emphasized that the connection point between our sound and light domains is DNA.

Practically, this means that *DNA must be activated from our position in space-time if we are to heal and transform our reality blueprint in time-space.*

This central topic is explored throughout the remainder of Part I, as we lay the conceptual groundwork for learning to potentiate DNA in Part II.

Bioenergy Fields as Ecosystems

A second critical discovery Leigh and I made while field testing was that the bioenergy blueprint for the vast majority of humans is composed of exactly nine fields (Figures 3 and 10a).

This came as something of a surprise, given that Vedic tradition recognizes only seven major bioenergy points known as the chakras. Then again, according to certain new age teachings, supposedly there are twelve chakras.

Many of these latter teachings also posit, without evidence, the existence of multiple human DNA "strands" ranging in number from as few as twelve to—somewhat comically—as many as hundreds or even thousands.

Simply put, even a cursory review of the esoteric literature reveals wide-ranging viewpoints as to the number of bioenergy centers humans possess.

For those unfamiliar with the term, as shown in Figure 3 chakras are bioenergy loci in the form of wheels aligned with the spinal column, starting with the first (or root) chakra at the sacrum and moving up.

In the 1980s, Japanese scientist Hiroshi Motoyama developed instrumentation capable of measuring bioluminescence emitted by the chakras of yoga masters.

The chakras differ from the bioenergy fields in that the former are composed of hyperdimensional *light* that operates in space-time, while the latter are formed by torsion *sound* waves functioning in time-space (Figure 3).

Acting as a counterpart to our sonic bioenergy fields, the light-based chakras match these fields in order and number and are responsible for distributing life energy originating in time-space to our physical anatomy in space-time.

The majority of elements regulated by a particular bioenergy field equally apply to the corresponding chakra. *Together, numerically matching fields and chakras form a "bioenergy center."*

Note that in these paired relationships, *the bioenergy fields govern the chakras*, not the other way around, just as at the torsion level sound directs the action of light.

I probably never would have become involved in the debate as to the exact number of our primary bioenergy centers—had extensive kinesiological data not clearly and repeatedly revealed the existence of nine chakras and nine bioenergy fields in the "unpotentiated" human.

Certainly, I had no preconceptions about this topic when Leigh and I began our research. At the time, like many people I barely knew what a chakra was.

Here, it is my sincere belief that my naïveté was helpful—allowing me to observe dispassionately simply what was, instead of seeing what I had been told should be.

This situation reminds me of an old shamanic tradition in which a task considered impossible by elder shamans is given to a novice. The idea is that since the novice does not know that the task cannot be accomplished, he somehow manages to accomplish it!

Shortly after our discovery of nine bioenergy levels, Leigh and I were gratified to learn that well-known medical intuitive Caroline Myss had picked up on the presence of an eighth and ninth chakra.

Since that time, various additional sources using SCIO and other subtle energy detection systems have confirmed the existence of nine bioenergy centers—as well as the transformation of this initial blueprint to eight centers that occurs during Potentiation as explained below.

Perhaps the reason the eighth and ninth bioenergy centers were glossed over in Vedic lore is that they are associated with the most subtle aspect of our being—DNA—in contrast to the other seven chakras that appear more directly situated within our physical anatomy (Figures 15, 16, and 17).

Be that as it may, there is a way to transcend theory and achieve an inner gnosis of our bioenergy blueprint. Beyond channeling, intuition, tradition, kinesiology and even technology, Potentiation allows you to *experience* these nine bioenergy centers in action as they are repatterned by torsion waves of consciousness.

Through Potentiation, as explored in greater detail in Chapter Seven, our inherently unstable and fragmented structure based on the number 9 is recalibrated permanently to a stable and balanced "infinity circuit" founded on the number 8 (Figure 10).

This occurs after the ener-genetic disruption constituted by the Fragmentary Body is sealed at approximately the five-month mark following the Potentiation session.

Also in Chapter Seven, while describing my personal experience of Potentiation, I offer a number of insights as to what the Fragmentary Body represents and why sealing it is so important to genuine healing and transformation.

For even more information on this subject, I encourage you to read *Conscious Healing*, where the Fragmentary Body is viewed from a myriad of angles that lie beyond the scope and purpose of this book.

Essential to grasping the role our bioenergy centers play in health and disease is to view them as "ecosystems" where various related factors function either harmoniously to maintain wellbeing, or disharmoniously to engender illness.

An ecosystem is defined as a biological community of interdependent organisms and their habitat.

In the case of our bioenergy blueprint, each field combines with a chakra to form a bioenergy center that regulates the activity of specific microorganisms in relation to particular "environments" in the form of organ systems and glands.

As an example, let us look at the second bioenergy center from the bottom, referred to as the Fragmentary Body prior to sealing during Potentiation.

In Figure 5, ignoring the blank categories (—), we see that the microorganisms governed by the Fragmentary Body are dental bacteria and parasites (with associated toxins), while the organ systems are the oral and reproductive, and the gland is the thyroid.

Linked to these material elements are the emotions of embarrassment, envy, jealousy and shame, in addition to a number of conditions.

Based on this bioenergetic ecosystem, consider the following scenario. In physical terms, dental bacteria obviously are linked to the oral system.

Bioenergy Structure of the Fragmentary Body

GENETICS: -

GLAND: Thyroid

ORGANS: Oral, Reproductive

TOXINS: Bacterial Toxins, Parasitic Toxins

MICROORGANISMS: Dental Bacteria, Parasites

EMOTIONS: Embarrassment, Envy, Jealousy, Shame

MIASMS: -

CONDITIONS: Dental Decay, Halitosis, Impotence, Parasitic Infection, Infertility, Periodontal Disease, Reproductive System Illness, Speech Impediment, Sterility

---

Figure 5: Bioenergy Structure of the Fragmentary Body

This chart shows the basic structure of the problematic bioenergy ecosystem known as the Fragmentary Body.

Distortion in the Fragmentary Body—brought on by, say, shame-producing sexual trauma in tandem with toxicity resulting from parasitic infection of the thyroid gland—increases the likelihood of breakdown in another part of the ecosystem: in this case, the oral system.

Such a situation can lead to proliferation of bacteria which, if left unchecked, eventually results in a number of possible conditions including dental decay, halitosis, and periodontal disease.

This example easily can be extrapolated to all nine levels of our bioenergy blueprint—giving rise to a novel and empowering way of understanding ourselves as bio-spiritual beings we will study more closely in Part III.

Digging at the Root

Before moving on to DNA and how to activate it with language to promote healing and transformation, I wish to point out that the above example of toxicity and trauma in the Fragmentary Body allows us to grasp how numerous spiritual and material disharmonies typically combine to produce a state of disease.

This example makes it clear that instead of being created in our space-time physical reality, illness grows out of sonic distortions recorded in our bioenergy blueprint in time-space.

Thus we can appreciate another dimension of Reciprocal System theory as applied to medical science:

The existence of time-space as a causal domain undermines the theory and practice of solely materialistic diagnosis, which only looks at effects.

The foregoing statement is far-reaching indeed. According to many native wisdom traditions, *there is a spiritual cause for everything,* including ostensibly physical dysfunctions.

For instance, a medicine man or woman virtually never looks at a broken leg as merely an unfortunate accident. Injury to the leg has archetypal as well as personal significance and may indicate that the injured person has failed to "stand up for herself" in some important way.

This line of thinking, in which even the most blatantly material effects of illness have a spiritual basis, informs the healing theory and practice of renowned author Louise Hay.

In fact, many conditions are so complex, being occasioned by multiple factors that distort the bioenergy blueprint, that trying to address them by treating each symptom individually—the approach adopted by allopathic medicine—more often than not fails in its objective.

Here, I am reminded of Henry David Thoreau's famous line that there "are ten thousand chopping at the branches of evil, for every one digging at the root."

As someone who endured years of expensive therapies that simply were chopping away at the branches, I deeply appreciate that in order to heal and transform ourselves, truly and lastingly, we must toss aside our axes, pick up a shovel, and dig for the root.

In the above analogy, the branches represent symptoms. Axes symbolize space-time (light-based) therapies for treating or managing symptoms.

The root is our bioenergy blueprint in the sound domain, where and only where disease-causing distortions can be restored permanently to harmony.

And the shovel is any modality capable of resetting the bioenergy blueprint via the only connection point through which such an activation can occur: DNA.

CHAPTER 5
Three
Perspectives on
DNA

To this point, we have established perspectives on the first two of the six questions necessary to understanding how to achieve and maintain true health and wellness asked in Chapter Three.

First, concerning our question as to the nature of bioenergy, we have determined that bioenergy is a form of consciousness. This means that, to varying degrees, any activity that raises our consciousness increases our bioenergy, and vice versa, encouraging healing as well as transformation across the body-mind-spirit continuum.

Secondly, in examining the structure of the Fragmentary Body in the last chapter, we began to paint a picture of what a map of our bioenergy blueprint might look like. This topic is explored in greater depth in Chapter Thirteen.

Questions three through six are still in need of being addressed. This chapter and the next two explore these questions from a variety of angles:

3. What is DNA?

4. Is there a relationship between the bioenergy blueprint and DNA?

5. What role, if any, does DNA play in mediating between our bioenergy blueprint and our biology?

6. How might it be possible to activate DNA so as to correct distortions in the bioenergy blueprint and thus facilitate healing and transformation?

While reminding readers that this is not a book about science and you do not need a scientific mind to grasp the ideas I present, it is worth pointing out that this and the following chapter are the two most intellectually demanding parts of the entire text.

I have simplified and streamlined this material to maximize its clarity and accessibility. Regardless of whether you fully comprehend every detail, you still can benefit greatly from Potentiation—which is *not* an intellectual technique and has proven, I reiterate, easy to learn and perform.

I encourage you to read this chapter as well as Chapter Six through to the end. Readers who resonate with new science, particularly as applied to biology, are likely to find these chapters quite engaging.

Those who experience this material as too "left-brain" are advised to move on without looking back to Chapter Seven. Here, the focus shifts from explaining the science and philosophy of DNA activation in general, back to a more narrative voice as the story of the development of Potentiation, specifically, concludes.

Three Eras of Medicine

In teaching the Regenetics Method to students from widely divergent backgrounds over the years, before even discussing DNA, I have found it valuable to lay out a historical framework for understanding the evolution of medicine. The rationale for doing so will become apparent momentarily as we establish three perspectives on DNA.

In *Reinventing Medicine: Beyond Mind-body to a New Era of Healing*, Larry Dossey, the former chief of staff at a major Dallas hospital, examines allopathic medicine in light of the principle of "nonlocality" often studied by quantum physicists.

Putting today's medicine in quantum perspective, Dr. Dossey asserts that we "are facing a 'constitutional crisis' in medicine—a crisis over our *own* constitution, the nature of our mind and its relationship to our physical body."

To help elucidate this "constitutional crisis," and to assist humanity in moving beyond it, Dossey outlines three main Eras in the history of Western medicine.

In practical terms, these Eras necessarily overlap to some degree. Conceptually, however, each clearly possesses a defining, exclusive focus (Figure 6).

While these three Eras are associated with specific historical time frames for reference, the characteristic thinking behind each Era appears transhistorical.

In other words, the Eras function almost like archetypes by tapping into distinctive evolutionary thought modes universally embedded in the human psyche.

This can, and does, mean that *outdated thinking from an earlier Era can be very much present during a later Era.*

In Dossey's model, the first medical Era initiated with Cartesian thinking in the 17th Century and was characterized by a mechanical view of the body. Era I medicine views the human body as a machine that can be manipulated.

In this rather primitive medical approach, which remains firmly entrenched at the center of contemporary allopathic medicine, there is no place for mind or consciousness—and certainly none for spirit. Surgery, drugs and vaccines are applications of Era I medicine.

Properly speaking, many often beneficial forms of so-called alternative medicine—ranging from herbs to bodywork to chiropractic—also are based on an Era I perception of the human body as an essentially mechanistic phenomenon.

The 19th Century, according to Dossey, saw the birth of Era II medicine with the acknowledgement of the placebo effect. Characterized by mind-body approaches, Era II thinking fostered the emergence of psychoanalysis and psychiatry.

Era II medicine is based on the fact that your mind and body are interconnected such that *your* consciousness can benefit *your* physiology in provable ways.

This is the "power of positive thinking," to borrow an iconic phrase from Dr. Norman Vincent Peale. Alongside Era I, Era II thinking is established solidly in today's medical paradigm.

The new kid on the block, which is expanding existing medical parameters at an exponential rate, is Era III medicine, also referred to as *nonlocal.*

The cornerstone of Era III thinking is that human consciousness, being nonlocal at its base, is capable of operating outside the confines of the physical body—and even outside the individualized mind—in order to facilitate healing in the self or others.

The well-documented evidence to prove this phenomenon is copious and staggering. I invite those interested in this topic to read *Conscious Healing* as a springboard to a fuller appreciation of the irrefutable evidence supporting Era III medicine and nonlocal healing.

Some Observations

Having sketched the basic historical outline of Eras I-III, we now can make a handful of important observations that will serve us well as we explore three complementary perspectives on DNA in the following sections.

As shown in Figure 6, we can conceptualize Era I medicine as *impersonal*; Era II medicine as *personal*; and Era III medicine as *transpersonal*.

In other words, Era I medicine, which treats the body as a mindless machine, seeks to heal without regard to individual identity.

Swinging to the opposite polarity, Era II medicine's therapeutic efforts, as developed primarily through psychology, center almost exclusively on the individualized mind.

A parallel framework sees Era I as a function of the *subconscious* mind; Era II as a reflection of the *conscious* mind; and Era III as emerging from the *super conscious* mind responsible for all creation (Figure 6).

Going above and beyond Eras I and II, Era III medicine is based on a novel understanding of three related truths:

1. Giving rise to the body as well as the egoic mind is a blueprint of consciousness;

2. By working with the consciousness blueprint, it is possible to transcend curing—the goal of Eras I and II—and embrace a new paradigm of permanent healing and radical transformation; and

3. Such healing and transformation ultimately are transpersonal, occurring nonlocally by way of the super conscious mind, or consciousness field, which connects us all because we all derive from it.

Era III medicine differs from Era I in that the former encourages healing and transformation on a level that is beyond and yet gives rise to our animalistic physical nature.

Similarly, Era III departs from Era II by grasping the fundamental unity behind all individuality as the domain where genuine healing and transformation must be initiated.

In fact, many Era III techniques, such as the Regenetics Method, do not even require that facilitators know anything about recipients' conditions or diagnoses in order to be of profound and lasting benefit.

This is because, viewed through the lens of Era III medicine, what is responsible for assisting the recipient to heal is not our individual, egoic mind, but the transpersonal, spiritual Mind—i.e., the consciousness field of our collective beingness where all is one, all is known, and all can be made well.

For this reason, it must be acknowledged that Era III healing occurs *through*, yet is not *of*, individual healers. This is why Leigh and I call ourselves developers—as opposed to creators—of Potentiation and Regenetics.

Central to this Method, as with any genuine Era III modality, is to allow oneself to be a vessel for hyperdimensional consciousness to flow through in order to assist the self or another on the evolutionary journey.

Three Eras of Medicine

ERA I Genetics	ERA II Epigenetics	ERA III Meta-genetics
body	**mind**	**spirit**
physical power	power of positive thinking	power of positive feeling
body	head (brain)	heart
body-based	local	nonlocal
impersonal	personal	transpersonal
subconscious mind	conscious mind (ego)	super conscious mind (Higher Self)
animalistic	individualistic	unitarian
domain of matter	light domain (space-time)	sound domain (time-space)
coding DNA	proteins (cell membrane)	potential DNA
nature (DNA)	nurture (environment)	consciousness
genetic fatalism	genetic self-determinism	"intelligent design"

evolutionary direction of medicine →

Figure 6: Three Eras of Medicine

The chart above outlines the evolution of the field of medicine through three Eras that correspond to the development of genetics, epigenetics, and meta-genetics.

As also shown in Figure 6, it can be useful to conceptualize:

1. Era I medicine as concerned with the *domain of matter*;

2. Era II medicine as focused on bioenergy in the *light domain* (space-time); and

3. Era III medicine as respecting the primacy of bioenergetic consciousness in the *sound domain* (time-space) in healing and transformation.

Stated otherwise, Era I ignores bioenergy altogether in its naïve belief that the material world is all that is worth considering for medical purposes. By contrast, Era II displays an appreciation of the role consciousness plays in maintaining or improving wellbeing.

Era II medicine, however, stops short of being able to activate our extraordinary self-healing potential to the extent that it restricts its operation to localized, individualized, light-based, predominantly mental techniques.

Here, I am coming from a shamanic perspective that views light and thought as equivalent energies. The new physics, as well, explains that the act of thinking produces electrical currents that generate torsion waves of light—much as audible sound waves produce torsion waves of sound.

Era II modalities function through light within the light domain and, thus, are restricted in their ability to reset and modify our consciousness blueprint without using sound to access and modify the sound domain.

The above observations relative to Era II therapeutic avenues illuminate why psychotherapy and counseling seem to go in circles; allergy elimination treatments never seem to end; and many forms of energy medicine seem to do so little.

From Light to Sound

Today's evolutionary, Era III movement from perception centered in the domains of matter and light, to a more holistic understanding of reality rooted in the sound domain, is beautifully expressed by Joachim-Ernst Berendt in his masterful exploration of music and consciousness, *The World Is Sound.*

"Many outstanding scholars, scientists, psychologists, philosophers and writers have described and circumscribed the New Consciousness," writes Berendt. "But one aspect has not been pointed out: that it will be the consciousness of hearing people."

To be clear: the "New Man will be Listening Man—or will never be at all. He will be able to perceive sounds in a way we cannot even imagine today."

Berendt explains that modern humans "with their disproportionate emphasis on seeing have brought on the excess of rationality, of analysis and abstraction, whose breakdown we are now witnessing [...] Living almost exclusively through the eyes has led us to almost not living at all."

In contrast, historically speaking, wherever

> God revealed Himself to human beings, He was heard. He may have appeared as a light, but in order to be understood, His voice had to be heard. "And God spoke" is a standard sentence in all holy scriptures. The ears are the gateway.

Emphasizing that humanity's collective Shift in consciousness will be realized only "when we have learned to use our sense of hearing fully," Berendt quotes from Isaiah: "Hear, and your soul shall live."

This line of reasoning is echoed by Dennis Holtje in a wonderful little book entitled *From Light to Sound: The Spiritual Progression.*

"The stunning simplicity of the Sound energy confounds the mind," explains Holtje. "We are conditioned to use the mind to solve all of life's dilemmas, unaware that the ... energy of Sound ... provides the permanent solution of awakened spiritual living."

Using sound to restore and evolve our consciousness blueprint in the sound domain, and thereby provide the "permanent solution of awakened spiritual living," perfectly describes how Potentiation and Regenetics have worked for many people. Literally, this Method is "for those with ears to hear."

Now, to avoid confusion, allow me to emphasize once again that the transformational sound energy being referenced is *hyperdimensional* in nature.

It is absolutely true that we can produce audible sounds here in space-time to stimulate repatterning—via DNA—of our sonic templates in time-space.

But please understand that much in the way thought creates torsion light waves, the sounds we make here generate subtle, torsion sounds that technically are inaudible to most people and must be "heard," energenetically, with the "inner ear."

The intimate relationship that unites sound, language and DNA is explored more fully in the next chapter. But first, let us outline three perspectives on DNA that correspond to the historical development of Eras I-III in the field of medicine.

Era I: Genetics

In this and the following sections, as we examine three distinct yet complementary ways of viewing DNA, it can be helpful to reference Figure 6.

So, what *is* DNA? The simplest answer is that in its typical form, DNA, deoxyribonucleic acid, is a two-stranded molecule shaped like a double helix and composed of various combinations of chemical structures called nucleotides formed from four unique bases.

The double helix of DNA is stabilized by hydrogen bonds between the bases attached to the twin strands like the rungs of a ladder. The four bases of DNA are named adenine (abbreviated A), cytosine (C), guanine (G), and thymine (T).

The discovery of DNA in 1953 by James Watson and Francis Crick rapidly engendered an elaborate genetic science devoted to studying the biochemical properties of the molecule of life.

Although there is much more that might be stated about DNA by way of introduction, for present purposes it is most important to recognize that *genetic science understands DNA as merely a molecular, biochemical phenomenon with no relation to bioenergy, consciousness, or spirit.*

Let us appreciate that DNA definitely *is* a molecule, or pairing of molecules. When you initially look at it, that is probably the first thing that stands out.

But let us acknowledge as well that such an understanding, being quintessentially Era I in its conception of DNA as a material matter, constitutes a superficial, Newtonian grasp of DNA—one that completely ignores the latter's nonlocal, quantum aspects.

Disregarding the energetic qualities of DNA has allowed mainstream genetic science, in true Era I fashion, to focus exclusively on DNA as a self-replicating machine for building proteins, cells, tissues, organs and, eventually, bodies.

This way of defining DNA, in turn, has led to crudely mechanistic, Era I attempts to manipulate DNA such as gene splicing and gene therapy.

Additionally, defining DNA solely in terms of biochemistry has fostered the problematic belief that DNA is the cell's "brain" and controls gene expression in a robotic, predetermined way.

In due course, this belief has spawned a widespread genetic fatalism, whose dubious assertion that most diseases are hereditary—and thus beyond our individual control—is used to peddle unnecessary pharmaceuticals and surgical interventions to the gullible masses.

In a nutshell, *mainstream genetics views DNA as, and only as, a physical molecule whose activity is primary* (Figure 8). If this were indeed the case, it would mean that "nature" is more directly responsible for our experience of reality than "nurture."

Fortunately, in recent years a second perspective has emerged that challenges the "Primacy of DNA" and the idea that nurture is less important to our health and wellbeing than nature.

Era II: Epigenetics

Enter the pioneering work of biologist Bruce Lipton, one of the developers of the science of epigenetics.

From the perspective of traditional genetics, epigenetics represents a radical departure that undermines the long-held assumption that DNA and nature are primary.

The following passage from Lipton's *The Biology of Belief* neatly summarizes the basic tenets of mainstream genetics. The "Central Dogma,"

> also referred to as the Primacy of DNA, defines the flow of information in biological organisms … only in one direction, from DNA to RNA and then to Protein … DNA represents the cell's long-term memory, passed from generation to generation. RNA, an unstable copy of the DNA molecule, is the active memory that is used by the cell as a physical template in synthesizing proteins. Proteins are the molecular building blocks that provide for the cell's structure and behavior. DNA is implicated as the "source" that controls that character of the cell's proteins, hence the concept of DNA's primacy that literally means "first cause."

Lipton's theory of epigenetics, which grew out of his longtime study of the effect of our individual thoughts and beliefs on our genetic function and overall health, effectively demonstrates that this "Central Dogma" is just that.

In contrast to the materialistic, mechanistic mindset of genetic science's Central Dogma, it is clear from the research cited by Lipton that our own consciousness always and inevitably impacts the function of our genetic and cellular expression—at least in limited ways.

Such is the case because, according to epigenetics, the cell membrane (not the DNA within the cell) is the cell's brain. DNA is merely the cell's reproductive system.

Lipton cites the fact that enucleated cells (i.e., cells whose nucleus and DNA have been removed) die as evidence that the "nucleus is not the brain of the cell—the nucleus is the cell's gonad!" Moreover, "[g]enes-as-destiny theorists have obviously ignored hundred-year-old science about enucleated cells."

According to the epigenetic model, genes in DNA simply store instructions for propagating a given species. In other words, the primary function of DNA is not to "think" or interact with the environment, but to pass on—automatically and brainlessly—the basic genetic coding that creates a human being or a chimpanzee.

In Lipton's words, "epigenetics, which literally means 'control above genetics,' profoundly changes our understanding of how life is controlled." Epigenetic research establishes that "DNA blueprints passed down through genes are not set in concrete at birth."

What is responsible for "thinking," epigenetically speaking, is the cell membrane—specifically, the various types of interlocking regulatory proteins in the membrane. These have been documented to reconfigure in response to environmental stimuli—including toxins, traumas, energies, thoughts, and beliefs.

Emphasizing that "[g]enes are not destiny," Lipton points out that "[e]nvironmental influences, including nutrition, stress and emotion, can modify … genes, without changing their basic blueprint. And these modifications … can be passed on to future generations as surely as DNA blueprints are passed on via the Double Helix."

Epigenetics explains how environmental signaling instructs chromosomal proteins to change shape, thus determining which parts of DNA are "read" and allowed to express themselves.

This theory contends that the activity of genes ultimately is regulated "by the presence or absence of … proteins, which are in turn controlled by environmental signals."

"The story of epigenetic control is the story of how environmental signals control the activity of genes," writes Lipton. "It is now clear that the Primacy of DNA … is outmoded." An updated understanding, in Lipton's view, should be called the "Primacy of Environment" (Figure 8).

As opposed to the old top-down genetic model that enshrined DNA and nature at the apex of the pecking order, the Primacy of Environment explains that "the flow of information in biology starts with an environmental signal, then goes to a regulatory protein," and then, and only then, passes to "DNA, RNA, and the end result, a protein."

From the brief overview above, we are in a position to make three critical observations about epigenetics.

First, it should be readily apparent that while genetics is invested in the power of nature, epigenetics sees nurture as even more central to life. Thus epigenetics provides a much-needed counterpoint to the formerly one-sided study of biology (Figure 7).

A second observation is that in providing greater balance to the biological sciences, epigenetics empowers people to move beyond genetic fatalism by embracing the fact that our own thoughts and beliefs play an important role in creating health or illness.

"Rather than being 'programmed' by our genes," writes Lipton, "our lives are controlled by our perceptions of life experiences!"

The third observation is that for all its impressive background science, in the final analysis epigenetics represents essentially a mind-body approach to understanding and interacting with our biological functioning.

The basic concept behind this "new paradigm" is anything but new, having been summed up decades ago by Norman Vincent Peale when he wrote, "Change your thoughts and you change your world."

One important corollary to this third observation is that, at its core, *epigenetics grows directly out of Era II thinking.*

In the final analysis, epigenetics is light-based and, therefore, limited in its ability to explain or promote thoroughgoing healing and transformation.

Before we introduce Era III's approach to the biosciences, "meta-genetics," let us take a brief moment to highlight some problems associated with epigenetics.

Problems with the Epigenetic Model

I am a big fan of Bruce Lipton and applaud his successes and efforts in elaborating a valuable avenue of inquiry in the biological sciences.

In pointing out that epigenetics is an Era II approach with some significant shortcomings, it is in no way my intention to belittle this helpful, necessary model.

Rather, by calling attention to the "gaps" in epigenetics, I wish to segue into an even more revolutionary approach to genetic science and healing that corresponds to the evolutionary current of Era III medicine.

If the power of positive thinking were the end-all be-all; if affirmations and visualizations were the final key to healing; if transforming our reality simply involved adopting a mental attitude of "Don't Worry, Be Happy," why have such Era II approaches failed to work for so many people—myself included?

I spent the better part of a decade unsuccessfully trying to get well through a combination of Era I and Era II techniques ranging from raw food diets to the Rife Machine to Process Oriented Psychology. But it was only when I embraced the transpersonal, transformational potential of Era III that my health was restored.

There are several problems with the epigenetic model that deserve mentioning.

For starters, as previously pointed out, epigenetics is restricted to the light domain, which curtails its ability to effect thorough healing and transformation to the extent that it cannot access or modify our consciousness blueprint in the sound domain (Figures 6 and 7).

Secondly, epigenetics is concerned with space-time and thus constitutes a "local" model that largely ignores the nonlocal basis for our being in time-space (Figures 6 and 7).

Here in particular, epigenetic theory can be misleading. While our own thoughts and beliefs do affect our space-time reality, they do not, in the strictest sense, *create* it.

Lipton has admitted as much, writing that "soul or spirit" represents "the creative force behind the consciousness that shapes our physical reality." Indeed, the "structure of the universe is made in the image of its underlying field."

Practically, however, epigenetics turns a blind eye to the consciousness field. While acknowledging that humans are "Earth Landers" in constant dialogue with our "controller/Spirit," Lipton's model fails to probe the profound "meta-genetic" ramifications of this concept.

Instead, Lipton zeroes in on epigenetic "control" over our lives. But here in space-time, we actually control very little.

Although we have free will to interpret and respond to events and situations however we like, our greater spiritual identity in the consciousness field—which can be conceptualized as our Higher Self—ultimately controls our life experiences.

Compared to the reality-engendering Consciousness in the sound domain that gives rise to our intuition, imagination and inspired thoughts, any so-called thinking rooted in the light domain is a variety of egoic, bodily consciousness whose ability to alter reality is quite circumscribed.

Rather than using the language of control to characterize the impact of our individual perceptions on our experiences, perhaps it would be more accurate to say that our own perceptions of events and situations help us epigenetically "manage" them.

Thirdly, a related point. In characteristic Era II fashion, epigenetics is largely individualistic, centered for the most part on the individual's thoughts and beliefs (Figures 6 and 7).

While this approach laudably encourages people to take responsibility for their lives, it can have the unintended effect of discouraging people from seeing themselves as spiritual beings on a human journey with a more collective, unified origin outside their immediate physical environment.

Just as critically, the idea that there might be functional applications, ones that could be understood and proven by way of the biosciences, to focusing outside our localized space-time to our spiritual templates in the nonlocalized realm of time-space is left hanging in the balance.

In other words, in the epigenetic model as elaborated by Lipton, the spiritual "creative force" that operates in the sound domain remains a nebulous, basically unusable concept that is—effectively if not entirely—dismissed.

Yet from the perspective of Era III medicine, this very creative force—which we have called torsion energy, bioenergy, and consciousness—is *the* key to healing and transformation.

Two additional problems with epigenetics, which are best understood in retrospect as we discuss the implications of meta-genetic theory in the following section and next chapter, need only stating here:

1. In discounting the role DNA plays in terms of consciousness and our conscious experience of reality, epigenetics does so while ignoring ninety-seven percent of the DNA molecule; and

2. Because it ignores the vast majority of DNA, where our meta-genetic interface with the consciousness field occurs, epigenetics cannot account for the origin and evolution of species any more than genetics can. Only meta-genetics can explain these two interrelated phenomena.

Era III: Meta-genetics

In order to grasp the basics of meta-genetics, how this revolutionary science goes above and beyond both genetics and epigenetics, it is necessary to be absolutely clear as to the manner in which Eras I and II view DNA.

According to the genetic model that grew out of Era I thinking, *only three percent of DNA is worth studying.* There was no misprint in the previous sentence. Decades ago mainstream genetics dismissed *ninety-seven percent* of the DNA molecule!

The three percent of DNA observed "doing something"—i.e., building proteins—is referred to as "exons" or "coding DNA." The rest—which from a materialistic perspective, appears to "do nothing"—is called "introns," "noncoding DNA," or simply "junk" (Figure 9).

Various theories have been proposed to account for "junk" DNA. According to some geneticists, these chromosomal areas could be what is left of archaic "pseudogenes" that have been discarded and broken up during evolution.

Another idea is that "junk" DNA represents the residual DNA of retroviruses. Alternatively, "junk" DNA might constitute a data bank of sequences from which new genes emerge.

Happily, more and more scientists who have asked how nature could be so mind-numbingly inefficient are beginning to rethink "junk" DNA. More on this topic in a bit.

When DNA is mentioned in the epigenetic theory of Era II, what virtually always is being referenced is the three percent of coding DNA whose activity has been studied by traditional genetics.

In this regard at least, epigenetics is basically no different from genetics: both theories discount the vast majority of the genetic apparatus. In fact, you will not find "junk" DNA mentioned anywhere in *The Biology of Belief.*

Nevertheless, recent findings have indicated that "junk" DNA has a number of vitally important functions. The very maintenance of noncoding DNA over eons of evolution, instead of signifying genetic detritus, provides tantalizing evidence of such functions.

More to the point, a wealth of Era III research in wave-genetics has shed light on extraordinary meta-genetic activity in "junk" DNA. This ninety-seven percent of the DNA molecule, which Leigh and I call *potential* DNA, appears to have much more to do with creating a specific species than previously acknowledged (Figure 9).

For instance, if we only examine the tiny portion of DNA made up of exons, there is practically no difference, in terms of genetics, between a human being and a rodent. There is also precious little at the level of exons that differentiates one human being from another!

Others who have studied the mystery of "junk," or potential, DNA have concluded that the three percent of the human genome directly responsible for building proteins simply does not contain enough information to build *any* kind of body.

Faced with this puzzle, many scientists have started paying attention to fascinating structures called "jumping DNA," or "transposons," found in the supposedly worthless ninety-seven percent of DNA.

In 1983 Barbara McClintock was awarded the Nobel Prize for discovering transposons. She and fellow biologists coined the term *jumping DNA* for good reason, David Wilcock has noted, as "these one million different proteins can break loose from one area, move to another area, and thereby rewrite the DNA code."

This mysterious, malleable majority of DNA that, based on reasonable observation alone, must carry out significant functions for the organism, is the focus of meta-genetics.

This emerging science, famously substantiated and applied through the work of Peter Gariaev in wave-genetics, understands that *potential DNA constitutes the biological organism's interface with a hyperdimensional "life-wave."*

The life-wave, originating in time-space, is responsible for giving rise to a particular physical species or individual identity in space-time by nonlocally directing the activity of the three percent of coding DNA to build species-specific, individualized bodies (Figure 9).

While epigenetics allows us to manage gene expression and cellular function to a limited extent from our local position in space-time, what more directly *controls* our collective and individual genetic blueprints is the meta-genetic consciousness field in time-space.

Because consciousness dictates our biological reality, not the other way around, I coined the term *meta-genetics* to highlight the ultimately *metaphysical* nature of genetic functioning.

We now are in a position to replace both the Primacy of DNA and the Primacy of Environment with that which subsumes both nature and nurture and resolves their apparent contradiction within the unified field: the Primacy of Consciousness.

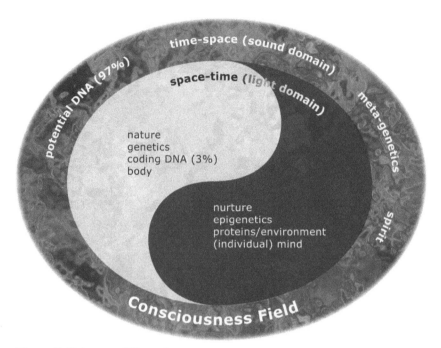

Figure 7: Primacy of Consciousness

This figure demonstrates that genetics and epigenetics are not mutually exclusive, but are subsumed and reconciled by meta-genetics, which understands that both nature and nurture are functions of consciousness.

The Primacy of Consciousness makes it easy to see that the real Brain behind the majority of our biological functioning resides neither in DNA nor in the cell membrane, but in the sound domain of time-space.

In the meta-genetic model of Era III, *the primary role of the vast majority of DNA is to mediate ener-genetically between our collective Mind in the consciousness field and our individual bodies (Era I) and brains (Era II) that exist as expressions of this bioenergy field in space-time.*

In the next chapter, we will examine just how DNA functions as a connection point between time-space and space-time, paying special attention to the lead role human language plays in activating DNA.

CHAPTER 6

DNA Activation

Thus far we have done a reasonable job addressing the question, *What is DNA?*

In this chapter and the following one, while broadening our understanding of DNA, we will explore the three remaining questions originally asked back in Chapter Three that are central to any discussion of authentic healing and transformation:

Is there a relationship between the bioenergy blueprint and DNA?

What role, if any, does DNA play in mediating between our bioenergy blueprint and our biology?

How might it be possible to activate DNA so as to correct distortions in the bioenergy blueprint and thus facilitate healing and transformation?

I wish to remind readers that, along with the previous one, this chapter is the most cerebral part of *Potentiate Your DNA*. While this material is essential to a mental grasp of the philosophy behind Potentiation and the Regenetics Method, it is in no way *necessary* to being able to perform and benefit tremendously from this work.

That said, the concepts I am about to share are among the most provocative and revolutionary you are likely to find anywhere in the biosciences.

A Quick Review

In the last chapter, it became clear that depending on one's perspective, DNA can appear to be several things.

According to the Era I version of the biosciences, genetics, DNA is the primary aspect of biological organisms that somehow drives the origin and evolution of species independently of other factors (Figure 8).

This viewpoint is contradicted by the Era II bioscience of epigenetics, which sees DNA as merely the gonad of the cell.

According to epigenetics, DNA is actually less important than cellular proteins. The latter are considered responsible for regulating DNA's expression and evolution through interaction with environmental stimuli (Figure 8).

In formulating their theories of how species evolve and replicate themselves, both geneticists and epigeneticists address only a small fraction of the DNA molecule: the so-called coding DNA that can be observed communicating with RNA to build proteins and, in the end, organisms (Figure 7).

At issue here is the fact that coding DNA constitutes only three percent of the DNA molecule. This scenario has led traditional genetics to disparage the other ninety-seven percent of DNA as "junk."

Such an erroneous perception of noncoding DNA is not called out by epigenetics for the simple reason that the latter is less concerned with DNA than with the activity of regulatory proteins in the cell's membrane.

"Junk" DNA, which I propose renaming potential DNA, is dismissed in both genetics and epigenetics because neither of these sciences can explain what it is or what it does.

In response to the mystery of potential DNA, genetics has relegated this vital part of the genome to the status of garbage, while epigenetics has ignored it altogether.

Only the Era III bioscience of meta-genetics has examined the nature of potential DNA without rearguard theoretical agendas and with a completely open mind as to the Primacy of Consciousness (Figure 7).

Meta-genetics—a term that encompasses a group of related fields including quantum bioholography, genetic linguistics, wave-genetics, and Regenetics—accepts two of the major premises of genetics and epigenetics, namely that:

1. The coding portion of the DNA molecule is physically responsible for building proteins; and

2. Regulatory proteins play an important role in interacting with environmental signals to determine which genes in coding DNA are silenced and which are expressed.

From the above, it should be obvious that meta-genetics subsumes crucial, irrefutable aspects of genetics and epigenetics and, thus, respects the relative importance of both nature (genetics) and nurture (epigenetics) in human experience.

By establishing the Primacy of Consciousness, meta-genetics provides an overarching conceptual framework under which the apparent duality between nature and nurture can be resolved (Figure 7).

Specifically, meta-genetics proposes that both nature and the reality conditions that allow for nurture emerge from—and are controlled by—conscious energy that constructs and directs our biological experience *intelligently.*

In so doing, meta-genetic theory calls attention to the blind spots of Era I and Era II, particularly with regard to the purpose and function of potential DNA.

According to meta-genetics, potential DNA is anything but "junk." Indeed, *potential DNA plays the truly primary role of interfacing ener-genetically with our bioenergy blueprint in the consciousness field* (Figures 7, 8, and 9).

In this way, potential DNA regulates cellular expression—and even the origin and evolution of species—in a manner that genetics cannot begin to account for and epigenetics cannot come close to matching.

In explaining the role potential DNA plays in the origin and evolution of species, meta-genetics reveals that genetics and epigenetics alike control our lives only relativistically, compared to the underlying spiritual energy that engenders, supports and develops life: consciousness.

Adaptation vs. Evolution

We could continue indefinitely to refine our understanding of the many elements that distinguish the three approaches to biology that correspond to the three Eras of medicine first outlined by Larry Dossey.

But to cut to the chase, one subject in particular sets apart genetics, epigenetics and meta-genetics like no other: evolution.

In true Era I fashion, genetics sees evolution from a Darwinian perspective, in which "random mutation" in DNA is responsible for the origin and evolution of species.

In most cases, what is thought to create such mechanistic genetic mutation—which is believed, incorrectly, to occur in the absence of environmental or conscious interaction—is the so-called law of "natural selection."

Somehow, according to the evolutionary theory of genetics, only the "fittest" qualities of a species "survive" by being passed on to new generations. Such is the logic behind the notion, so prevalent in genetics, of the "survival of the fittest."

The problems with this Era I model, which is seen by an increasing number of today's scientists as obsolete, are numerous. Here, I will share the three problems that are most relevant to our discussion of DNA activation.

For starters, the Darwinian interpretation of evolution is entirely deterministic—giving rise to the genetic fatalism and victim mentality that characterize the propaganda put out by the medical-pharmaceutical establishment to this day.

But as explained in the previous chapter, the Era II science of epigenetics clearly establishes that we have an appreciable level of ability to manage our own genetic expression.

Secondly, what genetics refers to as evolution should be called, in reality, environmental *adaptation*. On the one hand, it is a fact that species regularly adapt to environmental situations by developing new attributes.

In an oft-cited experiment demonstrating this phenomenon under laboratory conditions, lactose-intolerant bacteria were placed in a culture where their only food source was lactose.

What do you imagine these bacteria learned to do very quickly? Exactly. They adapted genetically, as a colony, in order to be able to feed on lactose.

On the other hand, the attempt to explain the *evolution* of species *into entirely different species* using the genetic model has failed monumentally.

Far surpassing the reach of step-by-step "evolution," which is just environmental adaptation, the fossil record reveals that species actually *evolve* in fits and starts—leapfrogging what would seem from a Darwinian viewpoint to be critical developmental phases.

At the top of a long list of species whose evolution has mystified geneticists is the human species. Although for more than a century a "missing link" has been assumed to exist based on fiercely upheld Darwinian concepts, many are convinced that not even the recent sensationalized discovery of a new type of hominid meets all the criteria for a direct human ancestor.

I share the view that Lee Berger's finding of a two-million-year-old hominid skeleton in the Sterkfontein region of South Africa is a false lead. Moreover, I offer that scientists never will uncover an indisputable missing link because *evolution of species occurs not incrementally, but more or less spontaneously.*

Recently, irrefutable evidence of spontaneous evolution was highlighted in the paradigm-shaking research of paleontologists David Raup, John Sepkoski, and Robert Rohde.

Their exhaustive studies of marine fossils revealed cyclical episodes of "punctuated equilibrium" unequivocally showing new creatures spontaneously appearing in the layers of the ocean's crust in regular cycles.

David Wilcock, who points out that these fascinating studies show that mass cyclical speciation usually occurs in the absence of cataclysmic events, puts it bluntly—and wittily—when he states that Darwinian evolutionary theory is "extinct."

Wilcock observes that the "probabilities that DNA could evolve by 'random mutation' are so minute as to be utterly laughable—akin to the idea that if you have enough monkeys tapping away on typewriters, one of them will eventually produce a complete Shakespearean play."

In a similar vein, biologist Elisabet Sahtouris has commented that the "history of evolution has repeatedly demonstrated that DNA is capable of rearranging itself intelligently in response to changing environmental conditions. Therefore, some types of mutation may not be random at all."

According to Dr. Sahtouris, "Clearly, we are moving toward a post-Darwinian era in evolution biology."

The third problem with the evolutionary model espoused by mainstream genetics that I will mention here is like the proverbial forest that, at first, you cannot see for the trees.

But if you simply step back and examine what genetics has to say about evolution from a distance, it soon becomes obvious that *natural selection and survival of the fittest describe not genetic, but* epigenetic *modes of environmental adaptation!*

Remember, DNA is supposed to be primary, which basically means "sovereign," according to mainstream genetic theory. There is no biological mechanism in the science of genetics that explains how a specific environment can foster a helpful adaptation in DNA, which then can be passed on to future generations.

Such a genetic "mutation" in a given species, however, is explained eloquently and redundantly by the Era II science of epigenetics.

In this model, so-called evolution occurs by way of environmental responses of regulatory proteins in cell membranes. These proteins, which react to localized environmental signals, direct the activity of genes—both electromagnetically and by utilizing RNA to communicate with DNA.

The problem with this model is that *while epigenetics offers insight into relatively limited adaptive responses, like genetics it sheds no real light on the mechanism behind the origin and evolution of species.*

In other words, epigenetics spells out how lactose-intolerant bacteria can adapt to a lactose-based environment. But epigenetics cannot explain, any better than genetics can, how a completely new species can evolve—more or less spontaneously—from a preexisting one.

With the above in mind, it is curious that Lipton's latest book on epigenetics is entitled *Spontaneous Evolution*. While I am thankful for, and resonate with, the general tenor of his positive and inspiring take on humanity's destiny, I am obliged to point out that his theoretical model simply cannot account for evolution—much less spontaneous evolution.

Only the Era III science of meta-genetics can explain the origin and (spontaneous) evolution of species. As will be discussed in-depth momentarily, *the related phenomena of the creation and development of species are driven by consciousness interfacing with potential DNA through a process that can be called DNA activation* (Figure 9).

In order to understand this process, first we must touch once more on genetics, epigenetics, and meta-genetics. Specifically, we need to grasp their relationship to the Flow of Genetic Information.

Flow of Genetic Information

Since the discovery of DNA in the 1950s, traditional genetic science has invested an enormous amount of energy establishing and maintaining a theoretical model in which genetic information flows from the top down (Figure 8).

According to the official theory of genetics, DNA passes on genetic information to RNA, the enzyme responsible for building proteins. In this dogma, where nature is considered primary, supposedly there is no information that runs from the bottom up—as in, from RNA or proteins to DNA.

In the 1960s, however, Howard Temin conducted experiments clearly indicating that information held in RNA can, and does, travel against the downward flow of genetic information so central to established theory (Figure 8).

As Lipton explains in *The Biology of Belief*, Dr. Temin, who was "originally ridiculed for his 'heresy'," subsequently "won a Nobel Prize for describing reverse transcriptase, the molecular mechanism by which RNA can rewrite the genetic code."

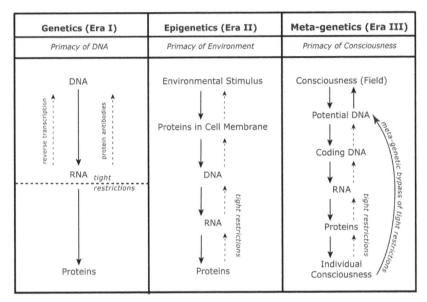

Figure 8: Flow of Genetic Information

The above chart summarizes the distinct ways in which genetics, epigenetics and meta-genetics explain the flow of information in biological organisms.

Pointing out that reverse transcriptase is used infamously by RNA in the AIDS virus to seize control of the infected cell's DNA, Lipton hypothesizes that proteins also must have the ability, despite the prevailing genetic theory, to "buck the predicted flow of information."

Logically, this must be the case, "since protein antibodies in immune cells are involved with changing the DNA in the cells that synthesize them."

There are, however, "tight restrictions on the reverse flow of information, a design that would prevent radical changes in the cell's genome."

Similarly, in a previously cited passage, Lipton was quoted as describing epigenetics as the science of how genes can be modified "without changing their basic blueprint."

These last two quotes provide clues as to what lies beyond the reach of epigenetics and nurture. The latter function with "tight restrictions" on the way our own localized consciousness, in response to environmental signals, can flow in reverse and rescript our "basic blueprint" (Figure 8).

Epigenetics is incapable of explaining evolution because it provides no mechanism allowing DNA to be rewritten, spontaneously, sufficiently to create "radical changes in the cell's genome" that transform a species into a new one.

Transcending both genetics and epigenetics, meta-genetics concludes that the origin and evolution of species are driven neither by coding DNA nor by regulatory proteins in cell membranes.

Rather, meta-genetics establishes that these two basically similar phenomena are controlled, via potential DNA, by what I have called a *life-wave*.

Meta-genetics & the Life-wave

The life-wave is best understood as a potentially infinite series of waves, much as an ocean is composed of an endless number of waves while remaining a single body of water.

The ocean in our analogy is the torsion, hyperdimensional sound domain of time-space, where individual waves act as sonic carrier waves for the genetic blueprints of past, present and future species (Figure 9).

Biologist Rupert Sheldrake's Morphic Resonance theory refers to this ener-genetic aspect of time-space as "morphic fields." Dr. Sheldrake's notion of "formative causation" stresses that these fields unite entire species universally outside space-time.

Sheldrake goes so far as to theorize that these nonlocal frequency fields can be expressed biologically if correctly "tuned into," even if a species is extinct.

In order for a particular life-wave in time-space to "go live" and become an actual, physical species in space-time, there is a specific meta-genetic protocol (Figure 9).

Recall that in biological organisms, potential DNA serves as the principal connection point between time-space and space-time. In other words, *potential DNA, far from being inactive, constitutes the hyperdimensional interface between the sound and light domains.*

In *Conscious Healing*, I described this interface as occurring through what I termed the *genetic sound-light translation mechanism.*

This phrase indicates the process by which chromosomes assemble themselves into different configurations designed to "translate" highly stable waves of sound into light (and vice versa).

The existence of the genetic sound-light translation mechanism indicates that the flow of information, or conscious bioenergy, through DNA is a two-way street.

Light becomes sound, and sound becomes light. Of course, given Dewey Larson's Reciprocal System of physical theory and the existence of sound and light domains, this must be the case.

The conception of the human body as a hologram, the basis of quantum bioholography, depends on such a mechanism, which has been validated empirically.

For an excellent overview of this paradigm-changing theory and the research supporting it, I recommend Iona Miller and Richard Alan Miller's article "From Helix to Hologram," which was republished in *DNA Monthly.*

For present purposes, we simply must grasp that, in addition to helping maintain the genetic sound-light translation mechanism at the level of chromosomes, potential DNA exists in both time-space and space-time—but in different ways.

Here in space-time, potential DNA appears as an inactive (noncoding) molecule, or part of a molecule. In this capacity, we can say that potential DNA is light-based, lacking any obviously transformational potential.

In time-space, however, potential DNA appears as a sound wave in continuous dialogue with the greater life-wave of the consciousness field (Figures 3 and 9).

The particle-wave duality—in which, say, an electron can be both a particle and a wave simultaneously—is an accepted phenomenon in quantum physics. Importantly, this duality can operate on much larger scales than the subatomic.

Named after Buckminster Fuller, the Fullerene molecule, or "buckyball," comprises sixty carbon atoms arranged spherically somewhat like a soccer ball. When propelled through a small enough "net," buckyballs have been demonstrated to transform into waves and back into particles again.

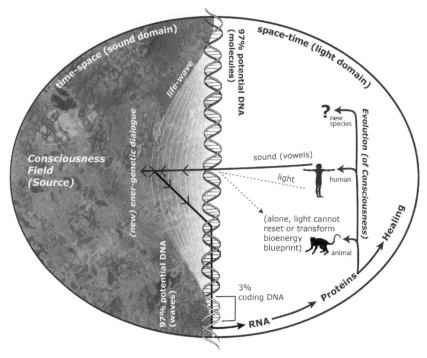

Figure 9: Sound, Light & DNA Activation

This illustration illuminates the ener-genetic interplay between the individual, DNA and the realms of space-time and time-space in personal healing and evolutionary transformation.

Of special interest to our discussion is that a Fullerene is roughly the size of a DNA molecule. Thus not only does DNA's network of chromosomes translate sound waves into light waves, and vice versa.

It is also reasonable to assume that potential DNA exists with "a foot in two worlds," exhibiting a molecular form in space-time and functioning as a wave in time-space (Figures 3 and 9).

Potential DNA's ongoing dialogue with the consciousness field allows for a constant, simultaneous exchange of information, in the form of sound and light waves, between time-space and space-time while bypassing any so-called tight restrictions on the flow of genetic information (Figure 8).

In one direction, as an example, light-based (holographic) traumas occurring in space-time are recorded as time-space distortions in our sonic bioenergy fields—which are, in effect, nested life-waves within the greater life-wave.

This example allows us to appreciate how, in a manner that challenges our notions of causality based on a perception of time as linear, *potential DNA both is projected by the consciousness field and simultaneously projects its bioenergy blueprint in the latter.*

In *Conscious Healing*, in fact, I emphasize that the bioenergy blueprint appears to be produced by potential DNA, as opposed to the other way around.

From the perspective of space-time, and considering that potential DNA translates local light waves into nonlocal sound waves in time-space, this interpretation is completely valid.

But as we have seen, there is another equally valid interpretation of the relationship between the consciousness field and potential DNA, in which sound waves from time-space manifest as light waves in space-time.

In this book, in order to sketch the basic outline of the meta-genetic model "through the looking-glass" from the vantage of time-space, I have chosen to focus on the way potential DNA appears to emerge from the consciousness field.

In a moment, we will explore just how human language can be used to correct sonic distortions, or disharmonies, in the bioenergy blueprint— allowing for information to flow from time-space back through potential DNA into space-time in order to actualize healing (Figure 9).

But before we do this, let us note that a similar protocol is utilized by the consciousness field in order to engender transformation—including the origin and spontaneous evolution of species.

Healing, Transformation & Potential DNA

In the meta-genetic model, potential DNA is both a *form* and *function* of the life-wave. In both cases, potential DNA can be theorized to exist as a consciousness blueprint in time-space *before* its physical manifestation in space-time.

As the primary connection point between time-space and space-time, *potential DNA's dialogue with the sound domain is directly responsible for producing the consciousness blueprint that gives rise to a specific species.*

The previous statement summarizes the basic mechanism behind the origin of species.

Any large-scale changes in this ener-genetic dialogue occurring nonlocally in time-space automatically result in commensurate changes to the wave frequencies in potential DNA. Stated differently, *a new dialogue produces a new consciousness blueprint.*

As shown in Figure 9, as this new nonlocal blueprint filters through potential DNA into local space-time, potential DNA becomes responsible for reorganizing the three percent of coding DNA into a novel configuration. Coding DNA, in turn, instructs RNA to build specific proteins and, ultimately, organisms.

Significantly, *a parallel phenomenon occurs during healing—only on a smaller scale.*

With the correct equipment, such as the quantum biocomputers used in wave-genetics, it is possible to observe at times subtle, but no less crucial, changes in potential DNA as the latter becomes activated "meta-genetically" during healing and transformation.

In both instances, transposons, or "jumping DNA," are instructed by potential DNA to shift their chromosomal positions—in small numbers when it comes to healing, but by the thousands during evolutionary transformation.

In the case of meta-genetic healing, while the observable molecular shift cannot be said to transmute one's basic DNA, nevertheless some genes necessarily are activated permanently even as others are switched off.

Regarding evolutionary transformation, such a massive molecular rearrangement fundamentally alters genes and creates radically new protein-coding sequences that produce distinct and unprecedented creatures.

The end result is the spontaneous evolution—which happens neither gradually nor adaptively, but as a veritable *metamorphosis* within a single lifetime—of an existing species into a new one.

Again, the evidence for this phenomenon is extensively present in the fossil record of our planet. Wilcock explains that the DNA molecule "is like a programmable piece of hardware ... so that if you change the energy wave that moves through it, the jumping DNA will encode it into a completely different form."

As Wilcock points out, this process—which can, and does, happen in regular, predictable cycles—explains why no "transitional" fossils can be found for so many species.

Moreover, meta-genetics neatly demonstrates that *evolution is driven by consciousness.* From a meta-genetic perspective, leaving behind new earth creationism, biology remains nevertheless a product of some kind of "intelligent design" (Figure 6).

Individually and collectively, there is only conscious evolution—or none at all. And such conscious evolution, personally and universally, occurs by way of DNA activation (Figure 9).

In addition to illuminating how evolution works, meta-genetic theory also explains why DNA appears to contain so little information distinguishing one species from another.

The life-wave in time-space, our real Brain, holds the consciousness blueprints for all species—which only manifest in DNA as, and to the extent, they are required for evolution.

Finally, the science of meta-genetics offers a sound intellectual scaffolding supporting the widespread belief that humanity as a whole may be on the verge of a genuinely spontaneous evolution.

University of Wisconsin anthropologist John Hawks' research, focused on genetic information in the fossil record, led to the declaration that for the last 40,000 years—and even more remarkably, within the past 5,000 years—the human species has experienced "supercharged evolutionary change."

Dr. Hawks is referencing measurable changes in DNA so exponential in the modern era that a human from 3,000 B.C. is more genetically comparable to a caveman than to someone strolling down the street today.

Likewise, the widely discussed Flynn Effect shows dramatic increases in human IQ over recent years that, having to do with abstract or symbolic thinking, simply cannot be explained by better education or improved technology.

What *can* account for these striking evolutionary developments is the concept of a meta-genetic life-wave in the process of changing its dialogue with—and thus *activating*—our potential DNA in order to evolve the human species into a new type of human (Figure 9).

Those who wish to delve deeper into the fascinating subject of spontaneous human evolution and how we can promote this process through DNA activation are encouraged to read *Conscious Healing*, where I greatly expand on the theory of meta-genetics as applied to the origin and evolution of species.

Genetic Linguistics

While the theory of meta-genetics is cogent, and even elegant, without research supporting it and documented practical applications, it would remain just that: a theory.

Fortunately, research and documentation that substantiate meta-genetics are available in abundance thanks to the pioneering work of Russian biophysicist Peter Gariaev, the father of wave-genetics.

Recently, a team of linguists headed by Dr. Gariaev, while studying a cutting-edge branch of semiotics known as genetic linguistics, discovered that the genetic code in potential DNA follows uniform grammar and usage rules virtually identical to those of human languages.

This groundbreaking research grew out of Jeffrey Delrow's stunning discovery in 1990 that *the four nucleotide bases of DNA inherently form fractal structures closely related to human speech patterns.*

As explained by Gariaev, a "group of scientists headed by M. U. Maslov and myself developed a theory of fractal representation of natural (human) and genetic languages."

This theory "postulates that the 'quasi-speech' of DNA possesses a potentially inexhaustible supply of 'words' and, moreover, that 'texts,' 'phrases' and 'sentences' in DNA transform into the letters and words used in human speech."

On the flip side, this theory supposes that *human language is "genetic" in nature and can be employed to interface with the genetic apparatus like a key fitting neatly in a keyhole.*

Gariaev's hypothesis that DNA is language-based (and vice versa) is bolstered by Gregg Braden's discovery, as described in *The God Code*, that the ancient four-letter Hebrew name for God is actually code for DNA based on the latter's chemical composition of nitrogen, oxygen, hydrogen, and carbon.

This assertion, with its enormous implications relative to DNA's universal role as a divine language spoken through the body, has been peer-reviewed and accepted by numerous scholars of Hebrew.

The research cited in this section establishes that the many human languages could not have appeared randomly, as is commonly taught, but reflect our essentially similar "genetically linguistic," or "linguistically genetic," blueprint.

As pointed out by linguist Noam Chomsky, human speech obviously does not exhibit a linear development from animal to human language patterns. "This poses a problem for the biologist," admits Chomsky, "since, if true, it is an example of a true 'emergence.'"

From a meta-genetic perspective, it is worth noting, *emergence* is an excellent term to characterize how biological species spontaneously evolve.

Furthermore, genetic linguistics reveals that DNA not only assembles proteins through RNA transcription, but also stores and communicates data in a patently *linguistic* fashion.

In fact, Gariaev's team found that the genetic code in potential DNA follows, for practical purposes, the same foundational rules as human languages (Mohr).

In a moment, we will explore how this new way of understanding DNA as an intrinsically linguistic phenomenon helped give birth to the many practical applications of wave-genetics. But before doing so, let us look briefly at another revolutionary discovery.

The DNA Phantom Effect

The theory of wave-genetics holds that potential DNA regulates meta-genetic, self-organization functions that occur in a hyperdimensional realm, which I have called time-space following Dewey Larson.

According to wave-genetics, *potential DNA magnetizes nonlocal streams of information from time-space to its physical location in space-time, then forwards this information to our consciousness*—including our "genetic consciousness" that manifests biologically.

Grazyna Fosar and Franz Bludorf, authors of an excellent summary of Gariaev's findings, *Vernetzte Intelligenz* ("Networked Intelligence") (summarized in English by Bärbel Mohr), refer to this data transfer process as *hypercommunication*, often experienced as intuition or inspiration.

In the next chapter, I share how hypercommunication played a pivotal and fascinating role in the final stages of the development of Potentiation.

When hypercommunication occurs, according to Fosar and Bludorf, an extraordinary phenomenon is observable in DNA. Gariaev irradiated a DNA sample with a laser until a typical light-wave pattern formed on his computer monitor. When the DNA sample was extracted, the pattern was still there, unaltered.

Control experiments proved that the pattern emanated from the absent sample, whose bioenergy field remained undisturbed for a whole month—even after being sprayed with liquid nitrogen—causing light to spiral on its own, as it were, tracing the outline of the physically removed double helix.

This meta-genetic phenomenon has become famous in new science circles as the *DNA Phantom Effect*. It appears that torsion waves from time-space continue to flow into space-time—where they manifest electromagnetically—for a month even after the DNA is removed.

The DNA Phantom Effect provides unambiguous evidence that:

1. Hypercommunication is an ener-genetic reality; and

2. DNA functions as a primary connection point between time-space and space-time.

"Most people tend to think that the DNA created the [phantom] energy field, and that the energy field is somehow just a 'shadow' of the DNA," writes Wilcock, who proposes a brilliant reinterpretation: "However, I believe that the wave actually exists before the DNA."

The "only logical explanation is that the phantom energy of DNA is actually the *creator* of DNA." Since this phantom spiritual energy pervades the galaxy, wherever the "materials that create life exist, the subtle, spiraling pressure currents of this energy will arrange the DNA molecule into existence."

Expounding on the subject of torsion energy and its relationship to DNA, Wilcock notes that for years he has "been saying DNA is a wave—spiraling 'nonliving' material together into a molecule. Now there's proof!"

Apparently, "loose inorganic materials can spontaneously and intelligently spiral together to form DNA … in the cold emptiness of space! One DNA molecule is as complex as an entire encyclopedia—so without a higher, organized intelligence guiding the process, we really cannot explain this."

The research Wilcock references involved experiments by Dr. Ignacio Ochoa Pacheco in which DNA emerged in a hermetically sealed container—containing only distilled water and sand heated to the point of killing any living organisms therein—when exposed to consciousness, or torsion waves.

If this evidence seems fantastical, consider the article "Dust 'Comes Alive' in Space" appearing in the *UK Times Online* in August 2007, where it was reported that an international panel from the Russian Academy of Sciences, the Max Planck institute in Germany and the University of Sydney found that galactic dust could form spontaneously into … double helixes […] and that [these] inorganic creations had memory and … power to reproduce themselves […] The particles are held together by electromagnetic forces that the scientists say could contain a code comparable to the genetic information held in organic matter.

Offering the simplest explanation of these related phenomena involving the spontaneous appearance of DNA and DNA-like formations, Wilcock concludes:

"DNA is a physical materialization of what torsion-waves look like at the tiniest level. Don't forget we are dealing with intelligent energy … This, of course, strongly suggests that life could form spontaneously from inert 'nonliving' material."

Wave-genetics

Meta-genetics provides a theoretical basis for understanding how biological life originates from so-called nonliving material.

From numerous pieces of hard evidence I barely have touched on, it appears that universal creative consciousness quite literally speaks the physical world, including DNA, into being.

Meta-genetics simply and logically explains why all human DNA is fundamentally linguistic in nature and why language can be understood and utilized from a genetic perspective:

The very energy that created DNA is language-based.

Stated differently, universal creative consciousness, or the Consciousness of Love, in order to utter life into being, generates torsion sound and light waves—in that order—whose hyperdimensional frequencies are inherently linguistic (Figures 1 and 4).

As pointed out in Chapter Four, the idea that "in the beginning was the Word" is central to the vast majority of the world's most venerable religions and mythologies.

Although it is just now coming into its own, this idea is also the key to the evolution of the biological sciences into their mature, Era III expression.

Beyond any reasonable doubt, based on redundant scientific data, behind the DNA molecule exists a template of linguistically sourced consciousness that directs the formation of organisms at the level of DNA.

By modifying this bioenergy blueprint meta-genetically through linguistic means, we can alter organic expression, facilitating both healing and transformation.

I have just provided the core rationale behind Potentiation and the Regenetics Method. This mode of human-potential-based DNA activation was inspired partly, on a theoretical level, by the Era III bioscience of wave-genetics.

One truly mind-blowing implication of Gariaev's research, which forms the backbone of Regenetics, is that to activate DNA and stimulate cellular healing as well as conscious evolution, we simply can use our species' supreme expression of creative consciousness: words.

This is possible because, as pointed out, the electrical energy involved in producing human speech automatically creates torsion waves of sound and light capable—when properly articulated—of accessing, resetting and transforming our bioenergy blueprint in time-space.

While Western researchers clumsily (and dangerously) splice genes, Gariaev's team developed sophisticated quantum biocomputers designed to influence cellular metabolism and stimulate tissue regeneration through sound and light waves calibrated to human language frequencies.

Employing pure linguistic frequencies embedded in radio waves and laser technology, Gariaev proved that chromosomes mutated by X-rays can be repaired; that a diseased pancreas in rats and missing adult teeth in humans can be regrown; and even more amazingly, that the genome itself can be rewritten.

Using sound and light waves keyed to human language frequencies to rescript DNA, as opposed to gene splicing, *Gariaev's team transformed frog embryos into perfectly healthy salamander embryos in the laboratory.*

Moreover, this was accomplished *noninvasively* by properly applying vibration and light, or sound combined with thought, or *words*, to DNA.

Gariaev's historic experiment in embryogenesis highlights the immense scope of meta-genetics—an area which has an obviously more primary influence on the origin and evolution of species than genetics or epigenetics.

Wrap-up

Make no mistake: I have synthesized and condensed a vast amount of information over the last two chapters.

Although ultimately self-evident, the theory behind meta-genetics and DNA activation can appear complex at first.

With this in mind, I will conclude the hardcore intellectual part of this book by responding briefly and directly (if somewhat simplistically) to our three outstanding questions:

Is there a relationship between the bioenergy blueprint and DNA?

Definitely. While three percent of DNA stays busy building our bodies, potential DNA (the other ninety-seven percent) is in constant meta-genetic interface with our bioenergy blueprint.

What role, if any, does DNA play in mediating between our bioenergy blueprint and our biology?

The meta-genetic dialogue between potential DNA and our bioenergy blueprint, or life-wave, determines which instructions for healing and evolving our bodies are passed on by potential DNA to the rest of our DNA for actualization.

How might it be possible to activate DNA so as to correct distortions in the bioenergy blueprint and thus facilitate healing and transformation?

As the science of wave-genetics has demonstrated, correctly applied, human language can be employed to access, reset and even transform our bioenergy blueprint.

Now, let us turn our attention back to some unfinished business: the development of Potentiation.

In the next chapter, we will investigate how—without any technology other than what nature gives us—we ourselves can adapt language, meta-genetically, to heal and transform our lives.

CHAPTER 7
Unfinished Business

When we paused the narrative of the development of Potentiation at the end of Chapter Four, my partner Leigh and I were busy field testing to substantiate the many ideas relative to DNA activation I was in the process of synthesizing from my voluminous reading.

In order to provide a philosophical and scientific foundation for Potentiation and the Regenetics Method, I outlined the most important of these ideas in the previous two chapters.

We now will pick up our narrative where we left off and chart the final, sometimes challenging, and always exhilarating stages of the development of Potentiation.

Surpassing the Teacher

As of late 2002, I had been offering a form of allergy elimination technique under the supervision of my mentor for about a year. My mentor had given me the keys to the office and permission to use the space and equipment after hours to perform allergy elimination on myself.

I saw some positive results in the many clients who showed up again and again for allergy clearings. But the fact that the clearings rarely culminated in a sustained state of wellbeing had started to weigh on me— all the more so, since I was still far from well myself.

Even as I became increasingly unsatisfied (personally and professionally) with this repetitious, light-based, Era II approach, my reading and field testing were revealing inspiring, new, Era III vistas for healing and transformation at the ener-genetic level.

In my heart, I knew there must be a way to transcend the therapeutic approach and help people achieve genuine wellness so that they could stop spending time and money on endless treatments and start putting energy and resources into living happier, fuller lives.

Unfortunately, my growing enthusiasm to rethink the field of allergy elimination was not shared by my mentor—from whom I had learned a great deal and for whose many insightful teachings I remain thankful to this day.

My gratitude does not change the fact that my mentor was uncomfortable with my ideas, and communicated as much. In unambiguous terms, she indicated that even if I was right about what I later would call meta-genetics, she had no intention of changing her therapeutic and business models.

Who could blame her? She had such a steady stream of allergic individuals fleeing from allopathic medicine desperate for anything that might help them, that until she trained and hired me, she had a long waiting list for new clients.

And she *was* helping people. This was true even though she admitted to suffering from lingering nutritional and environmental sensitivities—despite years of allergy elimination—stemming from her own chronic illness.

In many shamanic traditions, it is natural and proper for the student to surpass the teacher when the time is right. This indicates a good teacher and is a healthy sign that the shamanic lineage not only will be preserved, but simultaneously enriched.

Practically, however, this process is not always easy. In my personal experience, surpassing my teacher was unpleasant and even painful.

This episode constituted yet another example of breakdown and breakthrough—and I was better for it in the end, although at the time I would have welcomed smoother sailing.

Things came to a head when I mentioned to my mentor that Leigh and I were coming into the office after hours and using the homeopathic vials to conduct our own independent kinesiological research. Neither Leigh nor I saw anything remotely inappropriate in this—but my mentor obviously did.

Instead of discussing the situation with me, she reacted by taking the vials home with her when she left each day, which meant lugging several heavy boxes down the steps to her car and hauling them back up the next morning.

Not only was my research temporarily curtailed. Since now there were no vials when there were no clients in the office, I no longer could perform allergy clearings on myself.

This latter piece especially stung, since I still depended on clearings to keep my stubborn food and chemical allergies at bay. The implication was that if I wanted to receive a clearing, I should come see my mentor.

Never mind that, by her own admission, I was already beyond where she was in grasping and working at the ener-genetic level with the homeopathic frequencies contained in the vials.

And so, even though I had no savings and no prospects, I did the only thing I could do and still respect myself: I quit.

I am certain my mentor's intention was for me to do just that. Shortly thereafter, Leigh followed suit. Actually, it worked out just fine, for all of us.

My mentor's steady stream of clients never let up and, eventually, she trained another practitioner. And Leigh and I finally were free to develop our own ideas about true healing and radical transformation. The only thing we lacked was financing.

Unexpected Support

When my mentor and I finally parted ways, amicably enough, that December, I had no idea where the money to live was going to come from—to say nothing of the funds to continue my research.

Then when Leigh joined me in the ranks of the unemployed, the situation truly became laughable. We actually went out and shared an expensive romantic dinner to celebrate the absurdity of our impasse.

I long have considered myself highly adept at the leap of faith, an act that never has failed to produce remarkable serendipities and wonderful opportunities. This time was no different—except, perhaps, in scale.

Within days of Leigh's resignation, there was a knock on the door to the downtown apartment she and I were renting. It was our upstairs neighbor: a gentle, quiet woman in her mid-thirties with whom we had established a friendly rapport.

She had reported benefits from a couple of allergy elimination sessions with Leigh and myself; had expressed interest in our latest research in DNA activation; and knew we were both jobless.

Without a word, our neighbor handed me a brown paper bag with a lump inside.

I was aware that one of her parents had passed away recently and left her a tidy sum. This knowledge did nothing to mitigate my shock, when I opened the bag, at finding a wad of hundred-dollar notes!

"God told me to give this to you," she said. "Your work is important and needs to be completed. I believe it will help many people."

"But there's no way I can accept so much—"

She cut me off mid-refusal. "I'm going to go now before I change my mind."

And she did. She turned and walked straight up the stairs. Stunned, Leigh and I stared at each other. To say that we felt supported by unseen forces would be a huge understatement.

In less than a week after this miraculous event, two more unambiguous shows of universal support for our work occurred.

For starters, a mutual friend in the healing field who also knew what we were up to felt called to gift us an entire set of allergy elimination vials (in custom boxes) that must have cost a pretty penny. This allowed us to continue our field testing with hardly a hitch.

Around the same time, we were approached by one of our former clients to share our new work, which was just beginning to incorporate sound, with her and about fifteen of her students.

As it turned out, she was the leader of a mystery school and had a thing or two to teach us about sound, language, and DNA activation. Specifically, she called our attention to the supreme importance of vowels in activating DNA.

The Role of Vowels

The next two months, during which Leigh and I visited the mystery school to see clients twice a week, were a period of intense "downloads" of information.

I use the term *download* with a nod to Fosar and Bludorf's reflections on hypercommunication and how wave-genetics reveals that just as with the Internet, *one can upload data into the biological "Internet" that is DNA, download data from it, and even email others.*

In addition to synthesizing information with my rational faculties, for the first time I was fully engaging my intuition in accessing and integrating the reams of data that presented themselves daily to my consciousness.

In a world bloated with contradictory and often useless information, lacking faith in our intuition's ability to "separate the wheat from the chaff" represents a major evolutionary stumbling block for many people. It is easy to lose sight of the truth when trying to evaluate gigabytes of data using only the left brain.

To see clearly, it often is necessary to close our eyes and engage the right brain. At all times, as long as we are willing to listen to that "still small voice," our Higher Self is eager to guide us in making sense of things.

Here, I am reminded of Einstein's famous assertion that "the intuitive mind is a sacred gift and the rational mind is a faithful servant. We have created a society that honors the servant and has forgotten the gift."

In a similar vein, David Bohm's essays emphasize that there is little that is technically logical about scientific discoveries. Rather, scientific breakthroughs are inspired epiphanies that occur creatively in much the same way as do works of art.

When the leader of the mystery school shared her thoughts on vowels and DNA activation, I was digesting a fascinating book by French anthropologist Jeremy Narby entitled *The Cosmic Serpent: DNA and the Origins of Knowledge*.

The author spent years studying the extraordinary healing abilities of shamans in the Amazon rainforest. His account was riveting and proved particularly helpful in developing Potentiation.

In one intriguing passage, Dr. Narby points out that "DNA is not merely an informational molecule, but ... also a form of text and therefore ... is best understood by analytical ways of thinking commonly applied to other forms of text. For example, books."

Coming from my background in literary theory and fiction writing, this way of looking at DNA as a book was inherently attractive. More than anything, it just felt right.

Narby clearly says that we can learn to read DNA. By implication, he suggests that we also can learn to write, or rewrite, the genome.

In another inspiring passage that was enormously helpful in conceptualizing the interplay between light and sound in Regenetics, Narby states that according to

127

shamans of the entire world, one established communication with spirits via music. For [shamans] it is almost inconceivable to enter the world of spirits and remain silent. Angelica Gebhart Sayer discusses the visual music projected by the spirits in front of the shaman's eyes. It is made up of three-dimensional images that coalesce into sound, and that the shaman imitates by emitting corresponding melodies.

Throughout, Narby stresses that *in order to stimulate healing, shamans use sound—and to a lesser degree, light—because this combination allows them to change some aspect of the genetic code.*

Immediately and intuitively, I understood that Potentiation—a name that just recently had come to me—also would feature melodies of sound in tandem with light to activate DNA and permanently repattern the bioenergy blueprint.

With inspired clarity, in a manner that was similar to the way Narby describes the process of Amazonian shamans, I visualized how hyperdimensional light waves would guide paired sound waves to potential DNA.

I knew that light alone, in epigenetic fashion, would be unable to reset the bioenergy blueprint owing to the aforementioned tight restrictions on the flow of genetic information from the environment and our localized consciousness back to the genome (Figures 8 and 9).

Sound, however, could pass through the genetic sound-light translation mechanism into the nonlocal sound domain so as to correct distortions in the bioenergy blueprint meta-genetically (Figure 9).

But not just *any* sounds. In my mind's eye, I distinctly saw a grid of paired linguistic codes of sound and light very much like the two Potentiation grids I teach you to work with in Part II (Figures 12 and 13).

I may have seen a grid distinctly, but the codes between the lines were still out of focus. The only thing I could make out was that they were all *vowels.*

Not long afterward, at the mention of vowels and DNA activation, the proverbial light bulb came on in my head. Field testing had revealed that the five vowels in English—A, E, I, O, U—correspond energetically to the five nucleotide bases of DNA and RNA.

In a flash, I grasped that *vowels can be used here in space-time to "key" the genetic code in potential DNA to access, reset and even transform our underlying blueprint in time-space.*

My epiphany about the role of vowels in fostering wellbeing and conscious evolution found support in an impressive array of esoteric sources I will not burden the reader with here.

In written Hebrew, to cite but one example, vowels were omitted because they were revered as sacrosanct, the language of creation.

The "vowels were 'extras' in Hebrew," explains William Gray. "The vowels were originally very special sonics indeed, being mostly used for God-names and other sacred purposes. Consonants gave words their bodies, but vowels alone put soul into them."

Finally, I knew what Potentiation would look like, more or less. And I had a rough notion what it would sound like.

But I had no idea how to choose the right combinations of vowels so as to encourage the profound healing and transformation I believed were possible with this approach.

As if reading my mind, the mystery school leader looked deeply into my eyes and said point-blank: "You will return to Brazil, where I understand you have unfinished business. There, the correct vowels will find you."

Now, it is true that I had shared some of my travel experiences with her in polite conversation. But never had I referred to my time in Brazil as anything other than an extended vacation.

Certainly, nothing I had said suggested there was "unfinished business" for me in Brazil. But apparently, there was.

More Thoughts on the Fragmentary Body

Before traveling to Brazil, let us take a moment to revisit the Fragmentary Body, the problematic second bioenergy field from the bottom and related chakra whose basic structure was shown in Figure 5.

In previous chapters, we learned that the Fragmentary Body constitutes a major disruption in the bioenergy blueprint. It is related to parasites of all kinds, which often begin leaving after the Fragmentary Body is sealed at around the five-month mark following the Potentiation session.

Not surprisingly, in the shamanic tradition of the Toltecs of Mesoamerica, as popularized by medical doctor and author Don Miguel Ruiz, the Fragmentary Body is called the *Parasite*.

Another name for the Fragmentary Body stems from the bestselling writings of Eckhart Tolle, who refers to it as the *pain body*. Yet another name comes from David Wilcock, who calls it the *Original Wound*.

Regardless of the name we give it, *every spirit starting out his or her evolutionary journey as a human being possesses a Fragmentary Body.*

On the one hand, as suggested by its relationship to the mouth, tongue and reproductive organs, the Fragmentary Body is associated intimately with the meta-genetic creation of life as we know it.

On the other hand, the Fragmentary Body is linked to the "veiling," or forgetting, of our greater identity in spirit we undergo as we incarnate here in what poet John Keats famously termed the "vale of Soul-making."

Although it is not the ego, the Fragmentary Body is responsible for enlarging and distorting the ego by engendering shame and fear as egoic defense mechanisms against the embarrassing and frightful experience of separation.

In Judeo-Christian as well as Islamic sacred texts, the creation of the Fragmentary Body appears to be recorded in Adam and Eve's decision to eat of the forbidden fruit. Immediately after this event, feeling shame for the first time, the two fearfully cover their nakedness as best they can.

From the perspective we have just sketched, it makes sense that the Fragmentary Body is a bioenergetic reaction to—and marker of—our self-induced separation from the greater aspect of ourselves that is the Creator.

Adopting a truly cosmic perspective, we might go so far as to say that *the Fragmentary Body maintains the illusion of duality so that we can benefit fully from the experience of being human.*

At its core, this experience, with all its twists and turns, is designed to chart an archetypal trajectory from a sense of separation, to a gnosis surpassing mere intellectual knowing that we are—and always were—one with the Creator.

This trajectory is empowered at its beginning by the establishment of the Fragmentary Body, and near its culmination by the sealing of the Fragmentary Body (Figure 10).

Sealing the Fragmentary Body encourages not only physical healing, but also the truly transformative experience of conscious personal mastery.

Recall that the "wages" of Adam and Eve's act of disobedience involve death. The loss of vitality and eventual destruction of the physical vehicle directly result from the experience of separation (expulsion from the Garden) and, I would argue, the simultaneous creation of the Fragmentary Body.

It should go almost without saying that physical healing frequently results from "plugging up" the torsion "rift" caused by the Fragmentary Body, since this permits a free, uninterrupted flow of bioenergy throughout our systems (Figure 10).

Generating a more abundant and harmonious bioenergy flow encourages physical healing because, as Wilcock has observed, research in torsion physics and wave-genetics provides

> extremely convincing evidence that the DNA molecule is directly affected by outside energy sources. If DNA is actually assembled by an outside source of energy, then when we increase the flow of that energy into the DNA, we can also expect that the health and vitality of the organism will increase.

Sealing the Fragmentary Body also fosters conscious personal mastery as our sense of isolated *individuality* and corresponding *victim consciousness* are transformed through a process of *individuation* leading to a deeply felt reunification with the Creator and the experience of *unity consciousness*.

Sealing initiates the reintegration of the Higher Self—whose ostensible fragmentation appears to be a precondition for becoming human—and empowers us to love ourselves and others more completely through a bioenergetic gnosis of Oneness with all creation.

I have just provided a basic summary of a much longer and more detailed exposition of a subject that is central to *Conscious Healing*, where I examine the Fragmentary Body from a myriad of personal and transpersonal angles.

Leigh and I were aware of the Fragmentary Body from our earliest field testing, where it showed up again and again as a torsion distortion that drains people's life force and keeps their consciousness locked in self-limiting patterns of thought and belief.

It was obvious that the Fragmentary Body was what many have referred to as the "shadow self." Both of us intuited that in order to foster genuine healing, or wholing, across the body-mind-spirit spectrum, the Fragmentary Body had to be addressed.

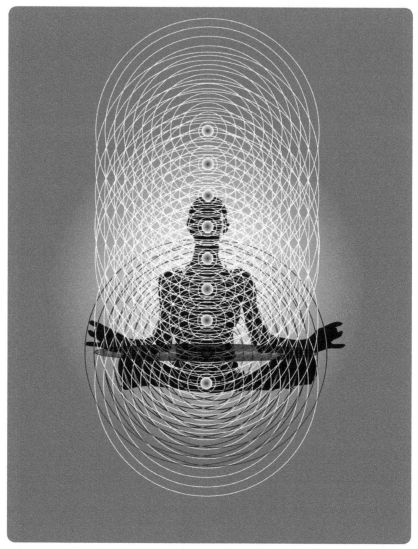

Figures 10a & 10b: Sealing the Fragmentary Body

The first image (Figure 10a) shows a typical human bioenergy blueprint with nine bioenergy fields/chakras and a Fragmentary Body, envisioned as an energetic disruption in the second field/chakra from the bottom. The second image (Figure 10b) shows a potentiated bioenergy blueprint with an infinity circuit of eight fields/chakras. Note how sealing the Fragmentary Body replaces fragmentation and duality with harmony and sacred geometry, allowing for the free flow of bioenergy throughout the body.

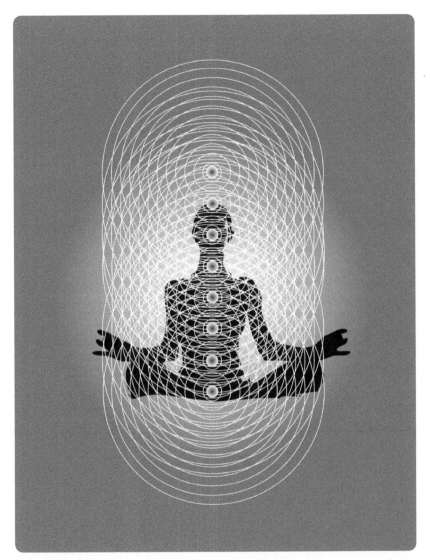

Figure 10b

And address it we did. Although there are other avenues theoretically capable of sealing the Fragmentary Body, I know of none as quick or effective as Potentiation.

When the Fragmentary Body came up in conversation with the mystery school leader, Leigh and I were delighted—if not exactly surprised—to hear her echo our own observations.

But one remark sowed the seeds for a new idea that would blossom a few months later in Brazil as the linguistic codes for Potentiation began to emerge.

"Just as the Fragmentary Body was spoken or sung into being by an aspect of ourselves," said the leader, "you will discover how to speak or sing it back into nonbeing. This will be the cornerstone of your work in DNA activation."

Intuiting a Geophysical Connection Point

There has been a misconception that I returned to Brazil to study with shamans, but this was not the case. By the time I boarded a plane for Rio de Janeiro early in 2003, I *was* a shaman heeding an intuitive call that was loud and clear.

Leigh was by my side every step of the way. Neither of us had any doubt we were supposed to travel to Rio or a second thought about using the funds our neighbor had given us to do so.

We simply put our belongings in storage; left our cars with family; packed our bathing suits and homeopathic vials for field testing on the road; and said *até logo* with no clear idea when we might be back.

The week before we flew out, the mystery school leader and her students insisted on performing a special ceremony of blessing for us. Never before had non-initiates been taken into the inner temple, as it was called, for any reason.

The ceremony was quite a sensory experience—complete with lots of powerful incense, unintelligible chanting, and ancient Egyptian rituals involving symbolically utilized knives to protect us on our journey.

I cannot say with certainty whether the ceremony did anything to protect us, but maybe it did. Halfway through our stay abroad, Leigh fell flat on her face in the middle of a busy intersection and, miraculously, all the cars speeding in from both directions stopped on a dime.

Not long after that, I nearly drowned when I was caught in a riptide on a beach with no lifeguard. I flailed with all my might to reach the shore even as it receded. Just as I was about to give up, I heard a voice distinctly urge, "Sidestroke, you fool!"

I instantly turned on my side and relaxed in the current, which I realized was swirling in a long crescent back toward the beach farther down the shore. Within thirty seconds, I was standing in the surf sucking wind like someone who had just finished a marathon, amazed to be alive.

I could write a travel book about the over-the-top adventures Leigh and I had for six months in Brazil. But for present purposes, let us zero in on a series of mystical (for lack of a better word) experiences that directly preceded our own Potentiation.

At the end of Chapter Three, I touched on Ivan Sanderson's studies of the major geophysical connection points between space-time and time-space. Although I was unaware of this research at the time, one of these connection points is in South America just off the coast of Rio de Janeiro state.

Instinctively, Leigh and I were drawn to the coastal town of Búzios about four hours by bus north of Rio. Ever since Brigitte Bardot visited Búzios in the 1960s, it has grown steadily as a tourist destination. But historically, Búzios supported itself through fishing.

I share this information because I believe it is significant that Búzios is one of the closer towns to the South American connection point mentioned above. In fact, I recall hearing stories from locals about fishing boats mysteriously disappearing and reappearing off the coast.

Now, I wish to emphasize that at the time Leigh and I were totally unaware of Sanderson's research. We found ourselves in Búzios because we intuitively sensed that the Potentiation codes would "find us" there.

That this would occur in the vicinity of a location with maximum permeability between the physical and spiritual worlds of space-time and time-space, respectively, was a fact we were able to appreciate only in hindsight.

How the Correct Vowels Found Us

Around nightfall of the March equinox, intuitively Leigh and I felt "summoned"—that is the best word to describe the sensation—to João Fernandes beach, one of numerous scalloped stretches of sand around Búzios.

Neither of us had been drinking alcohol or taking drugs. Given my allergies and precarious health, I was in no position to do either if I had wanted to; and Leigh typically was reserved in such matters.

Hearing an intuitive summons, we left our apartment with a sense of exhilaration neither of us had ever felt, walking along a cobbled road flanked by lush bogs vibrating with insect voices.

Twenty minutes later, we reached the dark horseshoe beach just as, seemingly out of nowhere, a storm blew in—lightning blushing an eerie blue while rain fell sideways and brushed our faces where we crouched sheltering under an *amendoeira*.

Eventually, the storm passed and the rain stopped, at which point we were "invited" to move down the beach to the vicinity of a CÔCO VERDE sign stuck in the sand, where we were to await another kind of "sign."

By this time, there was nobody except us on the beach. Three small fishing boats, all empty, were anchored in the middle of the little bay. Aside from the sound of the waves, there was no noise, not even the distant barking of dogs.

After maybe half an hour, the sign came. To our mutual astonishment, on each of the three unmanned boats riding the swells in the bay, a fantastically bright, perfectly round light suddenly appeared!

Some readers may be aware, through personal experience or otherwise, of the existence of mysterious light "orbs" that can pop out of the blue and have been captured in many photographs proven to be clean of dust specks or water drops.

The most thoroughly researched material on this fascinating subject is contained in *The Orb Project* by physicist Klaus Heinemann and theologian Miceal Ledwith, with a foreword by William Tiller, a professor emeritus from Stanford University.

Although their perspectives on orbs are nuanced, all three of these gifted thinkers and researchers agree in their conclusion that *authentic orbs appear to be spiritual beings, the majority of whom are here to help us if only we will allow them to do so.*

Graham Hancock, writing on shamanism from a scholarly angle in *Supernatural*, reaches the same basic conclusion relative to the beneficent nature of the vast majority of luminous "ancient teachers" encountered in visions by shamans and others engaged in visionary activities.

Addressing light orbs in their research on "networked intelligence," Fosar and Bludorf theorize that such balls of light—which are thought by many to be of extraterrestrial origin—are actually manifestations of some type of group consciousness operating through DNA by way of hypercommunication.

I believe that the swirling, brightly lit orbs Leigh and I saw that night on João Fernandes beach were, in fact, representations of our Higher Selves, who were contacting us ener-genetically in order to guide us in accessing the vowel codes for Potentiation.

Both the timing of this extraordinary event (the equinox) and the place where it occurred (a rare geophysical connection point between space-time and time-space) point to a conscious, premeditated decision on the part of the spiritual beings with whom we found ourselves interacting.

In many shamanic traditions, encounters with so-called paranormal forms of luminosity are so common as to be considered mundane. In a number of the world's religions as well, spiritual beings (such as angels) often are said to appear to human observers as lights.

Torsion physics and Reciprocal System theory combine to provide a compelling optic on how hyperdimensional life-forms from the sound domain might appear as light beings in the light domain—particularly when and where the connection is open enough to permit such a crossover.

After a moment of rapt interface with the orbs on the boats, Leigh and I both uttered a gasp of amazement as one of the lights abruptly projected a shimmering beam from itself—which seemed almost audible like electricity—across the opaque water to the CÔCO VERDE sign.

"Come on," I whispered, taking Leigh's hand and leading her down to the sign at the ocean's edge.

Simultaneously, the other two orbs added their own luminous, crackling streams to what now resembled a rainbow "bridge of light" stretching to us across the water.

At this juncture, the combined, prismatic light of the three orbs actually was shining on us. Physically, the feeling was one of warmth—as if all of our molecules were bathed in loud, beautiful concert music.

Emotionally, we both felt loved to such an overwhelming, unconditional degree that tears sprang from our eyes and cascaded down our cheeks.

Then the lights went out. Just like that. We stood in darkness with the surf lapping our ankles in complete silence for an unknowable length of time. Both of us understood that something exceedingly profound had just occurred, but for a while lacked the wherewithal even to discuss it.

Late that night, I awoke from a dream in which I was flying to find myself repeating a series of vowels that made no logical sense. Nevertheless, I got up out of bed and wrote them down in a row like a single word.

The next morning upon waking, Leigh yawned, stretched and said, "I had the strangest dream. I was flying. And then I heard this word in my mind made up of vowels."

"Me, too."

"I think I need to copy it down."

"I think the correct vowels are finding us."

"I think you're right."

For the next four days, that was how it went: we each woke up with a set of vowels that had come to us in our dreams.

We knew that dreams constitute their own interface between time-space and space-time. Neither of us had any doubt we were receiving sacred vowel sequences for healing and transformation.

We intuited that I was bringing through the "sound codes," which were to be chanted during Potentiation, and Leigh was bringing through the "light codes," which were to be thought silently in tandem with the sound codes. More on this technique in Part II.

After a mere five days, we had brought through the first Potentiation grid for in-person sessions (Figure 12). Later, we would repeat a similar process to establish the grid for distance Potentiation sessions (Figure 13).

It is my contention that Leigh and I were not "channeling" this information, so much as we were utilizing the power of hypercommunication to access universal data of a hyperdimensional nature.

Ken Carey, who similarly feels that the word *channeling* fails to capture the reality and immediacy of the "telepathic awareness," or "metapersonal thought," of his own higher consciousness behind his uncannily lucid transmissions, writes that after years

> of hearing the term *channeling* bantered about, I am convinced that it does not apply to the process through which I access this information. (I know many people who regularly tap into this awareness and I expect they would agree.) There is no trance involved in my reception of these thoughts, no loss of consciousness, no voice change or foreign accent. I am fully present throughout the experience ... [A]ccessing higher-frequency awareness is actually an organic process, a natural ability with which every child is born.

Significantly, in the case of adults who might suffer from intuitive "atrophy," the "ability to access higher-frequency thought can ... be reactivated," either be accident or intentionally. Recalling Berendt's notion of the "Listening Man," such an ostensibly "psychic" capability boils down to a fine-tuned capacity to *hear*.

It is worth quoting Dr. Jean Houston's excellent and scholarly Foreword to Carey's work, where in order to explain this clearly inspired form of "intuitive knowledge," she writes that the

> psyche is invested in matter and therefore matter can have access to psychic knowing. Thales of Miletus gave the first Western explanation in the sixth century B.C. when he said that "all things are full of gods," meaning that a sort of psyche, a divine emanation, is both complementary and co-extensive with matter and leads towards larger realities. Plato wrote of the Forms or Archetypes in all things, luring them to growth and becoming. Jesus speaks of the Kingdom Within and the immanence of the I AM nature of God in each person. The Sufi Islamic mystics refer to the *alam al mithal*, the *mundus imaginalis*, an intermediate universe that is thought to be as ontologically real as the sensory empirical world and the noetic world of the intellect.

This "intermediate universe," which I have called both time-space and the consciousness field, occupies a "metageography [that] can be experienced only by those who exercise their psychospiritual senses, and, through this special form of imaginal knowing (which is very close, if not identical to channeling) gain access to a visionary world that is not unlike the *mundus archetypas* of Carl Jung."

In a manner that speaks to the often difficult levels of shamanic initiation Leigh and I both underwent, in our own ways, to become vessels pure enough to reactivate our intuitive abilities and receive the Potentiation codes, Houston emphasizes that the brain and nervous system must

> be re-educated in order to open the doors of perception on the strange and beautiful country of channeled knowing. Otherwise one gets the great garbage heap of the unconscious, sanctified to the channeler and his duped disciples as the word of God. Indeed, a great deal of what passes for channeled information is just that—the flotsam and jetsam of the unconscious minds of inflated egos.

Fortunately, you do not have to take my word that the vowel sequences taught in Part II are particularly inspired, healing, or transformational. You are encouraged to experiment with them and decide for yourself.

DNA Activation & Love

Before we performed our own Potentiation that week following the equinox, Leigh and I returned to João Fernandes beach during broad daylight.

We had swum there on several occasions prior to the incident with the orbs, but neither of us had noticed that someone had gone to great pains to paint the Portuguese verb for love, *AMAR*, in huge white letters on the sheer rock face flanking the bay.

I still have a photograph of this remarkable feature snapped by Leigh that afternoon. It occurred to both of us that maybe the word had *not* been there before.

When I asked around, although I never got to the bottom of this mystery, I had a sense that—whether *AMAR* had been painted on the rock a day, a month or a decade earlier—nobody, not even the local vendors, had paid much attention to it.

Later, while considering the "love rock" in the context of what Leigh and I were doing, activating DNA, I experienced a series of related epiphanies.

DNA is a torsion field that manifests biochemically. It is basically energy. And what is energy really? Energy is consciousness. And all consciousness emerges from the Consciousness of Love (Figures 1 and 4).

There are, as we have seen, numerous external descriptions we can impose on DNA. But ultimately, DNA is simply a manifestation of what is. DNA is is-ness, and is-ness is love.

DNA is love in action. Activating DNA is just loving it back—with technique.

With the above in mind, there is decidedly a proper heart space to be in to perform or receive this work, one that is described more thoroughly in the next chapter.

Although Leigh and I required no additional signs in order to feel comfortable potentiating ourselves, we received one anyway—not five minutes before we started our session.

As we stood in silence getting ready to begin, we looked out our window toward the sea. To the best of my knowledge, it had not rained a drop that day—yet a colossal rainbow that encompassed the whole horizon hung in the pristine sky. It was easily the biggest, brightest rainbow either of us had ever beheld.

"Let's do this thing," I said. And we did.

Steady Unfoldments of Healing & Transformation

For me personally, as well as in Leigh's case, Potentiation empowered a steady series of at times subtle, at times dramatic ener-genetic unfoldments of healing and transformation.

During the first twenty-four hours after Potentiation, we frankly did not notice much of anything. Then we both started to detoxify through the most copious stools imaginable—a stunning release rivaling the best colon cleanse that went on intermittently for months.

I am not referring to diarrhea. Neither of us felt ill in that way or lost much weight in the process. For the most part, in fact, we were able to go on with our normal activities.

Even as our systems expelled previously unimaginable layers of pathogenetic and other toxic debris (the very elements, unmistakably, that had made me deathly ill and saddled Leigh with asthma and allergies since childhood), our physical strength and stamina began to increase.

Not all potentiators need to undergo physical purification to the extent we did after Potentiation—but many whose systems have been compromised enough to require cleansing and fortification do.

For those in need who do not experience such benefits from Potentiation, helpful detoxification and physical improvement often occur as a result of subsequent DNA activations in the Regenetics Method as explained toward the end of this book.

After weeks of regular but manageable cleansing, I realized I was beginning to crave foods I had been unable to tolerate for years. Many of these foods were starches: rice, pasta, potatoes, bread. All taboos, all like wrecking balls to my fragile system.

Tapping into her background in nutrition, Leigh theorized I was craving starches again because my body was purging and asking for foods capable of binding toxins from my cells and escorting them out of my system without further damaging my tissues.

This experience taught us that far from being evils, *cravings can be messages from a body in need.*

Especially in the case of potentiated individuals with a reset bioenergy blueprint, cravings can represent the body's innate wisdom as to what, on a daily basis, it requires for healing. More on this subject in Chapter Twelve.

Leigh suggested that I try some of the starchy foods I had been craving. Not without trepidation, I began eating them—like a mouse at first, but with growing enthusiasm as I realized they no longer were overrunning me with Candida or causing painful bloating!

Not only was it psychologically healing to be able to eat a wider range of foods again; a reasonable amount of starch intake undeniably "took the edge off" my ongoing detoxification.

As I have said many times before, if Potentiation had stopped there, Leigh and I both knew we had been given an extraordinary gift. But Potentiation did not stop there.

Over the next few months, I experienced greater and greater levels of vitality and was able to start exercising again. Within six months, I could swim a mile without stopping. I had been unable to perform anywhere close to this for years.

In addition, my environmental and chemical sensitivities gradually waned before disappearing completely. Years later, I can be in a moldy basement or beside a road being tarred without any reaction whatsoever.

My other symptoms and conditions, from hypochondria to migraines to muscle spasms, similarly faded over time into distant memories. To this day, I can eat and drink whatever I like, and work and exercise with remarkable stamina for my age.

Leigh also underwent a steady series of ener-genetic unfoldments with many palpable benefits that included the elimination of her allergies and asthma, as well as the partial straightening of her lifelong scoliosis that not even a back brace, regular chiropractic treatments and intensive Rolfing had been able to modify.

To this point, I have emphasized benefits from Potentiation of a material nature. And while these benefits were, from my perspective, life-restoring, in the long run it has been the strides I made in consciousness thanks to the Regenetics Method that have remained the most meaningful.

Specifically, I am referring to the unity consciousness—with its associated trust and faith in an ultimately benevolent universe—I now enjoy that has replaced my former "doom-and-gloom" feeling of victim consciousness.

Not that I consider myself perfect in any way, shape, or form. But as I have worked with Regenetics while walking my own path of conscious personal mastery, I have learned to forgive and love myself in profound ways despite my imperfections.

Just as importantly, I have begun to extend love and forgiveness to others who likewise are imperfect—even those with whose intentions or actions I may disagree vehemently.

One final note on the phenomenally transformational power of Potentiation, as Leigh and I continue to experience it with unwavering joy and gratitude.

According to two independent alternative health practitioners I saw prior to my Potentiation, probably owing to genetic damage from vaccines, I was sterile.

In fact, by the time we traveled to Brazil together, Leigh and I long since had dismissed the need for contraception because we sincerely believed I was incapable, biologically, of becoming a father.

You might recall that there was a third light orb that mysteriously connected with Leigh and myself that night on the beach in Búzios.

Apparently, that was the spirit of our child—who in all likelihood was conceived the evening of our Potentiation and entered the world as healthy as could be just over ninth months later, right as we were completing Potentiation's 42-week gestation cycle.

PART II

POTENTIATE YOURSELF

CHAPTER 8
Getting Ready

Now that you know how Potentiation came into being, it is time to learn to perform this life-changing DNA activation for yourself—and maybe others.

This chapter is designed, first and foremost, to help you prepare for your own Potentiation—materially, conceptually, and emotionally.

Additionally, if at some point you feel inspired to offer this work to family or friends, a number of the steps outlined herein are particularly worth sharing in advance.

To that end, while *Potentiate Your DNA* is copyrighted, you have the author's permission to photocopy the current chapter, "Getting Ready," for private, noncommercial use as a "preparation guide" for individuals whose Potentiation you will be facilitating.

Further guidelines and considerations for sharing Potentiation with others, from a facilitator's perspective, can be found in Chapters Nine, Ten, and Thirteen.

For individuals planning to be potentiated by someone else who find themselves reading this chapter by itself ...

More detailed information on Potentiation, the first DNA activation in the four-part Regenetics Method, is available at **www.phoenixregenetics.org** and **www.potentiation.net**.

In a moment, we will cover the things you definitely need to do prior to your Potentiation session. But first, let us call attention to a handful of things you do *not* need to do.

Things Not to Do

1. You do not need to have your aura cleared. I am aware of DNA activation practitioners who insist that you must clear your bioenergy blueprint, or aura, prior to having your DNA activated.

This view makes absolutely no sense since, as explained in Part I, *genuine DNA activation is what clears distortions in your bioenergy blueprint.*

On a related subject, many modalities calling themselves DNA activation are, at best, DNA *stimulation* of an epigenetic, Era II nature.

Remember, energetic techniques based exclusively in thought or light provide no direct access to our bioenergy blueprint and, thus, are limited in their ability to reset or transform it (Figure 9).

While it is possible that certain higher thought-forms using sacred geometry based on harmonics constitute an exception, this rule definitely holds for most current modalities—including touch-based ones—for working with DNA.

It is amazing how many stories clients and colleagues have shared over the years about starting out with mental or hands-on techniques— only to feel the need to incorporate sound to correct deeper ener-genetic distortions.

While epigenetic modalities can be beneficial, they are generally incapable of promoting the radical and permanent levels of healing and transformation encouraged by Era III techniques.

On the other hand, any DNA activation methodology that properly employs sound transcends Era II limitations and enters the meta-genetic, metamorphic realm of Era III medicine.

2. You do not need to have your polarity balanced. Polarity therapy is another Era II approach to healing that rarely is required when DNA is activated in an integrated, Era III manner.

Many clients who previously experienced problems with their energetic polarity have reported that such issues simply went away following Potentiation.

3. You do not need to do a cleansing program, fasting, colonics, ionized footbaths, Panchakarma, or the like. Given that Potentiation and other Regenetics activations can spur detoxification, the last thing you want to do is "add more fuel to the fire," before or after beginning this work.

Pushing yourself too hard, even when your body is screaming at you to slow down, is a particularly "Western" form of not loving yourself.

The same logic applies to taking fistfuls of vitamins and supplements—as well as pursuing intense bodywork or other forms of strong energy medicine—that force your eliminative system into overdrive.

If you do not feel one hundred percent certain that you should be doing something to assist your healing, just say no.

4. You do not need to have a complete understanding of the science and philosophy behind Potentiation and the Regenetics Method.

I recall a period of extreme waffling before I finally wrote my master's thesis. I kept insisting I needed to read "just one more" book or essay on this or that subject in order to collect my ideas.

To which my academic advisor eventually responded with this disarming question: "When do we ever *understand* anything completely?"

The not-so-subtle point was that even though I might not have read everything on or grasped every nuance of my topic, at some point I had to trust myself enough to sit down and start putting words on paper.

Potentiation is no different. There are perspectives you are likely to gain during or after this process that will open up previously unthinkable vistas. And even then, your level of "understanding" may only have just begun.

Having faith in your ability and intuition even in the absence of intellectual certainty is an important step on the path of conscious personal mastery.

I encourage you to get over any procrastination associated with low self-esteem or perfectionism, which are flip sides of the same dis-ease, and love yourself enough to move forward with your healing and transformation from wherever you are.

With the above things not to do in mind, let us move on now to the things you need to do before experiencing Potentiation.

Acquire Your Solfeggio Tuning Fork(s)

While the information contained in this section is likely to be of interest to most readers, *only self-potentiators and those facilitating Potentiation for others are required to procure the Solfeggio tuning fork(s).*

You may recall that my autoimmune illness was precipitated by toxicity and trauma from a series of hepatitis and yellow fever vaccines I received in 1995.

In Chapter One, it was stressed that so-called immunizations potentially damage, and even alter, human genetics through insertion of pathogenetic material into DNA.

In addition, and more disturbing still, kinesiological testing reveals that such damage and alteration can be inherited by children who never physically receive vaccines themselves.

After years of suffering and undergoing one expensive (and mostly ineffective) therapy after another, my turning point came when I realized that if I could reset myself ener-genetically, my thirty or so debilitating symptoms eventually would disappear.

I found myself on this path after reading Leonard Horowitz's *Emerging Viruses.* Basing his claims on meticulous research, Dr. Horowitz demonstrates that vaccines are a principal cause of a variety of autoimmune diseases, including AIDS.

He further exposes what is essentially profiteering and biowarfare conducted by the medical-pharmaceutical establishment against an unsuspecting populace in *Healing Codes for the Biological Apocalypse*, where a main theme is the use of sound to heal the body by restoring it to genetic integrity.

According to Horowitz, the specific frequencies used to restore genetic integrity derive from the ancient Solfeggio scale. This primordial six-note scale, which was dubiously "misplaced" by the Catholic Church centuries ago, was rediscovered by coauthor Dr. Joseph Puleo as described in *Healing Codes*.

The Solfeggio scale has become immensely popular in alternative medicine circles since the publication of *Healing Codes*. In a debatable move, Horowitz recently took the liberty of extrapolating three extra notes from the scale's intervals, forming a nine-note scale—which appears neither functionally necessary nor historically warranted.

Be that as it may, here it is simply necessary to point out that all DNA activations in the Regenetics Method employ one or more notes from the original Solfeggio scale, which some scholars believe to be the sacred set of six notes used by the Creator to fashion the world in as many days.

Specifically, Potentiation employs the foundational note "Mi," a frequency (528 Hz.) that has been utilized by leading-edge scientists to repair genetic defects.

You will need the Mi tuning fork to facilitate your own or another's Potentiation. But if you think that at some point you might pursue certification in subsequent levels of the Regenetics Method, which progressively introduce the full Solfeggio, or if you would like simply to experiment with this unique and beautiful scale, it may be worth considering the whole set of six tuning forks.

You can order either the single Mi tuning fork or the original six-fork Solfeggio scale directly from the Phoenix Center for Regenetics at **www.phoenixregenetics.org** or **www.potentiation.net**. We offer competitively priced, top-quality tuning forks.

For a worthwhile take on how to use the Solfeggio tuning forks by themselves for therapeutic purposes, you might enjoy sound healing pioneer David Hulse's entertaining little book *A Fork in the Road*, which thoughtfully describes his personal and professional journey with the Solfeggio.

Now, I am a firm believer in the beneficial qualities of the Solfeggio scale—which a musicologist friend of mine called the "real deal" in reference to its arguably sacred provenance, and which I maintain is an integral aspect of the Regenetics Method.

That said, I also contend that *the healing and transformational power of Potentiation and other Regenetics activations derives to an even larger extent from their vowel sequences.*

I can state this confidently for a variety of reasons—not least of which is that vowels always were the central focus of this work, whereas the Solfeggio was added at a later stage of its development.

While it may not have quite the effectiveness of someone performing Potentiation with perfect pitch, *it is possible to be slightly off-key—as long as the vowel sequences are handled correctly—and still achieve remarkable results.*

I emphasize this point because I know that most people reading this book are not musicians or sound healers, and some even may have difficulty carrying a simple tune.

You should do your best to stay on the Mi note throughout Potentiation. But if you find yourself straying, realize that you still are performing a linguistically based DNA activation with great potential for healing and transformation.

Virtually anyone who commits to mastering the Potentiation technique, particularly with relation to the vowels, and whose head and especially heart are in the right place, can perform this work effectively for him or herself—as well as others.

If for any reason you are uncomfortable performing your own or another's Potentiation, and do not know anyone you deem qualified to do it for you, there are certified Regenetics Method Facilitators worldwide who would be happy to assist—remotely or in person.

A complete and regularly updated list of certified Facilitators grouped by country is available at **www.phoenixregenetics.org** and **www.potentiation.net**.

Master Your Potentiation Technique

While this may seem self-evident to self-potentiators and facilitators, it is worth underscoring that you need to give yourself some time—a day or two, at least—to read the next chapter and familiarize yourself with how in-person Potentiation is performed.

Ideally, you will read the rest of this book first, then come back and read Chapter Nine again before practicing and performing your own Potentiation.

For those planning to share this work with others ...

Whether you will be doing so in person or at a distance, after your own session *I suggest giving yourself no less than a month* to get a feel for Potentiation before offering to potentiate your family and friends.

Know that All Healing Is Self-healing

We live in a global culture with such a skewed view of what healing actually is that this point needs to be highlighted.

Although healing often includes alleviating or eliminating symptoms, healing (wholing) must not be confused with simple curing. Whereas curing is designed to make the problem go away, no questions asked and no insights gained, healing is a very different activity.

True healing embraces the problem (which is actually a teaching tool employed by our Higher Self) as a way of integrating and being transformed by it.

Curing focuses on symptoms without realizing they are spiritual messages. By contrast, healing is a body-mind-spirit phenomenon involving an increase in awareness that takes the form of a transformational step on our evolutionary journey of conscious personal mastery.

At its heart, healing teaches us to love ourselves and others unconditionally and, moreover, to see others as ourselves.

This line of reasoning establishes that:

1. Healing is inseparable from loving; and

2. Loving leads to a higher state of awareness that has been called unity consciousness.

In this ultimately individualized process, very often the problem disappears, but not because we have ignored it or forced it to go away.

Rather, the problem is simply no longer of use to us because our dysfunctional relationship—which is always a variety of victim consciousness—to the underlying factors creating the problem has been healed *consciously*.

While we can facilitate healing in another through DNA activation, often with astonishing results, in the end we cannot *make* a person benefit from the transformational energies we offer.

If any part (conscious or otherwise) of the recipient's body-mind-spirit refuses to accept the DNA activation energies, to that extent the person will not experience healing or transformation.

This includes ourselves. In all cases, whether we perceive ourselves as the one doing the healing or the one being healed, *it is up to the individual to integrate, deeply and unconditionally, the ener-genetic reconfiguration that authentic DNA activation is capable of establishing.*

The view that all healing is really self-healing is strongly supported by Glen Rein's inspiring research in DNA's response to coherent emotions.

As mentioned in the Introduction, Dr. Rein found that positive emotions fortify DNA—making DNA more robust and arguably more available for activation, healing, and transformation.

On the other hand, negative emotions tend to damage DNA so that it cannot be easily activated through linguistically expressed consciousness.

It is up to us as individuals to determine—and if necessary, upgrade—which emotions we regularly experience as well as which emotionally charged attitudes we typically entertain so that our DNA can be activated successfully.

At the very least, *we must be receptive to the idea of healing ourselves in order actually to do so.*

Even a minimal willingness to undergo positive change can set the stage for remarkable benefits to unfold through Potentiation and the Regenetics Method.

To understand that healing is always self-healing is to grasp the primary role of free will in this process.

Nothing about healing is predetermined. To the contrary, *healing is a quantum unfoldment that at each instant respects our own myriad boundaries as to how fast—and how radically—we are willing to transform.*

Such boundaries can be conscious. They also can be subconscious, ancestral, and even karmic. Theoretically, we can heal and change overnight—and some people do.

But more often, healing is an incremental, cumulative and eventually exponential process that allows us to consciously integrate its numerous transformational lessons at a manageable rate.

Write down Your Intentions

For years now, Leigh and I have counseled clients to write down their intentions for Potentiation prior to the actual session.

Envisioning them in writing, clearly and creatively, is an excellent way to encourage your intentions for healing and transformation to manifest.

Working with your intentions in writing is one of several Era II, epigenetic tools for directing your Era III, meta-genetic unfoldment— other examples of which are explored in Chapter Thirteen.

Your flexible, heart-based intentions are exceedingly helpful in actualizing the energies of Potentiation. I suggest that you take an hour before your session to write down your intentions by specifying the areas where you seek improvement.

This document can serve as a fascinating and empowering retrospective as you move through Potentiation. Over the weeks and months following your session, you are likely to find yourself checking off, one by one, some or all of the very things you intended to manifest!

It is also a good idea to write down your intentions in a notebook that can be used after your session as a "Potentiation journal."

Keeping a Potentiation journal is an excellent way to stay intentionally focused on your healing and transformation. Even a brief notation when you experience a forward shift is enough to sketch a valuable outline of your evolutionary journey.

You can continue to clarify your intentions on a daily basis, by journaling or otherwise, throughout the 42-week Potentiation process. To the best of your ability, be sure to maintain an attitude of nonattachment relative to your intentions so that you avoid restricting or deflecting the desired outcomes.

The trick is to put out intentional energy with genuine feeling, then freely release it so that what you desire can come back to you.

It is also appropriate to remain open to serendipity and trust your intuition, as new situations and opportunities that present themselves may assist your healing and transformation.

Be in the Right Head & Heart Space

Writing down your intentions will go a long way toward putting you in the right head space to benefit from this work. Finishing this book can assist you further in feeling prepared mentally to perform and/or experience Potentiation.

By far, however, the most important thing to have in the right place is your heart.

There is a wealth of documented research from the Institute of Heartmath proving that *the intelligence associated with our heart profoundly impacts our experience of reality in ways that transcend mere intellectual processing.*

We are touching on the subject of Era II and epigenetics, which are associated with the head, versus Era III and meta-genetics, which center on the heart (Figure 6).

But for present purposes, let us call attention to the relatively unknown fact that the heart is technically a neural center—one that, according to Joseph Chilton Pearce, appears to be in a state of evolutionary development.

It seems that as a species, we finally are learning to tune out external "authority" designed to control our head and listen to our heart's unerring wisdom instead.

Berendt would explain this development as a move from seeing to hearing, from the eyes to the ears. Energetically, this movement parallels the evolutionary trajectory, introduced previously, from light to sound.

To put this discussion in the context of another earlier idea, humanity appears to be evolving—individually and collectively—so as to be able to connect with the Consciousness of Love on a more fulfilling and consistent basis (Figures 1 and 4).

What does all of this have to do with DNA activation? As Rein's research undeniably indicates, coherent emotions directly interface with DNA—positively or negatively.

Negative emotions like fear can be said to be "head-based" in a surfeit of mental processing. Positive emotions such as love, however, are "heart-based." Negative feelings "close" the heart, while positive ones "open" it.

Rein's work reveals that the position of the heart (open or closed) powerfully influences the health and activity of DNA—and similarly may facilitate or hinder DNA activation.

Recall what has been stated over the past two chapters relative to DNA activation, love, and healing:

DNA is love in action. Activating DNA is just loving it back—with technique. At its heart, healing teaches us to love ourselves and others unconditionally. Healing is inseparable from loving.

If your heart is not open to your healing, and your feelings with regard to your Potentiation are not love-based, it does not matter so much what you think because your DNA is closed to change.

By contrast, if your heart is open to your healing, and the emotions associated with your DNA activation are rooted in love, it matters comparatively little what you think because your DNA is available for transformation nevertheless.

The primary role of the heart in DNA activation is attested to by the fact that many skeptics with a positive enough feeling about Potentiation to try it anyway have reported terrific results.

On the other hand, some potentiators with a more metaphysical bent who are inclined to believe in energy medicine, but whose hearts appear closed through negative emotions and attitudes, have benefited substantially less.

Be sure to maintain a state of intellectual openness before, during and after your Potentiation.

But even more critically, make a concerted effort to open your heart—and DNA—with love and related emotions ... and keep them that way!

Readers inclined to worry should be aware that with even minimal positive intentions in place for healing and transformation, it is virtually impossible to negate your Potentiation.

Likewise, having a bad day, or even a bad phase, will not override a strongly heartfelt initial willingness to heal and change.

Choose a Time & Place

To recap, before performing your Potentiation session, it is your responsibility to:

1. Acquire the Mi tuning fork;

2. Finish reading this book;

3. Practice your Potentiation technique as taught in the next chapter;

4. Understand that all healing is self-healing;

5. Write down your intentions for this work in a Potentiation journal; and

6. Get your head and particularly heart in the right space.

At this juncture, the last thing to do is to choose a time and place for your Potentiation.

You want a quiet, private environment where you can avoid distractions and be present with yourself while honoring this special half hour as a time capable of seeding probabilities that can lead you to the realization of your potential in which you manifest the reality you desire.

You also will need enough light for reading the Potentiation codes and seeing what you are doing.

If you decide to be outdoors, too much wind can present a problem by blowing around your materials. And obviously, you want to be comfortable—so steer clear of intense heat and cold and inclement weather.

Beyond these basic considerations, the time and place for your Potentiation are entirely up to you.

CHAPTER 9

In-Person Potentiation

Ever since I started facilitating this work back in 2003, I have felt an intense desire to teach people to do it themselves. So I am extremely excited to have reached this stage, where we finally can focus together on mastering the actual Potentiation technique!

Before getting down to nuts and bolts, however, a handful of significant points are still in need of brief clarification.

Practicing Potentiation does not equal performing it. In order for Potentiation to initiate repatterning at the ener-genetic core of your being, your heartfelt intention to accept and integrate this DNA activation must be in place.

That said, when starting out practicing you may feel some "amping up" in your bioenergy centers that can manifest as anything from restlessness to mild dizziness to a sensation of being pleasantly "altered."

It is recommended that you remain seated while learning this technique and that, when standing up after practicing, you do so slowly and mindfully.

Some people also get an anticipatory "buzz" simply from reading about the Regenetics Method. Again, this is not the same as purposefully initiating your Potentiation when you are ready.

Nor is it possible to receive Potentiation merely through association with another person who is potentiating—although when people close to us experience this work, we often feel it on various levels.

In addition to ethical considerations relative to respecting other people's free will, the fact that Potentiation is designed to be experienced consciously whenever possible is a major reason why *you should not go around potentiating others without their awareness and explicit permission.*

Three exceptions to this important rule are specified in the next chapter on distance Potentiation. But for now, know that it is okay to practice your technique as much as you like before performing your session and embarking on your Regenetics journey.

As for sharing this work, since this often is done remotely, I will leave the majority of additional considerations regarding facilitating another's Potentiation for the next chapter.

The present chapter revolves around the in-person Potentiation grid shown in Figure 12. Each section that follows has the primary purpose of guiding you to work with these linguistic codes in the correct way.

To reiterate a previous point, while Potentiation's vowel sequences belong to a hyperdimensional "language" that interfaces with DNA in order to reset your bioenergy blueprint, you do not have to understand these so-called words.

There is nothing to understand. These linguistic codes are to be *experienced*—and only such experience can bring anything resembling understanding.

Last but not least, for those interested in hearing what Potentiation sounds like before trying it, there are numerous reasons why Leigh and I have chosen not to make a recording of this work available.

Many shamans insist that digital reproduction is essentially hollow— devoid of spirit and incapable of engendering healing and transformation. Under no circumstances would we wish for people to listen to a mechanical recording of Potentiation in place of experiencing it themselves through live human consciousness and voice.

Moreover, we insist that *Potentiation is simple to master using this book alone.* But if you have questions about your technique, you are urged to join the Regenetics Method Forum and ask them there. A special subgroup has been created just for readers of this book.

Membership guidelines and registration instructions are available at **www.phoenixregenetics.org** and **www.potentiation.net**.

Pronunciation Primer

Students and native speakers of the Romance languages descended from Latin—including French, Italian, Portuguese, Romanian, and Spanish— have a particularly easy time pronouncing Potentiation's vowels.

The five vowels used in all Regenetics activations—A, E, I, O, and U—are chanted roughly in accordance with Latinate pronunciation as shown in the chart below.

Before doing anything else, you need to practice these vowels until their pronunciation becomes automatic—if it is not already.

Pronunciation Guide for Potentiation

Vowel	Phonetic Pronunciation	Examples
A	short A (ah)	f<u>a</u>r, j<u>a</u>r, t<u>a</u>d<u>a</u>
E	short E (eh)	<u>e</u>bb, <u>e</u>gg, l<u>e</u>g
I	long E (ē)	<u>ee</u>l, m<u>ea</u>l, z<u>ea</u>l
O	long O (ō)	al<u>o</u>ne, cl<u>o</u>thes, n<u>o</u>se
U	double O (ōō)	b<u>oo</u>th, fr<u>ui</u>t, tr<u>u</u>th

Figure 11: Pronunciation Guide for Potentiation

This chart shows the pronunciation of the five major vowels used in Potentiation.

By far the most difficult pronunciation for native English speakers to perfect when learning Potentiation is the near transposition of the sounds for E and I.

In Potentiation I is pronounced as a long E as in "east," while E becomes a short E like that in "let." Practice these two vowels paying close attention to the tendency to mispronounce them.

Accurate pronunciation of Potentiation's vowels requires keeping your mouth rounded while chanting A, E, and O. When making these sounds, it can be helpful to imagine that you have a tennis ball in the back of your throat.

On the other hand, I requires an ear-to-ear grin to be pronounced correctly, whereas U needs slightly pursed lips like those used for a lazy kiss.

An important element to grasp right off the bat is that *these vowels are meant to be chanted together seamlessly*, one vowel flowing into the next without hesitation or interruption.

Except at the end of words and where there is a silent beat indicated by a —, Potentiation should be a continuous flow of vowel sounds blending together. The attentive ear can hear numerous other "vowels" in play as the primary vowels transition between themselves.

This phenomenon is a way of utilizing the "major" vowels on which many modern languages such as English are structured to articulate a number of "minor" vowels that are acknowledged in such ancient languages as Hebrew.

While chanting these sequences, *pay particular attention that no Ys (as in "yes") or Ws (as in "wow") come between the vowels.* Such "semivowels" detract from the purity of the vowels and their ability to activate DNA meta-genetically.

Ring, Breathe, Sing

Each vowel or silence (—) should last approximately one second. I say "approximately" because it does not matter so much how fast or slow you perform Potentiation.

The basic rule is that *a full chanting of Potentiation should be no longer than twenty-five and no shorter than fifteen minutes.*

With the addition of a total of five minutes for Opening and Closing combined (see below), *the entire Potentiation session should fall between twenty and thirty minutes in length.*

If you have one, feel free to use a metronome—when practicing only—in order to establish and maintain a regular pace. Having taught Potentiation for years, I have found that tapping a foot works just as well, and feels a lot less robotic.

The main consideration when pacing Potentiation is breathing. Ideally, *you should take one deep, diaphragmatic breath at the beginning of each line in Figure 12 and have it last until the end of the line.* For the longer lines especially, this can be difficult if you chant too slowly.

If you absolutely must take an occasional breath in the middle of a word, be quick about it and make every effort to stay on the beat. In such instances only, it is okay to take a fast, shallow breath in order to maintain your pace.

Otherwise, in diaphragmatic breathing there are four things to keep in mind. First, whether you are sitting or standing, *your back should be straight.*

The second guideline for diaphragmatic breathing may sound a little odd. But as my qigong teacher used to say, you should *breathe through your behind.*

When you arrive at this admittedly strange sensation while breathing with your diaphragm, the third thing to note is that your upper chest does not inflate and deflate. If it does, you are breathing improperly. Instead, *your lower abdomen should expand and contract visibly.*

Fourth and finally, if you are breathing correctly, *your shoulders should be relaxed.* If you tried to shoulder a purse or duffel bag while breathing this way, it would slip off and hit the floor.

Diaphragmatic breathing will help you get through the longer lines and keep you from becoming unnecessarily dizzy. It is also highly oxygenating for your system—as well as a wonderful way to relax and reduce stress.

Whatever pace you settle on, *at the start of Potentiation and subsequently at the beginning of each line you will ring the Mi tuning fork once.* This is to assist with your rhythm and help you stay on the right note.

(The two exceptions to this rule come at the end of the fourth and fifth "pass-throughs" of the Potentiation grid, as explained below under Sequencing.)

When ringing your tuning fork, be sure to hold it lengthwise away from your body parallel to the ground with the two tines arranged vertically, one above the other.

Strike the included rubber hockey puck solidly, but not too hard, with only the bottom tine to prevent double ringing. Allow the note to play out without dampening until time to strike it again.

I find it helpful to hold a clipboard to clamp down the Potentiation codes (which you have permission to photocopy for private, noncommercial use) as well as the hockey puck, leaving one hand free to ring the tuning fork. This becomes all the more important if you opt to include movement during Potentiation (see next chapter).

Immediately after ringing, breathe deeply but quickly with your diaphragm. This should take the same amount of time you spend on any given vowel or silence (roughly a second). Then without hesitating, begin chanting the next line in the sequence as outlined below.

You will repeat this protocol over and over as you work your way through Potentiation's repetitions:

Ring, breathe, sing. Ring, breathe, sing. Ring, breathe, sing.

Vowel Sequences for In-person Potentiation

Bioenergy Center	Line	Vowel Sequences											
Master	1a	E	A	E	E	I	O						
Master	1b	a	i	a	i	a	u						
9	2a	A	U	A	E	U	A	A					
8	2b	a	a	e	i	o	o	u					
7	3a	A	A	I	A	A	I	I	I	E	A	A	I
6	3b	u	u	i	i	e	i	a	-	-	-	-	-
5	4a	E	O	A	E	O	A	A	O	E			
4	4b	a	e	a	a	a	e	a	-	-			
3	5a	A	I	A	I	U	O	A	O				
1	5b	e	o	i	e	o	u	-	-				

one ring   three rings

4 pass-throughs down   1 pass-through up

two rings

Figure 12: Vowel Sequences for In-person Potentiation

The above grid's sound and light vowel codes are used for self-potentiating and working with others in person. Note the points relative to the number of tuning fork rings and the sequence of five pass-throughs.

Try it now. Using the first word that occupies line 1a of Figure 12, EAEEIO, practice chanting it as many times as you like. Remember to *ring* your tuning fork, *breathe* deeply, and *sing* the vowels together without interruption.

When you have spent one—and only one—beat on the last vowel (O), stop and then *ring, breathe,* and *sing* the line again.

Observe the tendency, which must be nipped in the bud, to hold the last vowel sound half a beat too long. Also, be aware that the EE in the middle of the word is chanted as two continuous beats of the vowel E.

Remember, each vowel occupies a beat. As an example, the three III's in succession in line 3a require the sound for I to be held—without syncopation or hesitation—over three consecutive beats.

A Word about Pitch

At 528 hertz, the Mi note from the original Solfeggio scale used throughout Potentiation is a frequency that most people love to chant. Neither too high nor too low for the majority of vocal ranges, Mi is like "comfort food" and gives one a sense of being "home."

This is because of all the ancient Solfeggio frequencies, the Mi note is related most closely to DNA's own harmonics. In fact, this wonderful note has been used by itself to heal damaged chromosomes.

Among Facilitators who have become certified in levels of the Regenetics Method beyond Potentiation, in which the other five Solfeggio notes progressively come into play, there is a general consensus that Mi is the easiest, most natural pitch to work with of the lot.

Most readers will no have difficulty staying on the Mi note when performing Potentiation for the simple reason that this frequency is so embedded in our ener-genetic makeup.

But as stated earlier, *even if you stray from the proper pitch occasionally, this will not negate your own or another's Potentiation.*

Now, there are a couple of things you can do to help you stay in tune. For starters, keep your back straight and practice diaphragmatic breathing as described above.

In addition, after you have rung your tuning fork and breathed, holding the vibrating fork like a microphone about an inch in front of your mouth while singing the vowel sequences can work wonders.

You actually should feel Mi's vibration on your lips. For many people, this is of great assistance in harmonically entraining the vocalized note to the Mi frequency emanating from the tuning fork.

Finally, for those individuals who find the Mi note too high or too low for comfort, *it is acceptable to chant the equivalent note in a higher or lower octave.*

Double Intoning

Alongside the distinctive vowel sequences used in Potentiation and other Regenetics activations, the act of "double intoning" is equally responsible for making this Method of DNA activation unique—and uniquely effective.

Somewhat like overtoning, a form of chanting practiced by many Eastern monks that allows two or more harmonically connected notes to be uttered simultaneously, double intoning is simpler to perform—particularly for Westerners and those with no voice training.

While double intoning can seem challenging to master at first, master it you most definitely can, with a little time and practice.

As Figure 12 demonstrates, Potentiation is divided into a series of five pairs of vowel-based words. *The top ("a") line of each pair, shown as a set of upper-case vowels, represents Potentiation's sound codes that are to be chanted audibly as taught above.*

During your first few rounds of practice, it is a good idea to focus solely on the top line, ignoring the bottom line completely until you are comfortable chanting each of the five audible words in the proper sequence.

Then you are ready to incorporate the bottom ("b") line of words. *These lower-case vowels are Potentiation's light codes—which rather than being chanted, are "sounded" in the mind only.*

Thus each vowel sound is accompanied by a silent vowel thought. Sometimes these paired vowels are identical, but more often they are different.

To be absolutely clear, *while you are chanting one vowel, simultaneously you will think the sound of another one—which may or may not be the same vowel.*

If the task of saying one thing while thinking another appears daunting, realize that most people do it all the time!

Seriously, after you have practiced the sound codes in isolation, spend half an hour doing the same with the light codes. Just sit down and think your way through the entire silent sequence, "listening" as the lower-case vowels blend together in your mind.

Note that at the end of lines 3b, 4b and 5b, the chanted vowels are accompanied by mentally created silent beats. Practice "hearing" a beat of silence for each —. Know that silence, the space between notes, is viewed by most musicians as an essential element of the music.

Now you are ready to combine the sound and light codes—which you can do by rehearsing one pair of audible and silent words together as many times as you like. When you have grasped how one pair goes together, move on to the next, until you have a good feel for all five pairs of words.

Using line 1a as an example, begin by chanting EAEEIO. Simultaneously, and *at the same pace*, think line 1b: aiaiau.

The first pair of words, composing line 1, combines audible E with silent a, audible A with silent i, audible E with silent a, audible E with silent i, audible I with silent a, and audible O with silent u.

When you are comfortable with these combinations, you can progress to the second line in which AUAEUAA (2a) is paired with aaeioou (2b), and so on.

Note that in line 2b, there are two points when sounds are to be thought back to back, without hesitation or interruption, as extended silent vowels: aa and oo. Similarly, line 3b starts with uu, and line 4b boasts a triple silent a.

When you have finished rehearsing all five lines independently, you are in a position to practice an entire Potentiation session using the double intoning technique following the rules for Sequencing outlined below.

Do not be concerned if at first you find it difficult to think the light codes while chanting the sound codes.

If I had to put a figure on it, I would guess that most people just starting out learning Potentiation are able to think the bottom line no better than twenty-five percent of the time while chanting the top line.

For whole stretches during chanting, it is common to think of anything and everything but the silent vowels.

With patience and dedication, however, your percentage gradually will increase until you are double intoning eighty or ninety percent of the time. Then you finally are ready to perform your own Potentiation session!

As you get better and better at double intoning, you will find yourself achieving a progressively deeper meditative state. You are not likely to enter a trance, and sometimes random thoughts still will occur— but even these rarely will interrupt the harmonious, integrated flow of sound and light codes.

Such a meditative state produces an abundance of theta brainwaves in your conscious mind. This is significant because research has demonstrated that theta waves have a powerful impact on healing and transformation.

When, and only when, you have reached this level of mastery with Potentiation, performed your own session and given yourself at least a month to feel it out should you consider potentiating others.

Sequencing

Besides showing in-person Potentiation's vowel combinations, Figure 12 also summarizes the overall sequence for working your way through the five lines of paired words.

When getting ready to start the session, feel free to ring your tuning fork and practice chanting some vowels to make sure you are on the right note. Think of this preparatory stage as the orchestra tuning up before the concert begins.

As soon as you are prepared and comfortable, ring the Mi tuning fork a single time, breathe and immediately double intone line 1 three times—using the *ring-breathe-sing* technique at the beginning of each additional line repetition.

Note that each line of paired sound and light codes always is double intoned exactly three times before the next line begins.

Following the third double intoning of line 1, when you have rung the tuning fork one time again and breathed with your diaphragm, begin singing line 2a while thinking line 2b.

After the third repetition of line 2, repeat the same protocol for lines 3, 4, and 5. At the completion of three repetitions of line 5, you have finished one *pass-through* of the Potentiation grid.

As you also can see in Figure 12, *Potentiation requires a total of five pass-throughs: four down and one up.*

The second pass-through starts with *ring, breath, sing* immediately at the end of the first pass-through. After ringing and breathing, simply revert to chanting line 1 at the top of the Potentiation grid and repeat the same process until you have double intoned line 5 again.

Repeat the entire procedure from the top down again for the third pass-through, and once again for the fourth pass-through.

Repetition plays three key roles in Potentiation.

First, it allows any significant gaps in your double intoning of the vowels—when you space out for twenty seconds after remembering you forgot to buy the dog food—to be filled in eventually.

Secondly, repeating these lines for the better part of half an hour slowly but surely entrains your consciousness into a more meditative state in which beneficial theta waves are produced with greater strength and regularity.

Third and finally, repetition is a way of mimicking and encouraging the spiraling movement of sound and light waves of torsion energy (bioenergy) you are creating by chanting and thinking these special vowel combinations.

Richard Hoagland, a former NASA scientist and one of the leading torsion energy researchers in the United States, famously rephrased the old real estate mantra as "rotation, rotation, rotation" to get at the dynamic movement of torsion energy.

When you have "rotated" your way via four pass-throughs down through the Potentiation grid as described above, you are ready to reverse direction and complete your fifth and final pass-through.

In direct antithesis to the first four pass-throughs, *this final pass-through starts with line 5 and works its way back up to line 1.*

Importantly, reversing direction requires that you *double intone line 5 a total of six times from the end of the fourth through the beginning of the fifth pass-through.*

In addition, the fifth pass-through initiates immediately following the fourth pass-through with *two rings* of the Mi tuning fork.

This is the only time during Potentiation you will ring twice in successive beats. For this one instance only at the end of the fourth pass-through, two beats of the tuning fork replace one beat to signal the directional shift.

Promptly following the second ring, breathe and start double intoning lines 5-1 again three times apiece—starting each repetition of a subsequent line with a single *ring, breathe, sing* as before.

When you have come full circle and double intoned line 1 for the last time, ring the tuning fork *three times* in successive beats and allow the sound to play out for a solid minute into complete silence.

Congratulations! You have made it through in-person Potentiation! You probably will notice that your entire body is buzzing at what feels like the molecular level. This is normal.

In the early stages of practicing, it is a good idea to *time yourself from start to finish.* As a reminder, the entire sequence of double intoning over five pass-throughs should fall between *fifteen* and *twenty-five* minutes, depending on your pacing.

Opening & Closing

When performing your own or another's actual Potentiation, before starting double intoning, then after you have finished five pass-throughs and allowed your tuning fork to taper off completely, it is recommended that you *take two or three minutes of silence to open and close, respectively, the session.*

There is no need to "quiet the mind" per se, as this should occur naturally, to a greater or lesser extent, over the course of double intoning.

During these "bookend" silences, the idea is to be fully present—with a positive mental attitude and a feeling of compassion and love for the spiritual being on a human journey experiencing this DNA activation.

In other words, on behalf of yourself or another, *open your head—and especially your heart—to the ever-present potential for permanent healing and radical transformation.*

In addition, any love-based emotions and attitudes—including gratitude, joy, bliss, trust, faith, excitement, adventurousness, and good-natured humor—are welcome guests when riding the ener-genetic wave that is Potentiation.

Throughout the session, from Opening to Closing, you are encouraged to *focus at least part of your consciousness on committing, either for the first time or again, to walking your highest path in life.*

That path, although uniquely yours, is certain to involve loving and serving the self in order to be of loving service to others. On this subject, to quote Berendt, "We cannot change the world if we do not change ourselves first."

Be particularly mindful of the areas you want to address and imagine infusing revitalizing energies into the places that need them most. Your goal should be to energize those areas that will allow you to reach your full potential.

As a final point of clarification relative to timing, after adding a combined total of approximately five minutes for Opening and Closing, the Potentiation session should last no more than *thirty* and no less than *twenty* minutes.

Be Patient & Release Mistakes

It is not unusual for people just starting to learn Potentiation to feel overwhelmed and make all kinds of errors in technique and execution.

My advice always is to be patient with yourself and let go of your mistakes. *Screwing up provides an excellent opportunity to love yourself more completely and unconditionally.*

This advice holds even when you perform a real Potentiation session. If you mess up, go back to that point and pick right up again without a second thought. If the session ends up taking a little longer than expected, so be it.

Again, with your flexible, heartfelt intention in place, even with some flubs, you are far more likely to benefit yourself or another with this DNA activation than your inner perfectionist might admit.

"Deleting" the Fragmentary Body

On the left side of Figure 12, you may have noticed that the paired line numbers align not just with the vowel sequences to be chanted and thought during Potentiation.

In addition, and quite significantly, these line numbers also indicate the various interrelated torsion fields that make up your bioenergy blueprint.

As explained in Part I, in the unpotentiated human there are nine bioenergy fields. These torsion fields increase in frequency from the first to the ninth and ultimately are subsumed by the Master (Source) Field (Figure 3).

Returning to a previous analogy, the Master Field can be conceptualized as the spiritual ocean of time-space, out of which our own bioenergetic structure, initially composed of nine levels, emerges like waves (Figure 9).

Lines 1a and 1b connect to the Master Field and are responsible for interfacing with it via potential DNA. Similarly, lines 2a and 2b link up with and activate the eighth and ninth bioenergy fields, respectively, and so on.

Critically, at the bottom of the grid note that lines 5a and 5b relate to the third and first torsion fields, respectively. Any reference to the second bioenergy center, the Fragmentary Body, has been omitted.

Recall that Potentiation sets in motion a repatterning of the bioenergy blueprint from nine to eight centers. This is accomplished not by force of will, but by simply *deleting* the ener-genetic liability constituted by the Fragmentary Body.

Potentiation empowers us to cease paying attention—and thereby giving life—to the illusion of separation that has manifested as the Fragmentary Body.

Deleting the Fragmentary Body is accomplished not by invasive physical manipulation, which would be Era I's approach (if it acknowledged spiritual energy). Nor are we discussing a psychological, Era II strategy for reasoning our way back to a more integrated state of being.

Instead, we simply can utilize vowel-based words to rewrite our blueprint in a fundamental way by changing the meta-genetic dialogue between our individual bioenergy structure and the greater consciousness field (Figure 9).

This phenomenon becomes all the more profound when one adopts a metaphysical perspective on the origins of our experience of so-called reality.

The basic metaphysical storyline is that our dualistic world—and the bio-spiritual vehicles we inhabit to experience it—were created by the insertion of *consonants* that fragmented the unified flow of creational vowels. *Thus we came to live in a divided self in a divided reality.*

But things do not have to remain that way. We have the ability—indeed, the responsibility—to become undivided.

And as we do so, by committing to our own conscious personal mastery, we progressively unify the world. This fascinating and far-ranging topic is covered in much greater detail in *Conscious Healing*.

In Potentiation we have a genuine Era III technique for naturally, permanently and radically upgrading our consciousness blueprint to a state of life-enhancing wholeness Leigh and I call an *infinity circuit* based on the number 8.

In this process, the inherently unstable ninth bioenergy center literally descends and fuses with the second bioenergy center approximately five months after the Potentiation session at the stage of repatterning referred to as sealing (Figures 10 and 18).

At this point, should you wish to go deeper in your journey of healing and transformation, you are eligible to experience Articulation Bioenergy Enhancement with a certified Regenetics Method Facilitator.

Figure 19 shows the complete Regenetics Method Timeline. You will find an updated list of certified Facilitators grouped by country at **www.phoenixregenetics.org** and **www.potentiation.net**.

Follow-up

A description of Articulation and other Regenetics activations is included in Chapter Fourteen.

For detailed information on the Time Frame for ener-genetic repatterning via Potentiation (Figure 18), as well as sealing the Fragmentary Body, you are encouraged to read and study Chapter Thirteen.

Chapter Thirteen also describes how you can muscle test to determine 1) whether your Potentiation session was successful; and 2) to which Electromagnetic Group you belong and which corresponding Schematic you should use to follow your process (Figures 15, 16, and 17).

Additionally, you can use this same kinesiological technique for others whose Potentiation you facilitate (Figure 14).

Part III as a whole is designed to provide the potentiator with a wide variety of tools spanning medical Eras I-III to maximize the entire range of body-mind-spirit benefits from Potentiation and the Regenetics Method.

But before we get there, let us have a look at some critically important guidelines and considerations for performing another's Potentiation.

CHAPTER 10

Distance Potentiation

After you have practiced enough to develop some mastery of in-person Potentiation, and performed your own session using the grid shown in Figure 12, once again you are encouraged to give yourself at least a month of integration time before offering this work to others.

At this point, you can consider potentiating your family, friends and even pets using either the in-person technique taught in the previous chapter or the distance Potentiation technique introduced toward the end of this chapter.

Just to be clear, in-person Potentiation is designed for your recipient to be within hearing of you. The remote technique is for people or animals you cannot be with physically.

In the case of in-person sessions in particular, given the prevailing climate in which many alternative healers find themselves harassed by the medical-pharmaceutical establishment, you might *consider asking recipients to sign the Potentiation Consent Form provided in Appendix B.*

You can photocopy this form and have the recipient sign and return it to you prior to the session. Alternatively, the recipient can download it at **www.phoenixregenetics.org** or **www.potentiation.net**, then print, sign and give it to you.

Other thoughts on avoiding running afoul of the establishment include refraining from touching recipients during the Potentiation session and *never, ever making medical claims* about Potentiation or the Regenetics Method.

These guidelines and many more are covered during certification for Potentiation and other Regenetics activations. If you are serious about offering this work to the public, I strongly recommend Facilitator training in the Regenetics Method. Information on seminars can be found at **www.phoenixregenetics.org** and **www.potentiation.net**.

When and if you offer to potentiate your family and friends, whether in person or remotely, please understand that you are *offering* to do so—and because people have free will, they may refuse to accept what you have to offer.

When facilitating this work for others, you have several responsibilities that are outlined hereafter. *But by far the most important thing, where human beings are concerned, is to acquire recipients' explicit, conscious permission beforehand.*

There are three, and only three, exceptions to this rule—embryos/fetuses, young children, and communication-impaired adults—that are covered a bit later.

Obviously, in most instances involving in-person Potentiation, when you literally are in the room with the recipient, permission is not a consideration. The moral gray line and ethical slippery slope typically come into play when performing distance Potentiation.

Not only does acquiring permission exponentially enhance Potentiation's benefits by establishing this DNA activation at a conscious level; permission also keeps you clean of any "negative karma" you would accrue by overstepping other people's free will without their knowledge.

I am aware that many people privately pray for and send "love and light" to others on a regular basis. Certainly, there is nothing wrong with these activities, and a good deal that is right.

But while Potentiation is similar to prayer and sending love and light, it often goes quite beyond these simple gestures by stimulating life-changing effects that can be physical, mental, emotional, and even spiritual.

If someone you care for declines your generous offer of Potentiation, do not take it personally. Eventually, the person may come around and be in a much better place to experience this work.

In such instances, it can be helpful to recall Ken Carey's wise words to would-be healers: "Where you are invited, you are empowered … Where there is no invitation, [you are assigned] not."

An alternative to offering to potentiate people close to you is to give them *Potentiate Your DNA* first. Naturally, this may not be feasible owing to factors such as age, language, physical condition, and mental state.

But in the case of English-speaking adults who are able and willing to read, perhaps sharing this book with them is the best way to "give the gift of Potentiation."

Of course, you still can offer to potentiate them after they have read the book—if for any reason they do not feel like activating their own DNA. Regardless of who performs the Potentiation session, reading this material can be both enlightening and empowering.

By providing a theoretical foundation for Potentiation in Part I, detailed instructions for performing it in Part II, and tried and true tools for maximizing it in Part III, *Potentiate Your DNA* is (as its subtitle indicates) a most useful companion for those experiencing the Regenetics Method.

Readers desirous to share this book with family and friends may be interested in our "Pay It Forward" program—which provides substantial discounts on orders of ten or more paperbacks. For more information, visit **www.phoenixregenetics.org** or **www.potentiation.net**.

For many readers, there will be appropriate occasions to perform Potentiation remotely. In a moment, we will examine the various considerations and guidelines for doing so.

But first, let us briefly touch on some of the new science that supports the reality and effectiveness of nonlocal DNA activation.

Scientific Foundation for Distance Potentiation

One does not have to look to rarified physics, whether quantum entanglement or chaos theory, to find a straightforward scientific explanation of how remote DNA activation actually works.

Whether we examine distance Potentiation through the lens of meta-genetics, hypercommunication, morphogenetic fields or wave-genetics, it becomes obvious—patently and even redundantly—that *remote DNA activation functions by way of ... DNA!*

According to the Era III, meta-genetic model outlined in Part I, distance DNA activation operates via the nonlocal sound domain of the consciousness field—with which we interface by properly activating DNA (Figure 9).

In the collective consciousness field of time-space, which we can access using the right sounds, everything is connected and the concept of distance is irrelevant.

That the hyperdimensional sounds utilized technically are not heard by the recipient is equally beside the point. With mutual intention in place, for one person to activate another's DNA in the unified realm of time-space is as easy as shaking hands.

Nor is there, based on the meta-genetic model as well as years of professional observation, any functional difference between a Potentiation performed in person and one done at a distance.

Citing well-known physicist Nick Herbert while discussing Era III medicine, Larry Dossey lists three principal qualities of nonlocal events. Such events are: 1) *unmediated,* 2) *immediate,* and 3) *unmitigated.*

This last quality is the one I wish to emphasize. The fact that nonlocal events (such as distance DNA activation) are "unmitigated" means that their strength and efficacy do not decrease because of distance.

"Many studies reveal that healing can be achieved at a distance," Dossey observes, adding that "modern scientists have discovered that nonlocal events, meaning events that don't happen where they're initiated necessarily, are not fantasy but are part of the fabric of the universe."

The concept of hypercommunication is also helpful in explaining distance DNA activation. In *Conscious Healing,* I define hypercommunication as "extrasensory communication similar to telepathy that transcends spatial and temporal limitations."

While discussing the DNA Phantom Effect in Chapter Six, we established that wave-activated DNA is designed to engage precisely in such nonlocal communication.

Fosar and Bludorf connected this realization to the behavior of a number of groups in the animal kingdom. When a queen ant is removed from her colony, for instance, construction normally continues.

It is a little-known but relevant fact that so long as the queen remains alive, even if she is miles from her colony, work goes on uninterrupted. But if the queen dies, all work instantly stops.

Apparently, the queen sends wave-activated "consciousness blueprints" even from great distances by accessing time-space in order to communicate meta-genetically with her subjects.

From this example, it does not require mental gymnastics to grasp that *distance Potentiation is a form of hypercommunication not unlike that utilized in nature.*

Rupert Sheldrake's notion of morphogenetic fields provides yet another scientific foundation to explain remote DNA activation. In

Sheldrake's model, these nonlocal, ener-genetic fields can be accessed for a variety of purposes, irrespective of time and space.

Similar to the theory behind wave-genetics, Sheldrake's theory of Morphic Resonance posits that *DNA constitutes a real-time network, a biological Internet that basically does away with distance.*

To reiterate a previous point, we can upload data into the DNA Internet, download data, and even send emails to others on the network.

Distance DNA activation is explained as a nonlocal transfer of morphogenetic consciousness in the form of torsion waves that interface with potential DNA.

As this ostensibly dormant portion of DNA is activated from our position in space-time, it goes to work in time-space to correct distortions in the recipient's bioenergy blueprint, which then modifies metabolic and replication functions in cells, facilitating healing (Figure 9).

Tangible evidence of this meta-genetic phenomenon is provided by such consistently observable effects of distance DNA activation as detoxification, increased metabolism, and resolution of acute and chronic health problems.

This is made possible because *our bioenergy blueprint controls the genetic and electromagnetic activity in our cells and organs.* When this blueprint resets, as occurs over the course of Potentiation, palpable improvement can occur in any damaged system.

On this subject, the majority of wide-ranging Testimonials provided in the next chapter come from distance Potentiation clients living all over the world, most of whom Leigh and I have never met.

The same holds true for the numerous Testimonials relative to the other three phases of the Regenetics Method—which normally are performed at a distance as well using the basic principles and methodology described in this chapter—at **www.phoenixregenetics.org** and **www.potentiation.net**.

On a final note, Peter Gariaev's extensive experimentation with the extraordinary healing applications of wave-genetics further—and definitively—substantiates the reality and effectiveness of distance DNA activation.

Over and over, wave-genetics has been documented to work successfully at a distance. This fact strongly supports the idea that DNA constitutes a network much like the Internet that, existing anywhere, is present everywhere—effectively negating distance.

No Telephone Necessary—or Recommended

Distance Potentiation, like all remote Regenetics activations, never requires use of a telephone during the actual session.

Even a cursory reading of the previous section should make it abundantly clear that *no type of external communication device is necessary for distance DNA activation.* Humans intrinsically are "hardwired" at the genetic level for this kind of activity.

From a practical perspective, you have enough to focus on just in performing the technique correctly—without holding a receiver to your ear, yelling into a speaker phone, or worrying if the recipient is still on the line.

If you decide to add Optional Movement to Potentiation as described below, fooling around with a telephone becomes even less practical.

Shamanically, there is also the problem of digital conveyance of your chanting mentioned earlier in reference to recording Potentiation. Given the probability that digital renderings of DNA activation are largely ineffective in promoting healing and transformation, I encourage you to *avoid the telephone even when using the in-person Potentiation codes.*

In fact, when Leigh and I performed this work for several thousand people at the same time on Global Potentiation Day in 2008, while allowing recipients to listen in via the Internet, we used the *distance* Potentiation codes to connect with them.

On the subject of facilitating Potentiation for groups …

Although certified Regenetics Method Facilitators potentiate whole families and groups on a regular basis, *it is suggested that you start out working with one person at a time.*

If you feel inclined to take things to a more collective level, please consider becoming certified in Potentiation at a minimum. Again, detailed information on Facilitator training in all phases of the Regenetics Method can be found online.

Of course, when potentiating individuals remotely, feel free to give them a quick follow-up ring to let them know how the session went on your end.

You also will need to provide Potentiation recipients with a copy of Chapter Thirteen. More on these subjects momentarily under Checking in after the Session.

No Photograph Required

Many energy healers who work with people at a distance require a photograph of the individual. Here again, with Potentiation and the Regenetics Method, no such external "prop" is necessary.

Nor do you need any other personal artifact associated with the recipient—whether a blood spot, a lock of hair, an article of clothing, a handwriting sample, or anything else.

We are far too networked—spiritually, energetically, and genetically—with each other to have to look outside ourselves for a connection that is by nature internal.

No Diagnosis, No Problem

In Chapter One, I explained in some detail why the Regenetics model eschews self-limiting diagnosis in favor of a more holistic perspective that invites the possibility of radical change.

Etymologically, *diagnose* comes from Greek and can be thought of as to "read through" in order to acquire knowledge, or *gnosis*. But as it usually is practiced in today's medicine, diagnosis ends up oversimplifying complex issues while "cementing" a problem in the sufferer's mind until it seems that nothing, or very little, can be done about it.

For years now, Potentiation and other Regenetics activations have been performed—often with mind-boggling results—with the specific intent *not* to focus on any diagnoses that might be brought to the table.

This approach grew out of trust in the ultimate wisdom of the bioenergy blueprint. As part of the consciousness field, when reset through DNA activation, *our bioenergy blueprint requires no intellectual diagnosis to know exactly what to do to promote an integrated healing and transformative experience.*

For facilitators of this work, maintaining an attitude of nonattachment relative to healing specific conditions is of vital importance. This applies not only to potentiating others, but equally to your own session.

A copious amount of scientific research indicates that *nonattachment to predetermined outcomes is a critical factor determining success or failure in bringing about healing and transformation.*

When facilitating Potentiation, it is perhaps best to know nothing about the recipient's health. This keeps diagnoses from becoming mental baggage from which we must detach in order to perform this work most effectively.

Clearly, especially in the case of family and friends, to say nothing of ourselves, maintaining nonattachment through intentionally ignoring diagnosis is rarely an option. Also, with people and situations close to us, nonattachment in general becomes more difficult.

But it *is* possible. Many facilitators of Regenetics have found it helpful to remind themselves that *nonattachment does not imply lack of love.*

To the contrary, *genuine nonattachment is born out of unconditional love* that respects and honors a spiritual being's human journey—regardless of whether that person chooses renewed health or continued illness as a learning path.

Preparing for the Session

When facilitating this work, once we ourselves 1) are in the right heart space, 2) can maintain nonattachment and 3) have been granted permission to perform Potentiation, it is best to *go into the session with the open-ended intent that this DNA activation be for the recipient's highest good in all areas*—physical, mental, emotional, and spiritual.

Naturally, before even scheduling someone else's remote session, it also is incumbent on you to *practice the distance Potentiation technique* as instructed toward the end of this chapter until you can pull it off more or less seamlessly.

Furthermore, well in advance of the session, you need to *provide the recipient with a hard or electronic copy of Chapter Eight, "Getting Ready," and emphasize that this preparation guide needs to be read and—where appropriate—implemented.*

A downloadable PDF version of Chapter Eight is provided for the convenience of all concerned at **www.phoenixregenetics.org** and **www.potentiation.net**.

Digesting "Getting Ready" will assist recipients in:

1. Embracing the self-healing paradigm on which Potentiation is based;

2. Writing down their intentions in a Potentiation journal; and

3. Getting their head and especially heart in the right place to maximize their benefits.

For individuals who are *unwilling* to read this material, perhaps it would be best to hold off on Potentiation until they are ready to engage more actively in this process.

For recipients who are *unable* to read the preparation guide themselves, it is okay to skip this step. Alternatively, you can read Chapter Eight to them to give them an idea of how to prepare.

As experienced Facilitators of the Regenetics Method, Leigh and I have performed sessions for babies, toddlers, autistic individuals, seniors with dementia, people with no access to Regenetics materials in their language, and even one person in a coma.

Even in instances when conscious preparation has been less than optimal or nonexistent, the results often have been surprising. Particularly in the case of young children, whose parents regularly report striking improvements, Potentiation has shown itself capable of doing without left-brain processing.

Below under Three Exceptions to the Permission Rule, I offer some tips for facilitating these anomalous kinds of sessions.

After you have done your own homework, and your best to help the recipient prepare, it is time to schedule the session. Thirty minutes should be sufficient for Potentiation.

Write down the recipient's first and last names in your planner, calendar or appointment book at an agreed-upon half-hour slot that suits both parties. If the individual prefers, it is okay to use a spiritual or chosen name.

You also should instruct the recipient to make a note of the Potentiation appointment—both to help in remembering the session, and to provide a starting point for charting the flow of torsion energy through the bioenergy blueprint as taught in Chapter Thirteen.

Make sure the recipient knows that you will *not* be using a telephone to perform the session. The individual is expected to remember the appointment and be in an intentional space at the scheduled time—and should not expect to receive a call as a reminder.

If you are asked what you will be doing during the session, the answer is that you will be performing Potentiation on behalf of the recipient in a ceremonial manner.

During the session, the recipient can be indoors or out. Chapter Eight provides some helpful advice for choosing a time and place to avoid interruptions while focusing on the healing and transformational potential of this work.

Unlike someone performing his or her own Potentiation, during distance sessions *recipients are free to 1) take a walk; 2) engage in other relaxing, introspective activities, such as a bath or massage; or even 3) fall asleep.* So be sure they are aware of these options.

After you have written down the recipient's first and last names, underneath in your calendar, planner or appointment book make a note of the person's date of birth, as well as his or her geographical location (time zone) if different from your own.

Scheduling people in other time zones can be tricky—and all the more so if they are in another hemisphere. By searching online, you should be able to find a number of websites to assist you in coordinating dates and times worldwide.

Finally, as a reminder, for sessions performed in person especially, please give thought to having the recipient sign the Potentiation Consent Form included in Appendix B.

Checking in after the Session

If at all possible immediately following, but certainly within a day or two after another's Potentiation, it is your responsibility as a facilitator to provide the recipient with several pieces of helpful information.

As above, in the case of individuals with whom you cannot communicate effectively, for whatever reason, use your best judgment at this point.

At a minimum, whenever feasible it is a courtesy to let the other person know how the session went from your perspective. It is a good idea to do so even for in-person sessions.

In Chapter Thirteen, I share a simple muscle testing technique (Figure 14) you can use to 1) get a sense of whether the Potentiation was delivered properly; and 2) determine the recipient's Electromagnetic Group and corresponding Schematic (Figures 15, 16, and 17).

You are advised to *test on these two points immediately following the session and pass on this information to the recipient at your earliest convenience.*

Also, be sure to record the person's Electromagnetic Group (1, 2, or 3) beside his or her name in your planner, calendar, or appointment book. This information can come handy if the person forgets this information or has questions about the Potentiation experience.

While testing as to the success of the session itself is basically a formality, nevertheless, it can bolster beginning potentiators with a sense of confidence as they embark on their journey of ener-genetic repatterning.

After years of experience facilitating and teaching this work, my perspective is that any Potentiation performed with permission, decent technique, a dash of love and a pinch of nonattachment is successful *as an offering.*

The real question is how well a given Potentiation will be *received* and *integrated* by the individual.

For readers new to Regenetics, the notion of muscle testing for the Electromagnetic Group and Schematic probably does not make a lot of sense at this stage. Chapter Thirteen delves into this fascinating and useful subject in detail.

When you have determined the individual's Electromagnetic Group and matching Schematic through kinesiology, make sure you communicate this information clearly.

In order to assist you here, you have the author's permission to *give the recipient a hard or electronic copy of Chapter Thirteen, "Era II Tools."* Alternatively, this chapter is available as a PDF download at **www.phoenixregenetics.org** and **www.potentiation.net**.

By elucidating the concept of Electromagnetic Groups and Schematics, Chapter Thirteen should answer many of the most common questions about the repatterning and consciousness aspects of this work before they are asked.

Finally, *make sure recipients know about the Regenetics Method Forum,* where individualized questions can be addressed by certified Facilitators.

If you are interested in performing this work for others, before doing so it is well worth joining the Forum yourself. As a reminder, a special subgroup has been created expressly for readers of this book.

Instead of via private correspondence with the Phoenix Center for Regenetics, potentiators and facilitators alike are urged to ask their questions relative to *Potentiate Your DNA* on the Forum. Membership guidelines and registration instructions are provided at the above websites.

Three Exceptions to the Permission Rule

As indicated toward the start of this chapter, there are three—and only three—exceptions to the permission rule when it comes to in-person or distance Potentiation for people: embryos, young children (under twelve), and communication-impaired adults.

The first exception is the least obvious because it involves a human being in utero. That we know a woman receiving Potentiation is pregnant is irrelevant—since we cannot very well ask her embryo/fetus for permission to perform the session!

Moreover, muscle testing and observation repeatedly have borne out that, even in cases when the mother is unaware she is expecting, *a child in the womb always is potentiated along with its mother.*

Actually, this is a good thing, because it usually means a healthy, happy baby. But it does raise the question of how we may or may not be infringing on the child's free will by potentiating it in the womb.

After much deliberation and consultation with others, years ago Leigh and I determined that *parents have the right to make an "executive decision" as to whether their children are potentiated until the latter enter puberty.*

Before children reach the age of twelve, our position is that the "soul contract" between them and their parents establishes a number of parental prerogatives where the free will of their children is concerned.

Through these prerogatives, parents are entitled to make certain crucial decisions—such as regarding Regenetics—with the potential to greatly impact the physical, mental, emotional and spiritual wellbeing of their children.

This line of reasoning led us to see that such prerogatives necessarily extend beyond strictly biological relationships to include *legal guardians* of children under twelve.

By contrast, *grandparents, godparents, aunts, uncles, siblings and cousins lacking legal guardian status should ask permission of a parent or legal guardian of their relatives under twelve before potentiating them.*

When children reach twelve, barring mitigating circumstances (such as autism) that effectively reclassify them as communication-impaired adults, whether to receive Potentiation is really up to them.

Obviously, most youngsters hitting puberty cannot be expected to grasp what this work is on an intellectual level. Simply telling them that Potentiation is a form of sound healing which works through their DNA to help them feel better is sufficient.

If they want to experience Potentiation, go for it! If not, give it some time and approach them with the idea again later. Whatever the situation, make sure you have their permission before proceeding.

Where adults with dementia or other conditions that impair their ability to communicate are concerned, the logic again is based on the idea of a soul contract. But here, the roles are reversed.

Instead of parents making use of prerogatives to potentiate their young ones, *adult children who have become primary caregivers of their communication-impaired parents are empowered to potentiate the latter without conscious, explicit permission.*

As with legal guardians of children, such a prerogative extends to any individual, whether another family member or someone outside the family, considered the primary caregiver of an adult who has lost the ability to think or communicate coherently.

On this note, while Potentiation was designed to improve physical health, given its powerful ability to heal mental, emotional and spiritual traumas, *this DNA activation can be used to help terminally ill individuals transition.*

I hesitated to share the above point because I would not wish for anyone to think that Potentiation can have a negative physical impact or that it is incapable of strengthening people who are very sick. Quite the opposite.

But for individuals whose time has come, and who consciously or otherwise have chosen to pass on, Potentiation has proven to be a tremendous blessing on numerous occasions in easing the psychological difficulty of passing.

By way of concluding this section, following are a couple of special tips for working with exceptions to the permission rule.

Before potentiating embryos/fetuses, young children or communication-impaired adults, feel free to exercise your prerogative as a parent, legal guardian or primary caregiver to *go through the appropriate steps outlined in Chapter Eight on behalf of the individual to be potentiated.*

In other words, empathetically stepping into the recipient's shoes, start by 1) embracing the fact that all healing is self-healing; then 2) write down your intentions for this work; and finally 3) make sure that your head and heart are in the right place to benefit from it.

You can think of this "surrogate strategy" as a way of "holding space," energetically and intentionally, in order for the recipient to experience the most positive and suitable results from this DNA activation.

Immediately after Potentiation, you can muscle test as you would with anyone to get a feel for how the session went and determine the recipient's Electromagnetic Group.

Over the forty-two weeks following the session, it can be enormously helpful to reference the recipient's Electromagnetic

Schematic (Figures 15, 16, and 17), which charts the flow of torsion energy through the bioenergy centers as explained in Chapter Thirteen (Figure 18).

By keeping this information firmly in mind, you will be in a far better position than you would be by ignoring it to make sense of any significant—as well as subtle—changes in the recipient's health and behavior.

Potentiating Animals

Most animals love Potentiation. Facilitators of this work who allow pets inside have reported that when a session is being performed, they hardly can keep their animals out of the room!

Animals possess the same basic bioenergy structure as humans. Potentiation can encourage animals to heal and evolve their consciousness much in the manner of humans.

Leigh and I have potentiated a wide range of farm and domestic animals over the years, and feedback from their owners has been overwhelmingly enthusiastic.

Just as with the three human exceptions to the permission rule outlined above, owners of pets and farm animals are considered to have a soul contract with the creatures they look after.

This special relationship empowers owners to potentiate their animal companions at their sole discretion—without acquiring permission or infringing on free will.

A similar surrogate strategy to the one described above for preparing another person to receive Potentiation can be used when working with animals.

You may or may not know the animal's date of birth, so this information is optional.

You also need to decide whether to perform the animal's session in person or at a distance. In terms of effectiveness, as is the case with humans, *it makes absolutely no difference whether you perform Potentiation for animals in person or remotely.*

Really, your decision should boil down to matters of personal preference, convenience, and feasibility. A number of factors might come into play here:

Are we talking about a house animal or one out on the range?

Will you be able to stay within hearing distance of the animal for a full half hour, or is it possible that the animal will head to the hills mid-session?

Is it just too darn cold in the barn in February for Potentiation?

Finally, one key factor distinguishing Potentiation for animals from working with humans is that *it is not necessary to determine the Electromagnetic Group and corresponding Schematic for animals.*

If you feel so inclined, it is okay to muscle test to get a feel for how the animal's session went. But obviously, there is no need to follow up with information and materials for animals.

It is sufficient to note that their Potentiation cycle lasts approximately forty-two weeks, with torsion energy following the same basic pattern through their bioenergy blueprint as with humans.

During this process, just as you would with yourself or another person, be on the lookout for detoxification, physical improvement, and positive behavioral changes.

Working with the Distance Potentiation Grid

Once you have mastered the technique for in-person Potentiation, learning distance Potentiation is a piece of cake.

Learning to perform this work remotely is as simple as replacing in-person Potentiation's vowel sequences with the distance Potentiation codes in Figure 13.

Clearly, practice is required. But this stage should not be nearly as long or hard as first wrapping your mind and mouth around pronunciation, rhythm, pitch, double intoning, and sequencing—which are all the same.

When starting out, you are encouraged to *reread Chapter Nine and simply substitute Figure 13 for Figure 12.* As with the in-person Potentiation codes, you have the author's permission to photocopy Figure 13 for private, noncommercial use.

After you have developed some technical mastery with the remote vowel sequences, reread this chapter to jog your memory of the various considerations and guidelines for distance Potentiation.

Congratulations once again! You now are ready to potentiate your family members, friends, and pets!

Vowel Sequences for Distance Potentiation

Bioenergy Center	Line	Vowel Sequences											
Master	1a	O	O	U	I	E	I	A	U				
Master	1b	e	i	o	u	a	e	a	a				
9	2a	I	A	A	I	A	E	E	I	E	-	-	-
8	2b	a	i	i	a	i	i	a	a	e	e	i	a
7	3a	I	O	A	I	I	I	O	A	I	I	E	
6	3b	i	e	a	o	u	o	u	-	-	-	-	
5	4a	A	E	O	U	A	E	I	E	-	-		
4	4b	e	u	u	i	i	e	i	a	i	e		
3	5a	A	E	A	E	A	E	U	O	U	O	I	
1	5b	a	e	o	a	e	e	o	a	-	-	-	

one ring   three rings

4 pass-throughs down   1 pass-through up

two rings

Figure 13: Vowel Sequences for Distance Potentiation

The above grid's sound and light vowel codes are used for distance Potentiation sessions. Note the points relative to the number of tuning fork rings and the sequence of five pass-throughs.

Optional Movement

We will conclude the "how-to" aspect of Part II with instructions for including movement while facilitating Potentiation—should you desire to do so.

Movement during Potentiation is completely optional. Some utilize it; others do not. Given the possibility of dizziness for inexperienced facilitators, *most people do not start out using movement.*

A potential positive impact of the suggested circular movement on the work itself is to help some facilitators enter a more meditative state in which more theta waves can be produced.

Again, many facilitators do not feel the need for movement in order to put themselves in a relaxed, deeply meditative place when performing Potentiation—and their results bear out that *movement is not required for this work to be one hundred percent effective.*

Some have theorized that walking in circles (rotation, rotation, rotation) might encourage the torsion waves produced when chanting and thinking the Potentiation codes to spiral more powerfully.

While this is an interesting hypothesis, I have witnessed such extraordinary results from Potentiation performed without motion that I tend to think *movement is really more about the one performing the work than the one receiving it.*

Whether to move or not during sessions is not a fixed, one-time choice. Some days you may feel like moving; other days you may opt to stay seated. You might prefer to utilize movement during in-person Potentiation and remain still for distance work, or vice versa.

At the start of the session, stand in a predetermined position facing either the recipient or, for distance sessions, an object that represents the recipient (optional).

Although a representative object is in no way required in order to establish a remote connection with another person, many facilitators find that using an object helps them focus.

Note that a representative object can be used without movement. Also, utilizing movement does not mean that you must do so with reference to an object.

When selecting a representative object on which to focus during distance sessions, endeavor to choose something that evokes a positive feeling in you. A lit candle is a good option. Or you might use a crystal, houseplant, or statue.

Using a photograph of or personal artifact belonging to the recipient is not recommended because of the potential for creating attachment to specific outcomes and thereby limiting Potentiation's effectiveness.

When opting for movement during Potentiation, hold your vowel sequences and hockey puck secured by your clipboard in one hand and the Mi tuning fork in the other hand.

As soon as you ring, breathe and commence singing, *start walking in slow, clockwise circles around the recipient or representative object without stopping until you reach the end of the fourth pass-through* as described in the previous chapter.

As you ring your tuning fork twice to signal the directional shift, *reverse direction yourself and walk in slow, counterclockwise circles until you reach the end of the fifth and final pass-through.*

Ideally, you will double intone the last line (1) right as you come full-circle to your original starting point. But if your timing is off, it is okay to finish chanting wherever you are on the circle and continue walking in silence back to your starting point.

When you have returned to your starting point, ring your tuning fork three times and do not mute it for a solid minute as the sound tapers off into silence.

For in-person sessions, having the recipient lie on pillows or a massage table in the middle of the room works great. Provided there is enough space, this setup allows you to move in circles around the individual.

Admittedly, there is something special, from a recipient's perspective, about being encircled by waves of sound and torsion energy. This approach is tailor-made for healthcare professionals seeing clients in a formal setting.

If you are working with a tight schedule of clients, *make sure you factor in enough time after the session for the in-person recipient to continue lying down processing the energies when necessary.*

In addition to spaciness, dizziness and sleepiness, the Potentiation session also can induce emotional release—so be prepared to offer a kind word in support of the recipient's expressing feelings and taking things easy for a bit.

Finally, while your starting point for movement is up to you, you might consider following a time-honored shamanic tradition and beginning at one of the four cardinal directions: north, south, east, or west.

The idea is to face in the direction that constitutes a "power base" for you personally at any given moment. If you are unsure of the cardinal points where you perform Potentiation, you can purchase a small portable compass inexpensively online or at your local mountaineering store.

CHAPTER 11

Selected Testimonials

Before shifting our focus to the various tools that can be implemented to maximize conscious personal mastery through Potentiation and other Regenetics activations, it seems appropriate to offer the reader a number of different perspectives on how this work can unfold.

In addition to revealing an impressive range of potential benefits spanning the body-mind-spirit spectrum, the following Testimonials also demonstrate that *the experience of Potentiation is highly individualized.*

Just as no two individuals are exactly alike, no two Potentiations are identical. Sometimes improvement occurs early in the process, while other times breakthroughs happen toward the middle or at the end.

To be clear, the established Time Frame for how torsion energy cycles through the bioenergy blueprint following Potentiation is relatively fixed at forty-two weeks—as explained and charted in Chapter Thirteen (Figure 18).

Of particular interest to individuals wishing to perform Potentiation for family and friends living far away is that *most of the Testimonials included in this chapter come from clients of distance Potentiation.*

Note that under no circumstances are these Testimonials intended to make medical claims with regard to Potentiation or the Regenetics Method. Please see the Disclaimer near the beginning of this book.

More Testimonials relative to Potentiation and other phases of the Regenetics Method are provided at **www.phoenixregenetics.org** and **www.potentiation.net**.

Addiction & Potentiation

"Before Potentiation I felt very weak and was experiencing strange headaches and higher than normal blood pressure. The day before my Potentiation session I quit smoking cold turkey and have not had a puff since. In the past 30 years, I've tried to quit smoking probably at least 20 times using all sorts of smoking cessation therapies such as acupuncture, hypnosis, etc., which helped during the initial withdrawal period but did nothing to overcome the lethargy and inertia that always followed. This is the first time I quit smoking without having the desire to break down and cheat once. Also, I didn't feel as lethargic as I normally do and feel my strength increasing on a daily basis. I'm not saying it was easy, but something was different this time. I feel as though I was ridding my body of all sorts of toxins, not only the nicotine. I'm one hundred percent confident that I've kicked the habit for good! And I attribute my success to Potentiation." JC, Woodstock, Illinois

Allergies & Brain Fog Disappearing

"I have completed my nine months for the Potentiation process and boy am I happy. I now have a life where before I had only restrictions. I can drive my car without wearing a mask. I can shovel shavings for my horse's stall without feeling dizzy and sick. I can stay on the computer 6 to 8 hours a day instead of less than one hour. I have a great boyfriend. I am well enough to work and earn a good living—something I've waited 15 years for. The person I was before Potentiation was so physically damaged by heavy metal and other toxicity it was just a matter of time before a nasty reaction would have sent me out with heart failure. It's difficult to describe in words, but I feel new and renewed, as if the best part of me expanded and everything else, including my brain fog, just disappeared. My heartfelt thanks." DM, Orcas Island, Washington

Better Personal & Professional Relationships

"As soon as I discovered the Regenetics Method and read about the Fragmentary Body, the missing piece for me, I contacted the Developers and booked my initial session. By supporting me through the release of two limiting relationships and the 'upgrading' of several more to healthier states, Potentiation helped me realize something I'd been unable to achieve before in all my spiritual and therapeutic pursuits: a sealed energy field with no more ongoing energy loss and no more vulnerability to compromising situations and relationships. In my estimation no amount of therapy or mental processing could have achieved comparable results. I actually felt the sealing of my energy field and, to this day, have no more problems navigating challenging circumstances, personal or professional. Regenetics has tremendously improved my work as a therapist as well as my personal relationships, old and new. As a fringe benefit, I'm often told I look ten years younger! Certainly, I feel younger, excited to be alive again, with consistently more joy." AW, London, United Kingdom

Closer to Realizing My Intentions

"While I have not fully gotten over all of my environmental allergies, I was pretty bad, and have much less attachment to them now. Rare is the day now that I wake up not breathing through my nose. Lately, I eat pretty normally, for me that is, and have virtually gotten over sugar cravings. I have a better understanding of my purpose, and more energy to carry it out. I had the most kundalini movement and most intense experience of awareness of everything around me from Potentiation; but I think that was because it initiated the most change in my case. I still have some back pain, but it is a lot better and it does not have the emotional impact it used to. A big step has been taken toward realizing my intention for the activations." BW, Goshen, Ohio

Consciousness Overhaul

"I can't believe it's been nine months already since Potentiation. There have been a lot of changes in my life, internally and externally. I'm starting a new career, and my health's never been better. But most importantly, my consciousness has gone through quite an overhaul. Life and the universe look totally different now, and I enjoy much more freedom and gratitude than I ever imagined before. I seem to encounter friends, teachers and inspirational materials on a constant basis. There is a strong sense that finally everything is coming together. Thank you so very much for the service you provide." LB, Little Rock, Arkansas

Emotional Release

"Thank you so much for last week's Potentiation session. I've been involved with energy work for a long time and have never experienced the kind of shift that has happened since connecting with you. I've already released a lot of emotional garbage. The amazing thing is that even though it was intense, I felt supported. Physically, in fact, I feel better than I have in years. Since the onset of my chronic environmental illness many years ago, any strong emotion would rattle my nervous system and make my allergies worse. Not now. I feel good. The emotional stuff has cleared. I never really expected to feel completely well again, and it's a little mind-boggling thinking about what I'm going to do with my life as a fully functioning person." SP, Orcas Island, Washington

Energy, Health & Wealth

"Unbelievable blessings have happened in my life since I began the Regenetics Method. I now have abundant energy, health, and wealth! The Regenetics activations have supported my spiritual growth and evolution in a relatively easy way. My body is no longer a burden, but more energized than ever. My energy sustains over time in a new way. I realize that I'm a creative Being with increasing amounts of blessing, joy and delight in my life. My finances have improved dramatically, as have my relationships. I find myself being able to help people as never before, with access to the right words at the right times, while no longer being 'caught' by my emotions as before. Finally, amazing 'coincidences' have become increasingly evident and common in my daily existence." AV, Pretoria, South Africa

Fewer Hot Flashes & Improvement with Arthritis

"Since initiating the Potentiation process 4 months ago, I've experienced several rather profound changes. My hot flashes have subsided, which is a real relief and allows me to sleep better at night. Most of the arthritis in my hands and knees has cleared up, reducing my dependence on glucosamine. I've gone through some detoxification and can sense more energy coming in through my chakras." PD, Myrtle Beach, South Carolina

Fewer Food Cravings, Less Anxiety & More Self-love

"Since Potentiation I generally have a sense of greater wellbeing, stronger workouts, less sugar and food cravings. I seem to be taking better care of myself, extending myself a certain tenderness, suffering less anxiety. It feels good!" CE, Asheville, North Carolina

Gradual Release of Food Allergies

"My experience of Potentiation was both subtle and powerful. During the early phase, the first few months, I felt an unusual sense of happiness and peace and an overall subtle shift inside. Then, as the process unfolded, I realized my food allergies had completely disappeared! I'd tried other treatments with limited success, but with Potentiation I gradually noticed I could enjoy food that would have normally caused headaches and spaciness. Very remarkable!" EL, Asheville, North Carolina

Healthier Relationships & Conscious Personal Mastery

"I am so grateful for Potentiation. It has really helped me turn the corner on emotional reactivity in important relationships. In the midst of conflict I am able to both understand the other person and have on-the-spot clarity about my feelings and the needs of the situation, and communicate it, with respect for myself and the other person. It has transformed conflict around here, with lovely effects that have radiated into my extended family, my daughter, my son and my mother." JS, Colorado Springs, Colorado

Healing Childhood Trauma

"My personal experience of Potentiation was powerful, initiating a great deal of emotional as well as physical (pain) release, especially in my head—which as a massage therapist, I found most interesting! As a child I had a lot of head injuries and also contracted meningitis at two and a half. Throughout my adult life, in therapy and elsewhere, I'd attempted to get to the core of the abandonment issues around my traumatic experience of meningitis (when I was quarantined away from my parents for days), but on some level I knew my cells were 'hanging on' to the memory. The very day of the Potentiation process when I entered the seventh field, which in my Electromagnetic Group regulates the musculoskeletal system as well as many emotions associated with abandonment, I was massaging a client. Halfway through I started sobbing and couldn't stop. I felt exactly the same sensation I felt during my meningitis episode: that of being catapulted into space, disconnected from everybody and everything, floating in a dark tunnel. Until Potentiation it wasn't possible to feel, at a body level, the full emotional impact of this experience. But now I was feeling it. Somehow I finished the massage and called two friends to be with me as I underwent the most extraordinary release over twenty-four hours during which I felt my cells were literally being cleansed biochemically of the hormonal residue of my childhood trauma. Within two days my lifelong fear of abandonment was merely a memory." SL, London, United Kingdom

Instant Improvement with Sensitivities

"Thank you so much for my Potentiation session yesterday. I definitely connected with you and it felt very powerful. While meditating during the session, I experienced tingling feelings which continue at times today— waves of energy moving through me, a very warm and expansive feeling in my chest/heart chakra area, and definite feelings of joy and an uplifted sense. I also started feeling shifts prior to the session after reading *Conscious Healing*, which is fascinating and inspiring. So much of it resonates with me. This may sound strange, but it feels like I'm absorbing essential nutrients as I take in your words. It is amazing work that you're facilitating. I already feel different: lighter, more clear-headed, energetic, and hopeful. I've had carb hangovers whenever I had even a little bit of carbs or sugars, and have thus had to totally avoid them for years, severely limiting my ability to eat out/socialize/travel. I do a lot of self muscle-testing and while I know it's early in my Potentiation, I'm AMAZED that I already test strong to healthy (organic) carbs and even straight sugar! Wow! As well, chemical sensitivities have dominated my life for 18 years. I'm already feeling shifts here as well and will keep you posted on my healing. Eliminating MCS and food intolerances will create a quantum leap of improvement in all areas of my life. Thank you again. I will spread the word to all those who can hear it!" JS, Cumming, Georgia

Less Depression with Structural Shifts

"What do I feel is different since last week's Potentiation? There will be a big layoff soon where I work, but I feel much lighter, calmer and more positive. A lot of my depression is gone. Also, for the last couple years I've felt the left side of my body tightening and I've constantly had the urge to stretch it. One doctor said I had Illio Tibial Syndrome and gave me stretches to do. A massage therapist/instructor said I had a fascia problem. Being treated by them helped very little. I underwent other unusual therapies, also with little results. But now I've had a major shift and tremendous release on my left side, especially in the left hip and leg. I really cannot believe it. My hip is so loose, lighter feeling and rounded out. I do massage therapy and for years have worked on myself. But now there is no need to work on these areas!" CH, Streamwood, Illinois

Less Insomnia & TMJ

"At the time of my Potentiation seven months ago, I was depressed and suicidal due to my inability to sleep. I'd often go whole nights and only get an hour of sleep. I still struggle somewhat with insomnia, but I no longer, or rarely, have the kind of nights I used to have before Potentiation. I've also suffered for years from TMJ, but in spite of braces and a mouth full of metal, I've improved in this area as well. I still have many challenges, but I now generally believe life is worth living and I even have feelings of happiness and joy. I also had a serious case of Restless Leg Syndrome when I began this process. I still have it at times, but lately it has been a lot less. I know this doesn't sound like much, but trust me, it's a big deal. I think of all the many things I've tried, Potentiation has probably been the best investment in my overall health and has helped me the most." KC, Atlanta, Georgia

Math Phobia Gone

"A subtle but very real thing occurred just three weeks after Potentiation. I'd suffered a math phobia for most of my life, ever since having my head thrown at a blackboard for getting a math problem wrong in grade school. (Prior to that, I was a math whiz!) So severe was the trauma that I cringed at anything that had to do with numbers. Years later, after Potentiation, it felt like tiny tiles were releasing from my brain and suddenly the calculator became my friend as I looked forward to numbers and calculations, and even to doing the financials in clients' business plans that I'd formerly farmed out to accountants. This was so exciting and freeing! Over time, my allergies and asthma also faded into a distant memory. The suffering was simply gone, and more and more vibrant health was becoming mine. As I went on to Articulation and then Elucidation, I experienced greater depths of living and loving. The separation I'd always felt changed to a oneness with everything and everyone. New possibilities and fresh insights arose. My entire being changed to a 'Light-ness' I'd never felt before. As an Interfaith Minister, counselor and coach, I've learned and shared many modalities to effect changes in clients. Some changes 'stuck' longer than others, but none ever deeply and profoundly changed the client at the core level and lasted like the transformations I've personally experienced through Regenetics DNA activations. This one modality directly and permanently promotes transformation at the physical, mental, emotional and spiritual levels. I am forever grateful I found Regenetics." MS, Wood-Ridge, New Jersey

Mental Clarity & Structural Benefits

"I must say that since my Potentiation over five months ago, I've become extremely clear and focused in a way that I haven't been before. Very frequently my body feels so light and erect—I feel as though I'm pure light in movement—can't quite describe it in adequate words. I just know that I wouldn't trade how I experience the world within for anything. As part of my experience I've literally felt torsion shifts—almost as though a chiropractor is working on me. Thank you." GP, Toronto, Canada

No More Chronic Fatigue or Fibromyalgia

"It's now 18 months after we first experienced Potentiation and I wanted to write about this first activation because in some ways it is the most important to me. My husband had been horribly sick with Chronic Fatigue (CFS) and fibromyalgia for nearly 3 years. We had tried countless therapies and moved to Hawaii from New York City in hopes that his 32-year-old body would recover. Every day was just pain for him; he couldn't think, had bad anxiety, heart palpitations, constant nausea, and couldn't sleep for more than 2 hours at night. We signed up for Potentiation. He felt visibly improved in the days right after. I was so happy! A week after Potentiation he was at his computer reading and interested in work again. He could think! The anxiety stopped. In the weeks that followed, he was able to get more and more sleep. As I'm writing this testimonial 18 months later, after completing Articulation and Elucidation, he is pain free. He sleeps like a log at night. He works out three days a week at the gym. While going through the DNA activation, we continued exploring ways to heal the physical body. There are many things that helped the detoxification process and some that didn't. In the end, many things contributed to my husband's recovery. Potentiation, however, in my mind, truly commenced the healing journey as well as provided a timeline that brought us both back from darkness." EK, Kamuela, Hawaii

No More Rash

"Up until the Potentiation session, I had been struggling with the most vile and crazy-making rash. The only thing that would relieve me of the severe discomfort was an over-the-counter antihistamine that left me feeling lousier than I did with just the rash. After the session I just knew that I could stop taking the drugs, so I went to bed drug-free for the first time in months. I woke up feeling refreshed with no itching at all. If this is all I have to look forward to, it would be enough. I know this is just the beginning, though." DP, New York, New York

Physical Improvement at an Advanced Age

"My daughter was so pleased with her Potentiation results I had to try it. I had severe food allergies that had escalated through the years to the point where I could barely eat anything without discomfort. Within the first month after Potentiation, I found myself able to add more foods to my diet. It has now been two months since my session, and I feel I've improved at least 70%. I'm 82 years old and to see my health improve so fast is thrilling." LH, Sylva, North Carolina

Removing Emotional & Mental Blockages

"Fascinatingly, Potentiation helped me overcome my eye disease—though indirectly. In a subtle but extremely important way, this work encouraged me to move beyond my duality and its resultant 'blockage' where the Western medical approach to this particular issue was concerned. Also, I believe that the enlivening process I experienced as Source energy tracking through my energy body after Potentiation helped prepare me on many levels to accept perfect success from my eye operation, when I finally got around to it. I most highly recommend Potentiation as well as the rest of the Regenetics Method to anyone who is looking for beneficial change in a variety of areas related to physical disease or pain, including discomfort and issues rooted in emotional or mental blockages. If you wish to have a greater conscious experience of yourself as a spiritual physical being, the Regenetics Method is definitely for you." DM, Montreal, Canada

Skin Healing & Personal Empowerment

"The past 5 months since my Potentiation have been amazing. What a process you have developed! I noticed the following ... I went on a HUGE house cleaning binge. I was tired but somehow had this incredible energy to clean everything in sight—like never before. I couldn't believe it. Later, a bump that I had above my eyebrow got itchy and burst open. I'd had it for over 15 years and thought it was just a part of me, but then it completely disappeared, healing without any scarring in just 3 days! Wow! I've also noticed that I have better tolerance for foods. My daughter has also greatly improved on the foods she can tolerate and her digestion. Finally, I've had an inner confidence that I never had before and am starting a private practice after hating my office job for many years. I'm really looking forward to the rest of the process to see where this will lead me!" AC, Ontario, Canada

Spontaneous Disappearance of Food Allergies

"I consider myself very open-minded and accept the power of spirit to heal physical and mental imbalances. Yet last year when I was suddenly confronted with severe food and chemical allergies after a trip to Haiti, I felt humbled by limitations I'd never personally experienced. A yoga and meditation practitioner for many years, I thought I was immune to chronic physical ailments. A close friend recommended Potentiation, and since I'd noticed significant improvements in her, I decided to try it. I prepared myself mentally for a week, drawing on my own knowledge of the power of intention to heal. My Potentiation session itself wasn't at first very different from deep meditation. Soon, however, the results were astonishing. In less than two days I felt my allergies completely leave my body, as well as mucus-forming food 'intolerances' to wheat and dairy that had plagued me since childhood. I could eat anything, though I'm still vegetarian for moral reasons, and could finally breathe through my nose again! I strongly recommend this healing process, but be very pure and strong in your intention as to why you're 'potentiating.' Don't forget it's your higher mind you're connecting with, and that healing starts in you." DR, Marshall, North Carolina

Total Life Transformation

"In 2000, I crashed. Suddenly I was having serious trouble sleeping, became severely bloated, had major digestive discomfort and distress, felt I would die each month before my period, experienced anxiety, depression, 'brain fog,' malaise, fatigue, aching muscles, fear, and despair. I experimented with practically every diet known to humankind, in addition to energy work, acupuncture, allergy elimination techniques, EFT, hardcore supplementation, sauna therapy, reiki, electrical cellular stimulation, IV therapy, reflexology, psychic detox techniques, acupressure techniques for emotional release, massage, heavy metal detox, German machinery, microscopy, and others. Although some alleviated my symptoms, I still did not feel a fundamental shift. One morning at 4 am, I was guided to do Internet research and found a commentary on a bulletin board about someone's boyfriend who had 'taken Potentiation' and healed his Leaky Gut Syndrome. Thinking Potentiation was a bottle of homeopathic drops, I contacted Sol and Leigh and began my journey through the Regenetics Method. The level of neuro-toxicity (caused by vaccine damage and compounded by other factors) I carried was quite high and Potentiation was the perfect avenue for its departure from my body. The process was intense at times, but I could gradually feel a lifting of the 'sludge' and knew I was headed for a life-affirming existence after years of extreme discomfort. This technique has helped transform my life beyond anything I could have imagined." CH, Dallas, Texas

Unity Consciousness

"Potentiation triggered/activated my great awakening to Self-realization, Galactic, Universal, Multi-Universal and Cosmic Consciousness and Oneness with life." JW, Wales, United Kingdom

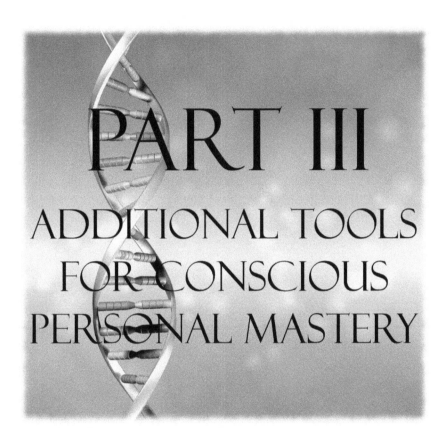

PART III
ADDITIONAL TOOLS FOR CONSCIOUS PERSONAL MASTERY

CHAPTER 12

Era 1 Tools

Having gleaned a basic theoretical understanding of Potentiation in Part I, and at some point potentiated yourself or received Potentiation as covered in Part II, you now are ready to learn to maximize and integrate the energies of this potent DNA activation.

It is worth mentioning that the first potentiators, including yours truly, were not provided with the full selection of powerful tools for enhancing Potentiation we will explore in Part III. Nevertheless, even the earliest results often were nothing short of amazing.

I also wish to point out that all of the suggestions—including ones having to do with nutrition and supplementation—offered in these last three chapters are just that. In no instance am I providing medical advice or prescribing or recommending any diet, supplement or activity for medical purposes.

The multifaceted "tool kit" outlined in Part III came into being over time, as various questions and situations arose with clients and students that led Leigh and myself to realize that offering such tools might make this work even more effective for some.

While facilitating and teaching the various phases of the Regenetics Method over the years, Leigh and I developed a set of tried and true tools for encouraging conscious personal mastery that correspond to the three Eras of medicine elaborated previously (Figure 6).

This book constitutes the first time these tools have been assembled in writing in one place—and we both are thrilled to pass them on to you!

Era I tools, the subject of this chapter, are designed to help the body harmonize with the energies of Potentiation as the bioenergy blueprint resets, damaged systems begin to detoxify and rebuild, and some of the old rules for nurturing yourself are replaced by other possibilities that belong to a new paradigm.

In the next chapter, Era II tools for conscious personal mastery are explored. *Era II tools encourage individual awareness of the process of healing and transformation* so that potentiators might interface productively with their own increasing ener-genetic consciousness over the 42-week Potentiation cycle and beyond.

Finally, Chapter Fourteen offers a look at the Regenetics Method as a whole in order to set the stage for additional *Era III tools capable of evolving the body-mind-spirit* to levels of conscious personal mastery that lie beyond Potentiation.

What Is Conscious Personal Mastery?

Before examining these comprehensive tools, let us take a moment to get on the same page with respect to the concept of conscious personal mastery.

In Parts I and II, various statements with considerable bearing on this subject were made. To recap, conscious personal mastery was said to:

1. Often utilize initiation as a catalyst for an internal experience teaching love (for self and others) and imparting compassion and wisdom as preconditions for healing and transformation;

2. Involve a student-teacher relationship with our Higher Self, complete with tough love designed to foster our spiritual development;

3. Require us to understand our own past dysfunctional creations—even to the extent of using detoxification to feel the energies of these old creations as they release—in order to create healthier, more functional situations for ourselves;

4. Transpose the roles of our Higher Self and ego, without submerging or destroying the latter, such that the ego relinquishes its attempts to control our lives and comes to serve the spiritual purpose of the Higher Self;

5. Seal the Fragmentary Body so as to replace our sense of isolated individuality and related victim consciousness with individuation leading to reunification with the Creator and embodiment of unity consciousness;

6. Teach us to forgive and love ourselves despite our imperfections—and just as critically, to extend forgiveness and love to others who also are imperfect;

7. Require us to trust our ability and intuition even when we lack intellectual certainty; and

8. Encourage us, via the healing process, to accept ourselves and others unconditionally and, moreover, to see others as ourselves.

In light of the characteristics just summarized, my definition of conscious personal mastery from *Conscious Healing* as "unconditional love of oneself as simultaneously the Creator and the created extended outward to all perceived others" should not seem particularly esoteric or farfetched.

With no exceptions, to pursue conscious personal mastery in our own way is why we are here in the first place.

Without conscious personal mastery providing a spiritual context for our bio-spiritual healing and transformation, healing and transformation are merely empty words divorced from any comprehension of why we even should desire such things.

The second we grasp that healing and transformation are integral aspects of a spiritual journey of conscious evolution, we can start to make use of this process—for the benefit of ourselves as well as others.

Conscious personal mastery of necessity begins with the self. There is nothing selfish about this fact. Quite simply, we cannot expect to create a better world if we cannot first heal and transform ourselves.

Logically, if we are to offer food to others who hunger, we first must feed ourselves. "Any other way," in the words of Joachim-Ernst Berendt, "would be absurd."

When we have recovered our strength, we can use it to assist others in finding their own inner fortitude. In reality, we cannot do this *for* them. As in the parable, rather than giving a fish, we teach the art of fishing. This is done by example.

In terms of conscious personal mastery, learning to fish starts with learning to connect with the Higher Self. At some point, it is accurate to say, on our evolutionary journey of reunification with the Creator, we *become* our Higher Self.

But in the initial stages of conscious personal mastery, just learning to listen to—and follow the guidance of—this spiritual aspect of our consciousness on a consistent basis is enough to keep us occupied.

As we engage our authentic spiritual purpose more and more, it is only natural that our own healing and transformation will begin to manifest in the people and circumstances around us.

Such is the case because, ultimately, conscious personal mastery reveals that we are inseparable from the people and circumstances around us.

Thus in a deceptively simple, absolutely effective way, our own progress in conscious personal mastery assists with the progressive healing and transformation of the world.

Feeding the Self

In terms of nurturing the self by taking care of the body during Potentiation, nothing is more important than eating right.

During this unique process when your entire bioenergy blueprint is recalibrating, rapidly and radically, your relationship with food can change just as often and as much.

Many former ways of approaching your personal nutrition suddenly can fall out the window as you undergo this DNA activation that reestablishes your body's inherent wisdom while typically altering and speeding up your metabolic processes.

For example, a lot of people come to this work so overrun with Candidiasis stemming from vaccine-induced genetic damage that they have been on alkalizing diets for years just to survive.

Often, such people have little or no starch intake. And for good reason—most of them are highly allergic, prior to Potentiation, to even simple starches such as rice and potatoes.

Understandably, these same individuals can be hesitant to modify their diet, even when they intuit profound systemic shifts occurring through Potentiation, and often cling to the idea that they must "alkalyze or die."

But the truth is that as the body's metabolism increases during Potentiation and more and more toxins are released from cells, *a little starch can go a long way in binding toxicity and mitigating symptoms of detoxification such as bloating, pain, and inflammation.*

In fact, many strategies that may have assisted prior to Potentiation, such as fasting and eating primarily raw food, become too powerful at this stage when the body typically needs more binding substance and less external prompting to cleanse and heal itself.

Leigh and I have observed that for many potentiators, *a balanced diet of mostly organic, mostly cooked food that includes regular starch intake combined with a decent amount of protein is the most beneficial.*

But keep in mind that as your relationship with food and your food needs change throughout the unfoldment of Potentiation, your diet will have to change as well.

Facilitators of Potentiation who provide nutritional counseling usually have to transform how they work with potentiators, as opposed to people who have not experienced this DNA activation, because of the extraordinary ability of Regenetics to render much of the old "wisdom" about food obsolete.

Once you begin to potentiate, the days for finding your ideal diet and sticking to it are probably over. With your body intelligently directing you to particular foods at particular times, say goodbye to eating solely for your blood type or consuming only meat and vegetables.

As your bioenergy blueprint becomes less distorted and your biological system starts to receive clearer ener-genetic instructions from the consciousness field, *your body will communicate which specific foods you require at any given moment via cravings.*

In the beginning, as an example, you may be able to tolerate very little starch (if any). But after a few weeks or months, it is common for potentiators to find themselves desiring some starch—and more food in general.

Regularly, to their delight and amazement, formerly allergic individuals discover that they suddenly can eat previously taboo foods with fewer—or even no—unpleasant reactions.

To be clear, listening to our cravings does not imply that we have carte blanche to binge. While making sure to feed ourselves well, moderation is still in order.

Happily, the tendency to binge—like many addictive behaviors— often dwindles and disappears over the course of Potentiation and the Regenetics Method.

The stronger, more insistent your cravings, the more your system needs the particular food in question. To ignore your cravings is to turn a deaf ear to the best nutritional advice available to you: your own.

The choice is ultimately ours whether to listen to someone else telling us what we should put in our bodies, at the expense of denying our own instincts and intuition.

Of course, most of us have been taught that our cravings are bad, things to be resisted at all cost—just as most of us have been indoctrinated not to trust our better judgment and to fear our own power.

Fortunately, the times are changing. In my opinion, *it is the correct, the evolutionary thing to be yourself and listen to your own inner voice.*

Diet should not be like religion where one must be right and all others must be wrong. In the eloquent words of M. F. K. Fisher in *The Art of Eating,*

> I cannot count the good people I know who, to my mind, would be even better if they bent their spirits to the study of their own hungers. There are too many of us, otherwise in proper focus, who feel an impatience for the demands of our bodies, and who try throughout our whole lives, none too successfully, to deafen ourselves to the voices of our various hungers. Some stuff the wax of religious solace in our ears. Others practice a Spartan if somewhat pretentious disinterest in the pleasures of the flesh, or pretend that if we do not admit our sensual delight in a ripe nectarine we are not guilty … of even that tiny lust! I believe that one of the most dignified ways we are capable of, to assert and then reassert our dignity in the face of poverty and war's fears and pains, is to nourish ourselves with all possible skill, delicacy, and ever-increasing enjoyment. And with our gastronomical growth will come, inevitably, knowledge and perception of a hundred other things, but mainly of ourselves.

For those concerned about their figure, bear in mind that with accelerated metabolism and detoxification, *an increase in cravings and food intake does not mean necessarily that you will gain weight.*

To the contrary, you may slim down while eating more during Potentiation. But even if you put on a few pounds, have faith that your body knows what it is doing and your weight will normalize when you are stronger and less toxic.

Have You Helped Your DNA Today?

There are some specific substances which support proper DNA activity in particular and good health in general and, thus, may be worth considering during Potentiation.

Whenever possible, rather than taking pills, capsules or liquids that your body may have a hard time integrating, it is suggested that you find ways to include such substances in your everyday diet.

According to an insightful article entitled "Have You Helped Your DNA Today?" by pharmacist Bryan Flournoy published in *DNA Monthly*, antioxidants such as vitamin C and vitamin E are "beneficial to DNA found in tissues all over the body; and vitamin A specifically blocks oxidation of DNA molecules involved with eyesight."

Flournoy points out that "omega fatty acids found in flaxseed, safflower and certain fish oils also provide antioxidant protection against free radicals."

In addition, trace minerals such as "iron, cobalt, chromium, copper, iodine, manganese, selenium, zinc and molybdenum work with amino acids (the building blocks of proteins) and enzymes to neutralize less harmful radicals created in the anti-oxidation process, and are only needed in small amounts."

Flournoy emphasizes that foods rich in folic acid contain critically important DNA-building materials: purines and pyrimidines. Such foods include fresh green vegetables like broccoli and spinach. Folic acid, sometimes called folate, also is provided by fruit, beans, whole grains, and starchy vegetables.

The list of foods particularly rich in purines and pyrimidines is topped by anchovies, sardines, yeast, herring, organ meat, legumes, mushrooms, asparagus, spinach, and cauliflower.

To be noted, Flournoy stresses that "over-consumption of these foods might aggravate gout (an inflammatory condition of the joints) or exasperate kidney stone formation in those predisposed."

Furthermore, "those who use anti-depressants or blood pressure control medications in the category called MAOI's (monoamine oxidase inhibitors) should check with their physician before intentionally eating more of these foods."

Finally, some dietary amino acids can assist with DNA synthesis. Be sure to "consume plenty of B vitamins, which can be found in the nutrient lecithin, usually isolated from soybeans, and the entire vitamin B group found in beef, brewer's yeast, and legumes."

More Food for Thought

Before we explore other Era I tools besides nutrition for maximizing Potentiation, let us quickly outline a handful of additional dietary concepts that might prove useful on your journey of healing and transformation.

Enzymes are magical substances whose potential benefits range from reducing pain and inflammation to stimulating the body's ability to digest food.

The most effective systemic enzyme Leigh and I have discovered, one we both have used on occasion to eliminate acute discomfort associated with detoxification, is Wobenzym N.

Alternatively, nature provides an unsurpassed enzyme product: *raw honey*. Nutritionist Aajonus Vonderplanitz observes that unheated honey—meaning honey that has not been so much as grazed by a hot knife during production—"helps replace missing enzymes for nearly all purposes throughout the entire body."

Not only that—many who are allergic to heated honey and other forms of sugar can eat as much truly raw honey as they like. Of course, some people experience allergic reactions even to raw honey. Because of this possibility, medical authorities generally do not recommend honey of any kind for children under two.

By asking around, you probably can find a local raw honey provider. Otherwise, the raw honey produced by Y. S. Organic Bee Farms is excellent. Visit www.ysorganic.com to check it out.

On the subject of *sugar*, an astonishing thing sometimes happens with potentiators. From being allergic to sugar, they suddenly can eat large quantities of it. In their case, *consuming sugar often seems to speed up metabolism and increase detoxification!*

Leigh and I both have felt sugar do this on so many occasions that we eventually dubbed it "rocket fuel." Needless to say, rocket fuel is not something you want to play around with. Even if sugar ceases to be problematic for you in an allergic way, it is probably best to go easy on it.

To this day, even though we occasionally enjoy desserts and drinks with sugar, Leigh and I often use *stevia* in baking and beverages. Stevia is a wonderful noncaloric sugar substitute, purportedly with antifungal and even insulin-balancing properties, obtained from the leaves of a South American plant.

An excellent variety, available in liquid and powder at many health food stores, is Kal brand. Since it is so much sweeter than sugar, and has different properties, getting used to stevia—to say nothing of learning to use it properly—may take time. Fortunately, there are some good stevia cookbooks out there (see Bibliography & Webography).

Another potential rocket fuel for potentiators is *alcohol*. When you are not allergic to alcohol and your metabolism can utilize it efficiently, drinking moderate amounts of wine, beer or even spirits can help reduce systemic pathogens by "solventizing" them somewhat like paint thinner and washing them out of the body.

Sometimes alcohol can make detoxification more intense. In other instances, *a little alcohol actually can help neutralize viruses and other pathogens involved in detoxification and help you feel better faster.*

Lest the skeptical reader dismiss this latter possibility as wishful thinking, chemist Gerard Judd, among whose credentials is a refutation of the bogus idea that fluoride promotes dental health, also authored a fascinating study called "The Alcohol Cure for Viruses."

Under no circumstances do I advocate that potentiators drink alcohol if they are underage or if for any reason they feel uncomfortable doing so. Always use common sense and trust your gut instinct. Realize that if you choose to consume alcohol during Potentiation, it can impact detoxification much like eating sugar.

Allergic individuals interested in incorporating a bit of alcohol in their diet might find that they can tolerate raw, unheated wine, such as Coturri, which can be purchased at many health food stores as well as online.

Most raw wines do not contain added sulfites, which is also good for allergies. And of course, red wine of any kind provides resveratrol, antioxidants, bioflavinoids and proanthocyanidins that, according to various studies, do everything from neutralize free radicals to inhibit cancer to strengthen blood vessels.

Another beverage with many potential benefits, one that has been much maligned for decades, is *coffee*. Once considered bad for health, in recent years caffeinated coffee in particular has undergone a major facelift.

According to Harvard Medical School, drinking coffee in moderation has proven to be beneficial in such wide-ranging areas as blood pressure, cancer, diabetes, and Parkinson's disease.

Alexandra Lupu, Health News Editor for Softpedia, adds gallstones, liver problems, bad breath, asthma, anxiety, depression and suicide to this list.

"The short-term effects of coffee upon our body are also extremely beneficial, as it helps us think faster and clearer, banishing drowsiness and fatigue," writes Lupu. Also, "coffee contains significant amounts of antioxidants … capable of counteracting the damaging effects of oxidation in the body's tissues."

In terms of Potentiation, *a cup of strong organic, caffeinated coffee or espresso in the morning can help you avoid constipation while facilitating the steady flow of toxins out of your system in the form of regular bowel movements and urination.*

Many potentiators previously made jittery by coffee have reported that this tendency decreases or simply disappears with Potentiation—yet another indication of real physiological shifts that often accompany ener-genetic repatterning.

Consuming reasonable quantities of quality *salt* also can fortify the body. While table salt—which has been stripped of nutritional value—is best avoided, Himalayan crystal salt (www.himalayancrystalsalt.com) is said to supply many beneficial trace minerals naturally.

The last dietary consideration I will mention here is particularly for individuals initiating this process whose physical health has been compromised tangibly.

In his landmark work *Nutrition and Physical Degeneration*, dentist Weston Price explained that in Western societies, where tooth decay and other forms of physiological deterioration are rampant compared to that found in many indigenous cultures, the missing nutritional ingredient is something called *Activator X*, now known to be vitamin K2.

Conspicuously absent from most "civilized" diets, Activator X is found primarily in the butterfat of grass-fed cattle and appears to be an essential element for keying the body to utilize minerals to repair even quite severe damage to itself.

Dr. Price discovered that *Activator X is especially restorative when consumed with cod liver oil*. In studies that Price conducted, even a small regular dose of Activator X in tandem with cod liver oil stopped cavities in their tracks and produced other extraordinary healing effects.

For detailed information on Activator X and how to combine it with cod liver oil for regenerative purposes through supplementation as well as diet, readers are encouraged to visit the Weston A. Price Foundation online at www.westonaprice.org.

A Word about Water

Any discussion of things to give the body during Potentiation would be incomplete without calling attention to the importance of water in the detoxification process.

The more toxicity you find yourself releasing, the more water you should be drinking. Below under Allergies vs. Detoxification, I offer some tips for identifying various kinds of toxic release.

It is okay to drink water all day long. And when you are doing so, it is just as okay to go to the restroom as often as you like.

Frequent urination when you are consuming lots of water and flushing out heavy metals, pesticides and parasites through your kidneys and bladder does not indicate, by itself, that you have a medical problem. Of course, if you have concerns, please consult a medical professional.

To avoid confusion, when I say water, I mean *water*. While moderate daily intake of organic juice, smoothies, teas and other drinks can assist with proper hydration, *the majority of your liquids should be in the form of pure water.*

Non-fluoridated filtered, reverse osmosis or spring water is preferable. As a general rule, stay away from any brand of bottled water that is not sold at health food stores, since there is little quality control with such varieties.

Naturally carbonated mineral water is acceptable for a change of pace—and can be tasty and refreshing chilled with a squirt of lime or lemon juice added. Both Perrier and Gerolsteiner are high in calcium, while citrus is a great source of vitamin C.

Last but not least, caution is urged when considering structured, clustered, ionized, energized or alkaline water. *Any water that has been altered molecularly in order to penetrate deeper into cells can be too strong and speed up detoxification during Potentiation to uncomfortable levels.*

For individuals experiencing this work whose health has been compromised substantially, I suggest sticking with plain old natural water most of the time.

Back to Nature

By now the reader probably is aware that the author prefers natural to contrived ways of doing things—especially where fortifying the body is concerned.

My sincere belief, founded on years of personal experience combined with professional observation, is that the body is profoundly capable of healing itself when prompted correctly in a natural manner.

While the previous statement applies generally, it becomes even more applicable during Potentiation and the Regenetics Method, when harmony has been reestablished in the bioenergy blueprint.

Rather than looking outside ourselves to other techniques or new technologies at this stage, it often is more effective—as well as empowering—to cultivate our own relationship with nature and natural ways of being.

There are numerous cost-free, perfectly natural things we ourselves can do on a regular basis with undeniable potential to assist in healing and transforming our body-mind-spirit.

For starters, and mostly obviously, make a point to *spend a decent amount of time in nature*. Following through here can be as simple as strolling in the park after lunch.

When you spend time away from noise and stress in a natural sanctuary of any kind, a noticeable increase in your overall sense of wellbeing is the norm.

An added perk of being in nature is that a degree of quietude typically is required when communing with our Higher Self. Nature is an optimal environment for learning to heed this soft-spoken inner guidance.

Gentle exercise (preferably in nature) such as gardening, walking or swimming is an excellent everyday activity to keep the blood and lymph moving during detoxification and rebuilding. Movement is good not only for the body, but also for the mind and spirit.

Moderate exposure to sunlight, in addition to providing the body with vitamin D3 and a corresponding boost to the immune system, similarly enhances mental acuity and lifts the spirits. There is nothing like a little sun on your face to make you feel refreshed.

Unless, of course, it is *air filled with negative ions from the ocean or a waterfall*, which a number of scientists claim to have health benefits ranging from better circulation to improved mood.

In addition to the above examples designed to connect us directly with nature, I wish to highlight several natural life-affirming activities that are just as effective indoors as out.

Laughter has been documented to provide body-mind-spirit benefits in virtually any situation. Be sure to engage in a good belly laugh at least once a day.

To this end, follow a comic strip that tickles your funny bone, or read comedic books, or watch movies that engage your sense of humor, or spend time playing with young children.

Touch also can be truly healing and transformative. In *The Continuum Concept: In Search of Happiness Lost*, psychotherapist Jean Liedloff advances the compelling theory that most Westerners and many others living in industrialized societies simply are not touched enough as babies to feel fully welcome in this world.

Conditions associated with this epidemic lack of human contact can range from low self-esteem and lack of confidence, to mental illness and depression, to decreased vitality and chronic health issues.

In order to fulfill your "continuum," it may be necessary to spend many hours over a number of weeks or even months in skin-to-skin connection with another person.

If you are in a relatively healthy relationship, romantic or otherwise, with someone willing to assist you, and possibly fulfill his or her own continuum in the process, problem solved.

To be clear, continuum contact does not imply or require sexual activity. Nor does it necessitate nudity. You can work on your continuum in a bikini or shorts.

Of course, *sex* with a loving partner is another completely natural activity with the potential to foster physical, mental, emotional and even spiritual wellness.

Dream On

It is impossible to overemphasize how important *sleep* is during Potentiation. Regular, uninterrupted sleep to the tune of at least seven or eight hours a night provides a number of important health benefits that nothing else—not even frequent naps—can replace.

Deep sleep time is deep healing time. During quality sleep, our systems naturally detoxify and rebuild to an extent that vastly exceeds what normally occurs during napping or waking hours.

Unfortunately, some people suffer from insomnia. The good news is that a common benefit reported by many potentiators is that sleep starts to come easier—and last longer—than ever before.

Yet similar to the experience associated with increased hunger, many potentiators feel guilty when their bodies demand even a little more sleep during periods of significant release and strengthening.

People make all kinds of excuses, personal and professional, when it comes to not getting enough sleep. But as with cravings, what are we really saying in terms of self-love if we refuse to listen to our genuine need for rest?

On the subject of listening to our inherent wisdom, much like being in nature, *sleep deep enough for dreaming can lead to revelatory experiences in which we directly commune with our Higher Self.*

In our dreaming state, we "cross over" to our mirror reality, time-space (Figure 2). Time-space, the consciousness field, is less "veiled" than space-time—which means we naturally see ourselves with more spiritual consciousness when dreaming than while waking.

David Wilcock shares two cardinal rules for learning to interpret the spiritual messages that our Higher Self encodes in our dreams:

1. Everyone we encounter while dreaming is an aspect of *ourselves*; and

2. Events and situations in dreams usually are meant to be understood *symbolically*, not literally.

Our dreams communicate vitally important information that can be interpreted and integrated retroactively by our waking mind. Usually, *such dreams have to do with practical steps we can take to live and embody our true identity and purpose.*

Naturally, DNA activation, if the real thing, can stir up all kinds of powerful dreams along these lines because what is being activated is, to use Arnold Mindell's wonderful term again, the Dreambody.

The Role of Serendipity

Paying attention to serendipity, defined as the ability to make fortunate and unanticipated discoveries as if by luck, is another way to interact with natural circumstances in order to stay connected with the Higher Self.

In the case of Potentiation, serendipity often occurs when someone experiencing this work "naturally" encounters another person, situation or technique that seems to make all the difference in terms of achieving health and wellbeing.

Other potentiators "follow their nose" along a complicated chain of serendipitous events—walking through a series of "doors," opened suddenly and inexplicably, that lead to an extraordinary healing or transformation.

Leigh and I contend that *raising our personal frequency by way of DNA activation often is responsible for generating more serendipity by increasing the rate of vibration of our bioenergy fields, which we sometimes call "attractor fields."*

Individuals "organically" magnetizing greater serendipity to themselves in order to achieve wellness may or may not trace their success directly back to the Regenetics Method.

DNA activation is a complex process that many times produces undeniable results, and other times lacks obvious causality with respect to its ultimate effects—like the proverbial butterfly flapping its wings and creating a hurricane on the far side of the world.

Leigh and I have adopted the mindset that it matters not at all what recipients of this work believe benefited them most on their evolutionary journey. All that really matters is that people are empowered to access whatever means necessary to become whole.

More Is Less, Less Is More

Someone once said that the definition of insanity is doing the same thing over and over while expecting different results. Many sources attribute this sentiment to Einstein, who certainly was an intelligent fellow.

On numerous occasions, I have remembered this trenchant definition while observing a certain "obsessive-compulsive" behavior in people trying to overcome chronic illness in particular. The typical profile of such individuals runs as follows:

They take a dizzying array and amount of herbs and supplements. They have a closet full of healing gadgets and gizmos. They see half a dozen therapists at any given time. Their weekly planners are filled with colonics, reflexology, acupuncture, EMDR, hypnosis, craniosacral therapy, lymphatic drainage—you name it.

Often, these people have been on their own version of this treadmill for years, having spent an enormous amount of time and money on Era I and Era II approaches in a laudable effort to reclaim their vitality. But nearly as often, they seem as unwell as ever, or worse.

I have just described myself in the years leading up to the development of the Regenetics Method. You might say I have a well-honed sense for picking up on similarly desperate, imbalanced behavior in others.

The only solution to the situation is to come back into balance—which often happens all by itself as distortions in the bioenergy blueprint are corrected over the 42-week Potentiation cycle.

Sometimes, however, people experiencing this work require additional encouragement in order to stop the "insanity" of continuing the same old ineffectual protocol day after day.

The first thing these potentiators need to grasp is that, quite often, *more is less.*

Trying everything under the sun in a panic to get well rarely results in a productive approach to healing. To the contrary, such a scattergun strategy can make you feel more miserable—as well as mightily confused as to what is doing what.

If you find yourself in a situation where more has become less, the next thing you need to realize is that, in all likelihood, *less is more.*

Without giving up anything you know in your heart you need, *start by paring down your regimen.* Ideally, you can let go of everything and establish a clean slate.

Obviously, before stopping any medications or medical therapies, you should consult your doctor. While it is possible to wean yourself off many unnecessary things during Regenetics, there may be medicines or therapies that will continue to be helpful for you.

As your body-mind-spirit harmonizes, detoxifies and strengthens over the course of Potentiation, *you are best served simplifying your daily routine in as many areas as possible.*

Once you have reestablished a clean (or nearly clean) slate, and have had time to listen to your inner guidance without the chaos and confusion of a patchwork regimen pushing the wrong buttons, you will be in a much clearer space to utilize serendipity for healing and transformation.

If you listen closely to and trust your intuition, your Higher Self will lead you unerringly to anything you truly need to support your wellbeing. You may be surprised how little extra you actually are directed to try.

The Higher Self never speaks through restrictive or self-limiting emotions. You can recognize its wisdom because it fills you with a decidedly expansive and uplifting feeling: confidence, happiness, excitement, love, etc.

Any lingering doubts, worries, fears or second guesses about a particular course of action usually indicate that your ego is still attempting to call the shots.

It is up to you to choose between bowing to the ego's old fear-based reasoning, which rarely worked in the past, or embracing the pure creative potential of a new, higher, more inspired evolutionary path.

Allergies vs. Detoxification

On the subject of allergies versus detoxification, the most important thing to keep in mind is that *detoxification can resemble an allergic reaction.*

Given that toxins and pathogens cause most allergies, it is only natural that during DNA activation, as our bodies release these temporarily mobilized allergens, the response can appear "allergic."

Therapies and drugs that suppress allergies by driving them deeper without inviting some degree of detoxification merely treat and mask symptoms, as opposed to undoing the underlying causes of allergies.

It is also crucial to grasp that *there are significant distinctions between allergic reactions and detoxification.*

Since it can be difficult for someone who has not experienced Regenetics to tell the difference between these phenomena, you must cultivate your own awareness in order to make sense of what is occurring in your body.

A major difference between allergies and detoxification is that whereas allergies are just vicious spirals going nowhere, *detoxification is actually productive.*

If after years of allergies, you suddenly find yourself releasing the very substances and microorganisms that have tormented you, that in itself is cause for celebration!

As a reminder, *many potentiators do not experience appreciable detoxification because it is not needed.*

But for others, especially those with a long history of chronic illness, signs to watch for following Potentiation that you might be detoxifying include:

• Your stools are more copious than usual, look different, or have a fouler odor than is customary.

• Your stools develop a different consistency—looser and "shaggier" with a tendency to float in the bowl indicating microorganism release, a hard "pebbly" look with an inclination to sink to the bottom resulting from heavy metals.

• Your number of daily bowel movements increases.

• Your regular time for having a bowel movement changes.

• Your urine becomes darker, smells more pungent than usual, stings slightly coming out, or bubbles in the bowl.

• You notice a "catty" or similar "animal" odor to your stools or urine, which means you are cleansing old, rancid hormones such as adrenaline.

• You start to perspire noticeably more.

• Your sweat has a stronger odor than usual.

• Your sweat smells uncannily like strong ammonia, indicating heavy metals releasing.

• Your white bed sheets visibly begin to turn brown or another color from the toxins (often pesticides) in your perspiration.

• You develop a runny nose, especially just after eating, meaning your system is using food to cleanse your head and sinuses.

• For no obvious reason, your breath suddenly smells bacterial, as if you have a cold when you do not.

• You sneeze three or more times in a row out of the blue.

• Your ears produce more wax than normal.

• Your eyes feel "gummy."

• You develop acne or a rash near problem areas that disappears as soon as your symptoms go away.

• You notice that your scalp becomes temporarily itchy or flaky.

• After vomiting or briefly experiencing other flulike symptoms, such as fever or diarrhea, you feel fine the next day.

• You experience heavier than normal menses.

When you observe any one of the above physiological shifts, it is possible that your body is releasing toxicity.

When several such signs are in play simultaneously, you almost certainly are detoxifying, rather than having an allergic reaction or immunological meltdown.

The very best approach to navigating a big release is to let your body's wisdom steer the course and allow yourself to sleep. Also, make sure to consume some starch, if possible, and drink plenty of pure water. Gentle exercise can be beneficial, but be mindful not to push yourself too hard.

Activities that speed up cellular detoxification—such as ionized footbaths, strong energy work, or consuming large amounts of raw fat—are to be strictly avoided during a difficult cleanse, as they only make things more intense.

Another huge difference between allergies and detoxification is that most allergies typically do not lessen or go away on their own, but *symptoms of detoxification can—and do—diminish and eventually disappear, typically resulting in greater wellbeing.*

Detoxification symptoms dwindle naturally as the body becomes cleaner and there is less need for cellular release. Of course, there can be ups and downs as the body pools enough bioenergy to purge the factors that have made it unwell.

It is an excellent indication when one who has been chronically ill suddenly feels uncharacteristically spry and chipper following a major release. Leigh and I call this a "window" and interpret it as a sign of returning strength.

Being stronger also means that when it is ready, the body will engage in yet more cleansing to restore even greater vitality and create even longer windows.

This cyclical process of detoxification followed by more pronounced stabilization can repeat a number of times, until one normally exists in a window—at which point symptoms associated with toxic release become rare and eventually cease altogether.

Because allergies and detoxification are so alike yet unlike, and most health professionals have no training in or context for differentiating between them, you might consider taking any diagnosis relative to allergies you receive during Potentiation with a grain of salt.

Clinical diagnosis, machine analysis and muscle testing are all prone to mistaking detoxification for an allergic response—and equally likely to send you down the Yellow Brick Road of more superficial therapeutic interventions.

In all three cases, the mentality is that because you appear to have problems, problems must be found—and you can bet they will be. And the blood work, computer readout or kinesiological testing will *prove* you have problems!

Not only might you be told that you have "allergies." You also might receive a fearful diagnosis to the effect that you are full of parasites or heavy metals, for instance.

But the fact is that many people's dangerous toxicity levels are so deeply embedded and immoveable as to be undetectable by any diagnostic technique—whereas your system, amazingly, has been empowered to purge these toxins from their hiding places on its own!

The reason toxins and pathogens often become detectable following DNA activation is that they have exited the deep cellular matrix and entered the lymph and bloodstream on their way out of the body.

That your system might be using the energies of activated DNA to cleanse and heal itself on a profound level never enters into the thinking about what is "wrong" with you—for the simple reason that the possibility that something might be "right" about you never is entertained.

Candida & Detoxification

Another misleading diagnosis potentiators sometimes receive is that they have Candidiasis, which can lead to recommendations for everything from hardcore pharmaceuticals to heavy doses of supplements to extreme elimination diets.

The fact is that *Candida albicans* is present in everybody's system. Candida is a critical scavenging microorganism in the yeast family—without which we would not last very long. Forming part of the intestinal flora, Candida's primary purpose is to clean up dead tissue and toxic debris.

When Candida proliferates in someone who has been damaged energenetically (usually by vaccines) and whose bioenergy blueprint remains distorted, it typically does so in an uncontrolled fashion.

In such cases, there is no guiding intelligence from the bioenergy blueprint to direct Candida's behavior in productive ways. The result is a wild, unmanaged struggle on the part of Candida to wrest toxins from cells that, for their part, have not been instructed by the consciousness field to release their toxins.

The upshot is basically internal biological warfare in which Candida wreaks havoc at the cellular level without accomplishing much of anything positive.

This impossible situation stirs up the besieged cellular matrix to a state of autoimmunity that begins to resist anything introduced into the body that is perceived as "foreign." Thus various types of often bewildering, debilitating allergies are created.

On the one hand, attempts to get rid of Candida when it is in desperation mode almost inevitably fail. Candida believes (with some justification) that it alone can save the body's cells from being destroyed by their internal poisons and returns immediately in the absence of medication or dieting out of pure survival instinct.

On the other hand, any Era I or Era II modality that tries to force cells to release toxins and pathogens without prompting the bioenergy blueprint to change its instructions to cells can do more harm than good.

Heavy metal chelation, parasite "zapping" and frequency therapy are just three examples of a myriad of techniques that ignore the bioenergy blueprint—to say nothing of how to reset it—in favor of coercing the body to detoxify without giving it the green light to do so.

When the bioenergy blueprint resets, the circumstances change radically. Cells are keyed to dump toxins in an organized, intelligent fashion, even as Candida starts to receive clear hypercommunication directing it to mop up the mess as gently and safely as possible.

As with so-called allergies, at this stage Candida overgrowth still may be detected through conventional diagnosis, especially during a major release.

But Candida's restored guiding purpose and renewed ability to help the body will be glossed over as you are handed an old-paradigm prescription or recommendation for destroying it.

Potentiation invites a new paradigm with regard to Candida that is collaborative, not antagonistic.

While seriously allergic individuals at first may need to limit their intake of starch and other foods capable of feeding Candida, over time it is common for potentiators to expand their diet and learn to work with, not against, this important microorganism.

As this symbiotic relationship develops, you are likely to discover that mild Candida overgrowth shows up in periods of tangible detoxification to latch onto and flush toxic debris from your system, then disappears during windows when you feel stronger.

Rather than trying to blast Candida out of your system with pills or starve it into submission, a generally more effective strategy is to *balance your intestinal flora through regular consumption of organic, sugar-free, cultured dairy products—such as yogurt and kefir—full of live, active, probiotic organisms.*

But as always, when it comes to eating, trust your cravings and intuition. And have some faith in your body's wisdom and ability to spiral slowly but surely up out of dysbiosis where Candida is concerned into a more normalized state of internal wellbeing.

The Homeopathic Effect

By way of wrapping up our discussion of Era I tools for promoting conscious personal mastery, let us examine another potential physiological change that potentiators can benefit tremendously from understanding.

One of the guiding concepts in traditional homeopathy is that *like stimulates like.* When addressing a health problem, it is common for homeopaths to have the patient take an energized remedy that closely mirrors the frequency signature of the problem itself.

For example, a patient suffering from overexposure to pesticides might be prescribed a benign homeopathic remedy that the body reads energetically as pesticides. The intended effect is to trigger the body to release pesticides and thereby remedy any associated symptoms through its own natural mechanisms.

Dating back to its development by Samuel Hahnemann in the early 19th Century, the Era II medical science of homeopathy has proven effective in addressing a wide variety of physical, mental and even emotional conditions.

But with many clients of the Regenetics Method, whose experience closely mirrors my own, homeopathy can be overmatched when it comes to serious genetic alteration caused by such modern plagues as vaccinations.

That said, knowing a thing or two about the principles behind homeopathy helped Leigh and myself get to the bottom of a fundamental, systemic shift that occurred in the aftermath of our Potentiation.

Not long into our process, as our "allergic reactions" began to feel more productive in terms of detoxification, we both realized that on many occasions, our immunological responses were triggered by environmental stimuli—although not in the former directionless, autoimmune manner.

Rather, a moldy hotel room prompted the tangible expulsion of fungus from our systems. Breathing hydrocarbons from roadwork near our apartment caused our lungs to dump petroleum-based toxins. Eating seafood with traces of mercury sent us into a heavy metal purge.

Grasping the fact that, on their own initiative, our potentiated bodies were starting to interact with our environment *homeopathically*, we coined the phrase "Homeopathic Effect" to describe this unprecedented development.

Not only did this new experience of being able to live in co-creative harmony with our environment promote a switch from victim to unity consciousness. It was also at this stage when we grasped that our so-called allergies, as defined traditionally, were gone.

Instead of being allergic reactions, responses on the part of our bodies to external factors appeared to be directed intelligently, and in homeopathic fashion, by the bioenergy blueprint—and inevitably led to detoxification followed by windows of greater wellbeing.

When experiencing the Homeopathic Effect during Potentiation and the Regenetics Method, it can make all the difference to shift your perspective—and language—from the old paradigm of allergic reactions to a new one of healing responses.

It is vital to trust that your body, in collaboration with a restored bioenergy blueprint, knows what it is doing. Keep in mind that over time as you become less toxic, the Homeopathic Effect should become correspondingly less frequent.

Finally, note that the Homeopathic Effect in particular, and detoxification in general, can encompass more than just material phenomena.

Mental, emotional and even spiritual detoxification and healing typically occur hand in hand with physical release. These more subtle (yet nevertheless quite powerful) aspects interconnect with the physical in numerous ways.

Over the course of our final two chapters, while introducing Era II and Era III tools to speed you on your journey of healing and transformation, we will explore the ultimate interconnectedness of the body-mind-spirit.

CHAPTER 13

Era II Tools

Era I tools are designed to assist the body in benefiting from the energies of Potentiation and the Regenetics Method. As noted, nurturing the physical vehicle of our spiritual identity is an important aspect of conscious personal mastery, or learning to embody unconditional love of ourselves and others as one.

At the close of the last chapter, while discussing the related subjects of detoxification and the Homeopathic Effect commonly experienced by potentiators, we began touching on Era II tools that center on one's conscious awareness of the inner workings of healing and transformation.

In this chapter, moving beyond genetics and the body, we will explore a number of epigenetic concepts for using the mind to maximize and integrate Potentiation's meta-genetic mechanism of bioenergy repatterning.

Remember, our individualized, localized mind is not meant to *control* anything with regard to experiencing DNA activation—which is directed by the collective, nonlocal intelligence of the consciousness field.

Tools associated with our personal awareness are to be employed epigenetically in order simply to *manage* the meta-genetic process of becoming whole.

The two foregoing paragraphs go a long way in explaining why Regenetics has proven to be extraordinarily helpful even for people who, because of age or illness, are incapable (mentally or physically) of utilizing any supplemental tools whatsoever.

That said, the Era I and Era II tools outlined herein absolutely can enhance the effectiveness of this work for those able and willing to implement them. As always, when deciding what to do and when to do it, listen to your intuition.

With regard to conscious personal mastery, trust in and surrender to the wisdom and ability of our Higher Self is just as important in mental matters as with physical ones.

Only by opening ourselves to the guidance of the Higher Self, which we access by listening to our heart, can we heal and transform sufficiently to fulfill our true purpose and live with authenticity as spiritual beings on a human journey.

Over the course of the following sections, detailed instructions are given for:

1. Determining your (or another's) Electromagnetic Group and corresponding Schematic;

2. Interpreting and utilizing your Electromagnetic Schematic (Figures 15, 16, and 17) ; and

3. Intentionally promoting your own conscious personal mastery on a daily basis.

Self-potentiators will need to determine their own Electromagnetic Group and matching Schematic. This should be easy after a thoughtful reading of this chapter.

If you still have questions, or wish to connect with others experiencing this work, please consider joining the Regenetics Method Forum by visiting **www.phoenixregenetics.org** or **www.potentiation.net**. Again, a special subgroup has been created for self-potentiators.

Potentiation recipients should be made aware of their Electromagnetic Group and Schematic by whoever facilitated their session.

Potentiation recipients also should be given a hard or electronic copy of this chapter, which readers have permission to photocopy for private, noncommercial use. Alternatively, this chapter can be downloaded at either of the above websites.

Individuals having received Potentiation from someone else likewise are invited to join the Regenetics Method Forum—where additional information on Potentiation and the rest of the four-part Regenetics Method is provided.

An Easy Way to Muscle Test

The main reason to use muscle testing, or kinesiology, in the context of Potentiation is to determine your own or another's Electromagnetic Group and corresponding Schematic.

This section applies mainly to self-potentiators and facilitators. If you have been potentiated by someone else, feel free to skim down to Determining a Person's Electromagnetic Group—where the central concept of bioenergy families is introduced.

The basic methodology behind most approaches to kinesiology, which is a veritable science employed by thousands of healthcare practitioners worldwide, is outlined below.

We will learn the O-ring Muscle Test (Figure 14). But if you are competent in and prefer another kinesiological technique, by all means use it!

Typically in muscle testing, you start by asking—either vocally or mentally—a "yes or no" question of yourself or another person.

Then you test yourself or another to produce an identifiable muscular response to the question. A strong response indicates a *yes*; a weak response signals a *no*.

With the O-ring technique shown in Figure 14, one hand makes a ring with the thumb and forefinger. The other hand tries to break the ring by inserting into it the thumb and forefinger and expanding them.

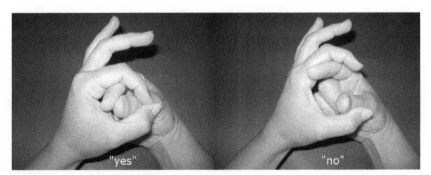

Figure 14: O-ring Muscle Test

The above images show a simple kinesiological technique for self-testing and surrogate self-testing.

When the thumb and forefinger of the first hand separate owing to the pressure of the second hand, this means the ring is weak and the answer to the question is no.

When the thumb and forefinger remain strong and together despite the pressure, the answer is yes.

Testing for yourself is called *self-testing*. Testing through yourself on behalf of someone else, which has been demonstrated to be just as effective as self-testing, is *surrogate self-testing*.

Although healthcare providers may choose otherwise, most readers of this book sharing Potentiation with family or friends are advised to use surrogate self-testing in order to avoid potential legal hassles.

In other words, unless you are a licensed and insured healthcare professional, *you should test through yourself and refrain from touching recipients during sessions*.

After performing your own or another's Potentiation, you can use the O-ring Muscle Test when asking a question such as, "Was this Potentiation performed correctly enough to produce significant positive results?"

If you have done your homework as a facilitator, the answer to this particular question almost certainly will be yes. A yes does not assure, however, that benefits automatically will be forthcoming.

As explained in Chapter Eight, the recipient plays a critical role in accepting and actualizing his or her own healing through the Regenetics Method.

Obviously, it is a good idea to practice muscle testing with questions to which you already know the answer until you feel that your testing is accurate most of the time.

No kinesiological technique is infallible, so learn to live with an occasional wrong answer. Practicing nonattachment to the outcomes of your tests increases their accuracy dramatically.

Muscle testing is a helpful tool for gathering information on its own. But it is most effective when used not in isolation, but in association with other methods of assessment—including instinct, observation, and common sense.

In the next section, we will walk through how to employ kinesiology in conjunction with other data points to identify your own or another's Electromagnetic Group.

Determining a Person's Electromagnetic Group

During the development of Potentiation, while Leigh and I were field testing as described in Chapter Three, we made an extraordinary discovery that literally changed our view of human nature.

Most writers on metaphysical subjects labor under the assumption that because human biology appears roughly the same across our species, human bioenergy must be uniform as well. But nothing could be more untrue.

On the basis of extensive kinesiological and experiential evidence, Leigh and I identified twelve different bioenergy families that together compose the larger human family.

These twelve different subgroups are not distinguished by race or ethnicity, but solely by their underlying ener-genetic blueprint.

In order to emphasize that we were discussing groups differentiated only by energy, at the time we decided to name these twelve families Electromagnetic Groups.

Never mind that the energy in question technically is not electromagnetic, but torsion energy—which I also have called bioenergy and consciousness (see Chapter Three).

Energetically, the twelve bioenergy families correspond to the twelve pairs of cranial nerves, with each group contributing to humanity's "collective Mind."

These twelve groups also align with the twelve acupuncture meridians, the twelve months, the twelve signs of the zodiac, and even Earth's twelve tectonic plates.

What unites these strikingly unique energetic families is their shared "operating system": DNA and, underwriting genetics, the meta-genetic consciousness field that subsumes all twelve groups.

Significantly, *each Electromagnetic Group possesses a specific arrangement in its bioenergy blueprint that applies to all members* (Figures 15, 16, and 17).

This is a truly consequential revelation because in the context of DNA activation, it renders individual diagnosis superfluous. One has only to ascertain the correct Electromagnetic Group and learn to read the corresponding Schematic in light of one's personal experience—and much is made clear on its own.

While potentiating thousands of individuals from different backgrounds and countries over the years, Leigh and I also discovered that—for reasons that lie beyond the scope of this book—Figures 15, 16 and 17 apply to the overwhelming majority of people attracted to the Regenetics Method.

The rationale for including Schematics for only three of the twelve Electromagnetic Groups is based on the fact that *there is virtually a one hundred percent chance that if you find yourself reading these words, one of the three Schematics in the next section applies to you.*

Additionally, the need to simplify and streamline this material for readers new to the field of DNA activation also has been taken into account.

Now, if you recently have performed your own or another's Potentiation, it is time to use the O-ring muscle test described above to determine the correct Electromagnetic Group.

The most straightforward way to do this is to muscle test, either for yourself or the person you have potentiated, the following three questions in order:

1. Is the recipient of this Potentiation a member of Electromagnetic Group 1?

2. Is the recipient of this Potentiation a member of Electromagnetic Group 2?

3. Is the recipient of this Potentiation a member of Electromagnetic Group 3?

Often, you will receive a clear yes to one of these three questions and clear no's to the other two. But sometimes, you will get two or more yeses, or even three no's—which means you should retest all three questions, in reverse order, to see if a definitive response emerges.

Having established your Electromagnetic Group, putting in some time to learn to interpret and work with your Schematic is the next step (see below).

If you have determined the Electromagnetic Group of someone you have potentiated, make sure that, whenever appropriate, you provide the person with this information along with this chapter at your earliest convenience.

On very rare occasions, muscle testing can fail to reveal the right bioenergy family. This possibility, however slight, highlights the importance of employing additional methods of assessment in order to ensure the accuracy of your findings.

Here, by far the most important thing you need to know is that Electromagnetic Groups are always matrilineal. In other words, *children automatically belong to the same Electromagnetic Group as their biological mothers.*

Be aware that *the same does not apply to fathers and their children*, who can be—and often are—members of different Electromagnetic Groups. Similarly, *the rule of matrilineality has no bearing on adopted children*.

If you ever have doubts about someone's bioenergy family after testing, you can repeat your questions for the person's biological mother (regardless of whether she is still living). Alternatively or additionally, you can test for the Electromagnetic Group of a mother's child.

By comparing the results of more than one test while looking for patterns of similarity, usually it is easy enough to identify the correct Electromagnetic Group of the entire maternal line.

Another form of assessment that can help you sort through any fuzziness in your testing is to listen to your gut instinct. Especially when you have no preconceptions relative to the Electromagnetic Group, in many instances your intuition will be right on the money.

Finally, as we explore the similarities and contrasts characterizing the three Schematics below, you will acquire even more fine-tuned assessment tools owing to the fact that different Electromagnetic Groups exhibit marked predispositions to particular kinds of illness.

Reading Your Electromagnetic Schematic

Once you know your Electromagnetic Group, understanding your underlying bioenergy blueprint is an essential tool for maximizing conscious personal mastery through Potentiation and the Regenetics Method.

Without this information, many important body-mind-spirit shifts that can occur as a result of this work might make little sense, be downplayed, or even go unnoticed.

In the case of individuals you have potentiated who are unable to familiarize themselves with their Electromagnetic Schematic, such as young children, be sure to keep this information in mind on their behalf while observing any changes that take place in them during the 42-week Potentiation cycle.

Your Electromagnetic Schematic matches your Electromagnetic Group in number, so start by identifying the blueprint (Figure 15, 16, or 17) that corresponds numerically to your bioenergy family.

Initially, you are encouraged to focus on learning to read your own Schematic. But over time, especially if you begin potentiating family and friends, it can be interesting, useful and even necessary to develop some skill in interpreting all three Schematics.

Since I belong to Electromagnetic Group 1 and know it like the back of my hand, I will use Figure 15 in teaching you the basics of reading any Electromagnetic Schematic.

The structure of the Schematic in Figure 15 is that of a simple grid chart, with a horizontal and vertical axis showing various points of intersection between the bioenergy centers and the elements connected to them.

The horizontal axis contains information relative to eight different categories ("Genetics," etc.) listed across the top that are discussed momentarily. Blanks (—) indicate no applicable information for a given category.

The vertical axis indicates the number and position of the bioenergy centers, starting with the Master (Source) Field and descending through the other centers from the ninth to the first.

The Master Field can be thought of as the collective ocean of the consciousness field, or the Consciousness of Love made up of pure torsion energy in the form of love and related feelings of creativity, empathy, gratitude, and the like (Figures 1, 4, and 9).

From the universal creative consciousness that is love, humans' own nine bioenergy fields emerge like sound waves, before being translated by potential DNA into equivalent light frequencies that manifest as the nine chakras (Figures 3 and 10a).

In the Regenetics model, the interface between a sonic bioenergy field and a light-based chakra is called a *bioenergy center*. A bioenergy center, composed of a field and its chakra, constitutes an ener-genetic *ecosystem*— the nature of which is defined in the next section.

As explained in Part I, the bioenergy fields control our various physiological functions. The chakras are merely torsion processors that distribute bioenergy, as instructed by the fields, to the appropriate organ systems and glands.

The numbers in the left-hand column (vertical axis) refer to both the bioenergy fields and the more well-known chakras, with 1 indicating the first field and root chakra, 2 indicating the second field and sex chakra, 3 indicating the third field and solar plexus chakra, and so on (Figures 3 and 10a).

Electromagnetic Schematic 1

Bioenergy Centers	Genetics	Gland(s)	Organ(s)	Toxin(s)	Microorganism(s)	Emotions	Miasms	Conditions
Master (Source) Field	-	-	-	-	-	-	-	-
9	DNA	Salivary	Nervous, Gall Bladder, Liver	-	-	Creativity, Empathy, Gratitude, Faith, Inspiration, Joy, Love, Trust, Unity	-	Anemia, Cirrhosis, Gallstones, Jaundice, Multiple Sclerosis (MS), Neurosis, Parkinson's Disease
8	Mitochondrial DNA	Hypothalamus, Lacrimal	Sinus/Limbic, Olfactory	-	-	Atonement, Deprivation, Resentment, Sense of Being Trapped, Unforgivingness / Despair, Grief, Guilt, Melancholy, Yearning	-	Depression, Sinusitis, Seasonal Affective Disorder (SAD)
7	Cytosine, RNA	Parathyroid	Bladder/Kidney/Urinary, Musculoskeletal	Antibiotics, Fluoride, Root Canal Toxins, Vaccines	Intestinal Flora (includes Candida)	Apathy, Despair, Disappointment, Discouragement, Disillusionment, Frustration, Helplessness, Hopelessness, Lack of Faith, Stress	Vaccination, Will	ADD/ADHD, AIDS, Arthritis, Autism, Candidiasis, CFIDS (CFS), Fibromyalgia, Incontinence, Kidney Stones, Leukemia, Lupus, Multiple Chemical Sensitivity (MCS), Osteoporosis, Scoliosis
6	Adenine	Sweat	Auditory, Dermal, Mucous Membrane, Respiratory	Airborne Allergens, Bacterial Toxins, Heavy Metals, Metallic Dental Materials	Bacteria, Mycobacteria, Mycoplasmas, Spiroplasmas	-	Psora, Tuberculosis	Acne, Asthma, Bronchitis, Dandruff, Eczema, Environmental Allergies, Hearing Loss, Inner Ear Infection, Psoriasis, Tinnitus, Vertigo
5	Thymine	Pituitary	Circulatory, Endocrine	Chlorinated Hydrocarbons, Hydrocarbons	Homeostatic Soil Organisms (HSOs)	Ambition, Desire, Greed, Lust	Syphilitic, Thuja Focal	Addiction, Arteriosclerosis, Bipolar Disorder, Co-dependency, Counter-dependency, Endocrine Imbalances, Heart Disease, Hemophilia, Hot Flashes, Hypertension
4	Guanine	Pineal	Brain, Central Nervous, Optical	Artificial Sweeteners, Food Additives, Food Colorings, Genetically Modified Organisms (GMOs), Processed Sugars	Yeasts	Abandonment, Arrogance, Betrayal, Confusion, Pride, Rejection	Gonorrhea, Psychotic	Alzheimer's Disease, Cataracts, Diabetes, Dyslexia, Encephalitis, Food Allergies, Glaucoma, Hypoglycemia, Insomnia, Migraine, Obsessive-compulsive Disorder (OCD), Psychosis
3	Uracil	Adrenal, Thymus	Immune	Chemicals, Mechanized Fields, Microwaves, Pharmaceuticals, Radioactive Metals, Recreational Drugs, Smoke, Solvents	Viruses	Anxiety, Fear, Lack of Trust, Panic, Terror, Worry	Cancer, Radiation	Cancer, Hepatitis, Herpes, Influenza, Lowered Immunity, Paranoia
2 (Fragmentary Body)	-	Thyroid	Oral, Reproductive	Bacterial Toxins, Parasitic Toxins	Dental Bacteria, Parasites	Embarrassment, Envy, Jealousy, Shame	-	Dental Decay, Halitosis, Impotence, Parasitic Infection, Infertility, Periodontal Disease, Reproductive System Illness, Speech Impediment, Sterility
1	-	Parotid	Digestive, Pancreatic	Mycotoxins (from fungal overgrowth)	Fungi	Anger, Disgust, Hatred, Rage	-	Acid Reflux, Colitis, Crohn's Disease, Fungal Infection, Hemorrhoids, Irritable Bowel Syndrome (IBS), Leaky Gut, Pancreatitis

Figure 15: Electromagnetic Schematic 1

This chart provides useful information, spanning the body-mind-spirit spectrum, for understanding the bioenergy blueprint of the first Electromagnetic Group identified during the development of Potentiation as a series of ecosystems.

239

Electromagnetic Schematic 2

Bioenergy Centers	Genetics	Gland(s)	Organ(s)	Categories Toxin(s)	Micro-organism(s)	Emotions	Miasms	Conditions
Master (Source) Field	-	-	-	-	-	Creativity, Empathy, Gratitude, Faith, Inspiration, Joy, Love, Trust, Unity	-	-
9	DNA	Salivary	Nervous, Bladder/ Kidney/ Urinary	-	-	Atonement, Deprivation, Resentment, Sense of Being Trapped, Unforgivingness	-	Incontinence, Kidney Stones, Multiple Sclerosis (MS), Neurosis, Parkinson's Disease
8	Mitochondrial DNA	Hypothalamus, Lacrimal	Sinus/Limbic, Olfactory	-	-	Despair, Grief, Guilt, Melancholy, Yearning	-	Depression, Sinusitis, Seasonal Affective Disorder (SAD)
7	RNA Thymine	Parathyroid	Digestive, Musculoskeletal, Pancreatic	Airborne Allergens, Bacterial Toxins, Fluoride, Heavy Metals, Metallic Dental Materials, Root Canal Toxins	Bacteria, Mycobacteria, Mycoplasmas, Spiroplasmas	Abandonment, Betrayal, Confusion, Rejection	Psora, Tuberculosis	Acid Reflux, Arthritis, Asthma, Colitis, Crohn's Disease, Environmental Allergies, Hemorrhoids, Irritable Bowel Syndrome (IBS), Leaky Gut, Osteoporosis, Pancreatitis, Scoliosis
6	Cytosine	Pituitary, Thymus	Immune	Artificial Sweeteners, Food Additives, Food Colorings, Genetically Modified Organisms (GMOs), Processed Sugars	Intestinal Flora (includes Candida)	Anxiety, Fear, Lack of Trust, Panic, Terror, Worry	Gonorrhea, Psychotic	Diabetes, Food Allergies, Hypoglycemia, Lowered Immunity, Obsessive-compulsive Disorder (OCD), Paranoia, Psychosis
5	Adenine	Sweat	Auditory, Dermal, Mucous Membrane, Respiratory	Chemicals, Mechanized Fields, Microwaves, Mycotoxins (from fungal overgrowth), Pharmaceuticals, Radioactive Metals, Recreational Drugs, Smoke, Solvents	Fungi	-	Cancer, Radiation	Acne, Asthma, Bronchitis, Cancer, Dandruff, Eczema, Hearing Loss, Inner Ear Infection, Psoriasis, Tinnitus, Vertigo
4	Guanine	Adrenal	Circulatory, Endocrine	Chlorinated Hydrocarbons, Hydrocarbons	Viruses	Ambition, Desire, Greed, Lust	Syphilitic, Thuja Focal	Addiction, Arteriosclerosis, Bipolar Disorder, Co-dependency, Counter-dependency, Endocrine Imbalances, Heart Disease, Hemophilia, Hepatitis, Herpes, Hot Flashes, Hypertension, Influenza
3	Uracil	Pineal	Brain, Central Nervous, Optical	Antibiotics, Vaccines	Homeostatic Soil Organisms (HSOs)	Anger, Disgust, Hatred, Rage	Vaccination, Will	ADD/ADHD, Alzheimer's Disease, Cataracts, Dyslexia, Encephalitis, Glaucoma, Insomnia, Migraine, Obsessive-compulsive Disorder (OCD)
2 (Fragmentary Body)	-	Thyroid	Oral, Reproductive	Bacterial Toxins, Parasitic Toxins	Dental Bacteria, Parasites	Embarrassment, Envy, Jealousy, Shame	-	Dental Decay, Halitosis, Impotence, Parasitic Infection, Infertility, Periodontal Disease, Reproductive System Illness, Speech Impediment, Sterility
1	-	Parathyroid	Gall Bladder, Liver	-	Yeasts	Disappointment, Discouragement, Disillusionment, Frustration, Helplessness, Hopelessness	-	Anemia, Cirrhosis, Gallstones, Jaundice

Figure 16: Electromagnetic Schematic 2

This chart provides useful information, spanning the body-mind-spirit spectrum, for understanding the bioenergy blueprint of the second Electromagnetic Group identified during the development of Potentiation as a series of ecosystems.

Electromagnetic Schematic 3

Bioenergy Centers	Genetics	Gland(s)	Organ(s)	Toxin(s)	Micro-organism(s)	Emotions	Miasms	Conditions
Master (Source) Field	-	-	-	-	-	Creativity, Empathy, Gratitude, Faith, Inspiration, Joy, Love, Trust, Unity	-	-
9	DNA	Parotid, Salivary	Nervous, Digestive, Pancreatic	-	-	Atonement, Deprivation, Resentment, Sense of Being Trapped, Unforgivingness	-	Acid Reflux, Colitis, Crohn's Disease, Hemorrhoids, Irritable Bowel Syndrome (IBS), Leaky Gut, Multiple Sclerosis (MS), Neurosis, Pancreatitis, Parkinson's Disease
8	Mitochondrial DNA	Hypothalamus, Lacrimal	Sinus/Limbic, Olfactory	-	-	Despair, Grief, Guilt, Melancholy, Yearning	-	Depression, Sinusitis, Seasonal Affective Disorder (SAD)
7	RNA Thymine	Adrenal	Brain, Central Nervous, Musculoskeletal, Optical	Fluoride, Root Canal Toxins	Homeostatic Soil Organisms (HSOs)	Ambition, Desire, Greed, Lust	Syphilitic, Thuja Focal	Addiction, Alzheimer's Disease, Bipolar Disorder, Cataracts, Co-dependency, Counter-dependency, Diabetes, Dyslexia, Encephalitis, Glaucoma, Hypoglycemia, Insomnia, Migraine, Obsessive-compulsive Disorder (OCD)
6	Cytosine	Pineal	Bladder/Kidney/Urinary	Antibiotics, Vaccines	Intestinal Flora (includes Candida)	Apathy, Despair, Disappointment, Discouragement, Disillusionment, Frustration, Helplessness, Hopelessness, Lack of Faith, Stress	Vaccination, Will	ADD/ADHD, Arthritis, Incontinence, Kidney Stones, Osteoporosis, Scoliosis
5	Guanine	Parathyroid	Gall Bladder, Liver	Artificial Sweeteners, Food Additives, Food Colorings, Genetically Modified Organisms (GMOs), Mycotoxins (from fungal overgrowth), Processed Sugars	Fungi	Abandonment, Arrogance, Betrayal, Confusion, Pride, Rejection	Gonorrhea, Psychotic	Anemia, Cirrhosis, Diabetes, Hypoglycemia, Food Allergies, Gallstones, Jaundice, Psychosis
4	Adenine	Sweat	Auditory, Dermal, Mucous Membrane, Respiratory	Airborne Allergens, Bacterial Toxins, Heavy Metals, Metallic Dental Materials	Bacteria, Mycobacteria, Mycoplasmas, Spiroplasmas	-	Psora, Tuberculosis	Acne, Asthma, Bronchitis, Dandruff, Eczema, Environmental Allergies, Hearing Loss, Inner Ear Infection, Psoriasis, Tinnitus, Vertigo
3	Uracil	Thymus	Immune	Chemicals, Mechanized Fields, Microwaves, Pharmaceuticals, Radioactive Metals, Recreational Drugs, Smoke, Solvents	Viruses	Anxiety, Fear, Lack of Trust, Panic, Terror, Worry	Cancer, Radiation	Cancer, Hepatitis, Herpes, Influenza, Lowered Immunity, Paranoia
2 (Fragmentary Body)	-	Thyroid	Oral, Reproductive	Bacterial Toxins, Parasitic Toxins	Dental Bacteria, Parasites	Embarrassment, Envy, Jealousy, Shame	-	Dental Decay, Halitosis, Impotence, Parasitic Infection, Infertility, Periodontal Disease, Reproductive System Illness, Speech Impediment, Sterility
1	-	Pituitary	Circulatory, Endocrine	Chlorinated Hydrocarbons, Hydrocarbons	Yeasts	Anger, Disgust, Hatred, Rage	-	Arteriosclerosis, Endocrine Imbalances, Heart Disease, Hemophilia, Hot Flashes, Hypertension

Figure 17: Electromagnetic Schematic 3

This chart provides useful information, spanning the body-mind-spirit spectrum, for understanding the bioenergy blueprint of the third Electromagnetic Group identified during the development of Potentiation as a series of ecosystems.

Figure 15 highlights a fascinating point about the chakras that has been obscured much like the actual number of chakras possessed by unpotentiated humans—which is exactly nine, not seven, twelve, or any other of the numbers bandied about—namely, that:

Just because a chakra is located in a particular part of the body does not mean necessarily that the chakra in question is involved directly in regulating the activity of that part of the body.

As an example, it is clear from Figure 15 that in the case of Electromagnetic Group 1, the fourth (or heart) chakra does not have anything specifically to do with the actual heart organ.

Rather, in Electromagnetic Group 1 the fourth chakra is associated with the brain, central nervous system, and eyes. The circulatory system, which includes the heart, is paired with the fifth (or throat) chakra.

Take a moment to locate the circulatory system in Figures 16 and 17. For Electromagnetic Group 2, note that the heart indeed is paired with the fourth chakra. But in Electromagnetic Group 3, the circulatory system is associated with the first chakra.

Now, choose any gland and determine which bioenergy field and chakra connect with it in all three Schematics. Mostly likely, as with organ systems, you will find major differences in the location of glands.

Finally, have a look at the emotions associated with the three Schematics. Note how the positioning of groups of emotions relative to the bioenergy centers can change dramatically from one Electromagnetic Group to another.

Are you starting to grasp how the Electromagnetic Groups are quite distinct, bioenergetically speaking?

Obviously, and contrary to popular belief, *human beings are not all the same.*

In only three instances are all Electromagnetic Groups identical: the Master Field, the eighth field/chakra, and the second field/chakra (the Fragmentary Body).

In these three aspects of the bioenergy blueprint, information relative to the eight horizontal categories is always consistent. Otherwise, when it comes to real distinctions among Electromagnetic Groups, expect many!

Bioenergy Centers as Ecosystems (Revisited)

In Part I, the concept of ecosystems as applying to the bioenergy centers was introduced. Here, we revisit this key idea, paying close attention to how to read the bioenergy centers as ecosystems.

Recall that an ecosystem is a biological community of interdependent organisms and their habitat. As shown in Figure 15, in physical terms the bioenergy centers regulate the activity of particular microorganisms in relation to specific "habitats" in the form of organs, glands, and related elements.

By locating the categories associated with the seventh field and chakra in Electromagnetic Group 1, you can begin to see how this intersection constitutes a unique ener-genetic ecosystem comprising RNA, the parathyroid gland, the urinary and musculoskeletal systems, intestinal flora, and toxins ranging from antibiotics to vaccines.

In addition to these physical elements linked to the seventh bioenergy center, Figure 15 also provides information relative to this ecosystem's:

1. Bioenergy (the vaccination and will miasms from homeopathy);

2. Emotions (apathy, disappointment, discouragement, etc.); and

3. Potential health conditions ranging from AIDS to incontinence.

Before we examine some of the ramifications of this especially intriguing ecosystem, spend a minute or two perusing the elements connected to the seventh bioenergy center in Figures 16 and 17.

Observe the many major distinctions. The Electromagnetic Groups do not simply represent different kinds of apples. We are talking apples, oranges and grapefruits here!

The same bioenergy centers in different Electromagnetic Groups can contain quite distinct ecosystems with a direct bearing on the physical, mental, emotional and spiritual health of group members.

The foregoing statement helps explain why some people are made ill by certain toxins, for instance, while others appear to tolerate the same toxins without any problem.

Returning to the example of the seventh bioenergy center in Figure 15, this ecosystem leaves little room for argument as to why members of Electromagnetic Group 1 tend to suffer genetic damage from vaccines resulting in a wide variety of autoimmune conditions.

Copious research detailed by Leonard Horowitz reveals that vaccines are capable of hijacking the genetic transcription process involving RNA and using it to rewrite the DNA code with pathogenic sequences from diseased animal tissue (Figure 8).

When this occurs, DNA, which is designed as a "repair enzyme" for the body, becomes a "disrepair enzyme"—instructing the body not to heal itself, but to damage its own systems in a manner similar to the way the altered code of a computer virus can lead to degeneration of computer systems.

What Horowitz fails to realize, however, is that for this haywire situation to arise in an individual, he or she must have an ener-genetic susceptibility to being rescripted genetically by vaccines.

Homeopathy is to thank for identifying just such susceptibilities to particular types of induced illness. *Miasms, a term coined by Samuel Hahnemann, describe genetic predispositions to particular diseases that are energetic in nature.*

Below, we will have a closer look at the different miasms. But for present purposes, it is simply necessary to grasp that *with certain exceptions, for an illness to manifest, the miasm that allows the illness to come into being must be open and positioned in the correct ecosystem.*

In the seventh bioenergy center of Figure 15, the vaccination miasm is present. And all that is required to open it is … a vaccination! This can be a vaccine that one has received personally, or one that has been inherited.

Having said this, receiving or inheriting a vaccination does not *automatically* open the corresponding miasm. But if this miasm does activate, you can be certain it was opened by a vaccine.

To be perfectly clear, miasms have nothing to do with genetic fatalism, but simply indicate possible predictable responses on the part of the body-mind-spirit to specific traumas, toxins, and pathogens.

When a member of Electromagnetic Group 1 is vaccinated, the disease-producing potential of the vaccination miasm can be switched on. But more than just opening this miasm is required to cause serious genetic damage.

In Electromagnetic Group 1, the fact that the vaccination miasm is located in the seventh bioenergy center is of critical importance because RNA is also in this ecosystem.

This situation allows reverse transcription to occur from the seventh to the eighth field, which regulates mitochondrial DNA and grants access to the other parts of DNA governed by the ninth field, thereby rewriting the genetic code in a potentially devastating manner (Figure 8).

Genetic alteration from vaccines on this scale cannot occur in members of the other two Electromagnetic Groups because, as shown in Figures 16 and 17, neither of these bioenergy families pairs the vaccination miasm with RNA in the seventh bioenergy center.

While harmful toxins such as mercury and squalene contained in vaccines certainly are bad for everyone, members of Electromagnetic Groups 2 and 3 are incapable of the types of vaccine-induced autoimmune illnesses regularly observed in members of Electromagnetic Group 1.

Instead, members of Electromagnetic Group 2 typically are more robust while being prone to acute situations appearing seemingly out of nowhere, such as heart attack, while individuals belonging to Electromagnetic Group 3 can suffer from environmental and nutritional sensitivities without any clear signs of autoimmunity.

But in the case of Electromagnetic Group 1, the seventh ecosystem with an open vaccination miasm can be a recipe for interminable trouble.

The result is often one or more debilitating autoimmune conditions combined with dysbiosis of intestinal flora (Candidiasis) as well as kidney, bladder or musculoskeletal problems, topped off by an array of self-defeating negative emotional states.

Learning to interpret your own Schematic as a series of ecosystems can clarify many mysteries having to do with your health and wellness, or lack thereof.

Also, as you acquire more experience in reading all three Schematics, grasping differences in disease patterns and other distinctions related to the positioning of ecosystems in the bioenergy blueprint can assist you tremendously in determining another person's Electromagnetic Group.

Additional Notes on the Eight Categories

The eight categories forming the horizontal axis of all Electromagnetic Schematics were handpicked by Leigh and myself out of dozens of categories that emerged during our intensive field testing and mapping of the human bioenergy blueprint.

The categories included in this book represent the most tangible and verifiable elements of the various ecosystems—i.e., the ones you yourself already may know or intuit or, alternatively, can feel being activated with healing energy as described below under Time Frame for Potentiation.

Genetics refers to which aspects of biochemistry are present in and governed by particular bioenergy centers.

Most likely, you will not be able to sense genetic positioning at the level of ecosystems, in contrast to more palpable aspects of physiology such as glands and organs.

Nevertheless, as demonstrated above in our discussion of miasms and the seventh bioenergy center, this information can be illuminating indeed.

Glands are organs that secrete powerful substances, called hormones, with a wide range of critical functions in the body. Some people suffer from too much glandular activity, while others experience too little.

Since the presence or absence of specific hormones produced by glands biochemically impacts everything from sex drive to hot flashes to metabolism and energy levels, potentiators often are aware when their hormonal levels change.

In addition, individuals undergoing this work frequently smell old, rancid hormones—which are about as healthy for the tissues storing them as battery acid—being expelled through their urine, stools, and even sweat.

By identifying which bioenergy center you are in (see below) when experiencing any phenomenon possibly related to glands and their hormones, often you can pinpoint which glandular system is speeding up, slowing down, or detoxifying.

Organs are systems in an organism designed to carry out specific vital tasks. As examples, the reproductive system (male or female) and oral system are positioned in the second bioenergy center of all Electromagnetic Groups.

Keep in mind that organs are, in fact, *systems* composed of a number of interrelated body parts and functions. To illustrate this point, the oral system includes the mouth opening, teeth, tongue, gums, oral mucosa, and even vocal cords.

Since it is impractical to list all the elements that make up the many different organ systems, use common sense when determining whether a particular aspect of your physiology about which you may have questions belongs to one system or another.

At first glance, for instance, the jawbone might seem to be part of the oral system. But since it is a bone, and operates in tandem with other bones, it technically forms part of the musculoskeletal system.

If you are unable to tell to which organ system a body part belongs, the answer often becomes apparent the instant torsion energy moves into a particular ecosystem during Potentiation.

Returning to Figure 15, if you are Electromagnetic Group 1 and your tonsils suddenly swell up and turn bright red when you hit the third bioenergy center, you have just been given an indication that the tonsils are part of the immune system, which belongs to the third ecosystem.

The fact that your tonsils—in our hypothetical scenario—respond to bioenergy tracking into their ecosystem probably signifies detoxification.

As Figure 15 indicates for the third bioenergy center, the most likely pathogens being released in our theoretical detox are viruses, while toxins being expelled by the immune system can include chemicals, radioactive metals, recreational drugs, smoke, and solvents.

Your immune system is being stimulated to remove pathogenic and toxic elements first from itself and its ecosystem, then from other body parts and ecosystems that require housecleaning.

Toxins are poisonous substances (or less frequently, harmful energies such as microwaves and radiation) that usually are allowed to accumulate to dangerous levels in the body only as a direct result of the opening of a miasm linked to the same ecosystem.

The exception to this general definition that applies to artificial, externally introduced substances is organic toxins (parasitic toxins, mycotoxins, etc.) occurring due to internal microorganism overgrowth.

Once again using the example of the seventh bioenergy center in Electromagnetic Group 1, the opening of the vaccination miasm can "open the door" to the non-release and cellular accumulation of antibiotics, fluoride, thioethers from root canals, and the toxic cocktail mix stirred into vaccines.

As with organ systems, it is impractical to list every potential toxin that might apply to an ecosystem. On this subject, note that there are often categories within categories—as is the case with heavy metals and hydrocarbons—which subsume an array of more specific toxins.

Microorganisms indicate either 1) harmful pathogens along the lines of viruses, parasites, and fungi; or 2) microscopic organisms that normally exist in harmony with the body, such as intestinal flora and homeostatic soil organisms (HSOs).

Similar to the way in which toxins can build up when given the energenetic green light, it is possible for both pathogens and beneficial microorganisms to proliferate when their corresponding miasm has been opened. This is precisely what occurs in the case of Candida overgrowth.

Bacteria and yeasts are broad categories that take into account both purely pathogenetic and naturally helpful microorganisms. Like pathogens, normally beneficial microorganisms can multiply and cause disease as a result of a miasm turning on in their ecosystem.

But as demonstrated by the second ecosystem, which regulates parasitic activity in the absence of any miasm, it is not always necessary for a miasm to open for pathogens to spiral out of control.

Emotions are (with the exception of those pure states listed for the Master Field) self-limiting feelings that, like their physiological and energetic counterparts, arrange themselves in familial groups in particular ecosystems.

It is impossible to index all potential emotional permutations in a single Schematic. If you experience an emotion that is not listed verbatim, find the emotion closest to it and add your emotion to the same ecosystem.

For example, happiness is closely related to joy and, thus, belongs in the Master Field. The same could be said for exaltation, ecstasy, and similar blissful feelings.

A blank (—) indicates a lack of any emotion whatsoever in a given ecosystem—which is just as potentially compromising for the health of the body-mind-spirit as harboring negative emotions.

Emotions (including their absence) are extremely powerful energenetic phenomena that resonate so strongly in the bioenergy blueprint that it can be difficult to assign causality in their case.

While it is possible to understand specific emotions as arising from corresponding physiological dysfunctions that belong to the same ecosystem, it often makes just as much sense to view physical problems as stemming from harmful emotional attitudes.

If you have a health condition listed in a particular bioenergy center, you might benefit from doing some soul searching as to the related emotions. You are likely to discover that some or all of these emotions have contributed to your situation.

Making a commitment to overhaul any negative or defeatist attitudes you identify in yourself constitutes an important stride in conscious personal mastery as you learn to "follow your bliss," to quote Joseph Campbell, while coming to love yourself and others more fully.

The result is often a more consistent, transformative experience of positive, life-affirming emotions—specifically, the ones linked to the Master Field which are integral to the Creator in all of us—combined with a marked increase in your overall wellbeing.

The core idea here—that positive emotions are essential to good health—is substantiated scientifically by the aforementioned research performed by Glen Rein on the transformational effect of such emotions on DNA.

The more time you spend feeling the energy of universal creative consciousness and unconditional love represented by the Master Field, the more you can get out of your head (ego) and into your heart (spirit).

Connecting through our heart with our Higher Self allows us to go beyond using the power of positive thinking in managing our lives epigenetically—and begin experimenting as co-creators with the *power of positive feeling* to master our experience of reality on a far more conscious, meta-genetic level (Figure 6).

The process of mastery I have just described is promoted quite naturally by Potentiation and the Regenetics Method for those willing to surrender their emotional limitations during the profound metamorphosis from victim to unity consciousness.

Miasms were introduced above as ener-genetic predispositions to specific patterns of illness related to the positioning of ecosystems in particular Electromagnetic Groups.

A quick review of Figures 15, 16 and 17 yields three interrelated observations concerning the ten major miasms acknowledged by most contemporary homeopaths:

1. Miasms always come in pairs within ecosystems;

2. Miasmic pairs are always the same across all Electromagnetic Groups; and

3. Miasmic pairs only occur in bioenergy centers 3-7, which means the first, second, eighth and ninth ecosystems lack miasms.

Without exception, the following five miasmic pairs are "tied at the hip" in whatever ecosystem of any Electromagnetic Group they occupy:

vaccination and will

psora and tuberculosis

syphilitic and thuja focal

gonorrhea and psychotic

cancer and radiation

Years of studying these dyads in the context of Regenetics has revealed that *miasmic pairs are complementary—with the first miasm inducing mainly physical disease, and the second miasm playing the lead role in engendering mental or emotional illness.*

The vaccination miasm, when open, might lead to any number of autoimmune conditions—whereas the corresponding will miasm can encourage sustained emotions of helplessness and hopelessness leading to a perpetual state of despair.

This complementary structure repeats as an open psora miasm can result in palpable skin and mucous membrane problems, while the tuberculosis miasm often produces conditions some believe to be mentally or emotionally induced (or even created), such as asthma.

An open syphilitic miasm typically is involved in heart or endocrine problems. Its counterpart, the thuja focal miasm, often is linked to emotional imbalances running the gamut from co-dependency and counter-dependency to addiction and bipolar disorder.

When active, the gonorrhea miasm can lead to eye disease, brain and central nervous system dysfunction, food allergies, and difficulty processing sugar possibly resulting in diabetes. The paired psychotic miasm usually is implicated in severe mental illness such as psychosis.

Finally, cancer of any kind typically results from an open cancer miasm—while the radiation miasm can produce mental states such as anxiety and emotional conditions characterized by paranoia.

More often than not, when one half of a miasmic pair opens in a given ecosystem, its other half opens as well.

As was the case above with regard to negative emotions and physical disease, causality here is hard to assign. Does the "physical" miasm cause the "mental/emotional" miasm to open, or vice versa?

Whatever the case, the fact that two miasms tend to kick in more or less simultaneously in an ecosystem sheds light on:

1. Why often there is a deep and abiding mental or emotional aspect to most physical disease; and

2. How mental or emotional dysfunction resonates energetically with potential physical problems that can appear as a result.

By observing miasmic pairs in the context of particular ecosystems, the complex interplay between the material and the energetic in creating health and disease becomes patently obvious.

You know when a miasmic pair has opened in a given ecosystem when you can identify with any of the conditions (or related ones) listed below that belong to the same bioenergy center.

Also, be aware that if two miasms open in one ecosystem, the next mostly likely miasmic pair to open and start causing problems will be found in an adjacent ecosystem, either above or below.

With members of Electromagnetic Group 1, for instance, when the vaccination and will miasms become active in the seventh bioenergy center, a common scenario is for the psora and tuberculosis miasms to open subsequently in the sixth center.

This scenario illuminates how people genetically damaged by vaccines enough to exhibit symptoms of autoimmunity often begin accumulating heavy metals, particularly from their dental work.

A toxic overload of mercury and other metals from so-called silver fillings, crowns and bridges used in mainstream dentistry is both a function of the psora miasm and a desperate attempt on the part of the body to stop vaccine pathogens from proliferating systemically.

Precisely such an "unzipping" of miasmic pairs starting with the seventh bioenergy center occurred during my own chronic illness, when kinesiological testing combined with self-assessment revealed that eight out of ten of my miasms—spanning the seventh through fourth ecosystems—where open and wreaking havoc!

Thankfully, over time Potentiation and the Regenetics Method went beyond traditional homeopathy in closing my miasms and healing the vast majority of damage they had caused.

Since the same can be said of a large number of individuals who have experienced this work, keep your chin up when contemplating your miasms and have faith that you are capable of using DNA activation to heal and transform your life.

Conditions comprise possible verified or intuited health problems across the body-mind-spirit continuum that, in the typical manner of ecosystem elements, form familial subgroups within a bioenergy center.

As with a number of categories explored previously, there is simply no way to list all the conditions nuanced ad absurdum by allopathic medicine that potentially relate to a given ecosystem.

Use logic when determining that your extremely rare skin disease with a polysyllabic Latin name (which is basically a rash) probably belongs to the same bioenergy center as the dermal system.

A crucial fact to grasp right off the bat when discussing the conditions indexed in the Electromagnetic Schematics is that these *conditions do not constitute or imply diagnosis.*

In no case is the information provided in Figures 15, 16 or 17 intended to diagnose any medical problem or recommend any medical treatment or course of action.

If you have been diagnosed by a healthcare professional, you can use this information in assessing:

1. Which of your miasms might be open;

2. What other factors—toxins, microorganisms, negative emotions, and so forth—might be contributing to your problem in a particular ecosystem; and

3. Which related glands and organs might be compromised and in need of fortification through proper diet and possibly other means.

If you have not been diagnosed, you still may know that you have an issue in a given area that needs addressing. If so, find the ecosystem that fits your situation and use this integrated perspective on the potential causative factors to your advantage in healing.

A second fact to keep firmly in mind here is that some people—who nevertheless may benefit greatly from Potentiation—do not have any conditions at all.

Just because various conditions are listed for a given ecosystem that may attract your attention does not mean necessarily that you have any of these conditions.

Third and finally, to individuals inclined to view any discussion of health conditions as focusing on the problem versus the solution, I offer that sticking your head in the sand when you know something is wrong does not by itself make anything better.

If you just ignore something that is intended by your Higher Self as a teaching tool for spiritual growth, such as an illness, you can bet that it probably will do anything but disappear.

The real challenge—and the real opportunity for conscious personal mastery—is to acknowledge the problem, understand your own involvement in creating it, and commit to using this information not to blame yourself, but to heal the issue en route to transforming your body-mind-spirit.

Time Frame for Potentiation

Although the Potentiation session very well may reset the recipient's bioenergy blueprint instantaneously in the fluid domain of time-space, a reasonable period of time is required in our comparatively fixed space-time reality for repatterning to play out.

Potentiation initiates a wave pulse of torsion energy, which emanates from the consciousness field (Master Field) and immediately begins to track through the nine levels of the recipient's bioenergy blueprint over a specific gestational Time Frame (Figure 18).

It can be helpful to view the Master Field as the quantum biocomputer ("hardware") ultimately running the show, as the "software" associated with the consciousness field's meta-genetic intelligence keeps the energy on pace and moving in the right directions.

As bioenergy flows down and up through your ecosystems, it removes distortions from, raises the vibratory frequency of and repatterns your bioenergy centers.

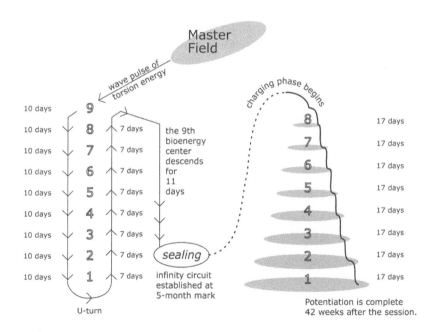

Figure 18: Time Frame for Potentiation

The above diagram outlines the various stages of the 42-week Potentiation cycle, which starts in the ninth bioenergy center and ends just over nine months later in the first bioenergy center.

253

Figure 18 shows that starting in the ninth ecosystem, potentiators spend an average of ten days in each bioenergy center on the way down (9-1), then approximately seven days per center on the way back up (1-8).

This means you will spend a total of seventeen days (10 + 7) in the first ecosystem as the bioenergetic pulse reaches the bottom of the blueprint, makes a U-turn, and begins going back up.

When the energy comes full circle and the ninth ecosystem is reached again, the latter instantly begins to descend, somewhat like a cake falling, through the bioenergy centers. Note that *the second time you hit the ninth ecosystem, you do not spend any time in it.*

As shown in Figure 18, there follows a transitional period of eleven days or so as *the bioenergy centers—which, to reiterate, subsume both the bioenergy fields and corresponding chakras—recalibrate from nine to eight in number.*

During this normally eleven-day period, as the ninth ecosystem drops and fuses with the second ecosystem, a more stable bioenergy blueprint called an *infinity circuit* is created, making possible the roughly four-month "charging phase" of Potentiation.

The infinity circuit—which comes into being as the disruption known as the Fragmentary Body is sealed by the incoming bioenergy of the ninth ecosystem—is in place approximately five months (based on thirty-one days each) after the Potentiation session.

At this point, potentiators become eligible to experience Articulation Bioenergy Enhancement, the second DNA activation in the Regenetics Method, which further energizes what once was the Fragmentary Body, but now represents an important power source for ongoing healing and transformation.

Additional information on Articulation is provided in the next chapter. If you find yourself reading this chapter by itself, you can learn more about Articulation at **www.phoenixregenetics.org** or **www.potentiation.net**.

During the charging phase that follows sealing, also illustrated in Figure 18, each bioenergy center from the eighth down progressively fills with torsion energy like a tiered fountain. You can expect to spend approximately seventeen days in each of the eight ecosystems during charging.

When you add up the time spent in the various stages of Potentiation outlined above, allowing for very small individualized differences, *the total time spent potentiating comes to just under nine and a half months, or roughly forty-two weeks: a human gestation cycle.*

I suggest that this is no coincidence. Indeed, a profound ener-genetic rebirth occurs over the course of Potentiation that is quite beyond anything most people have ever experienced.

Some potentiators have wondered whether it is possible to speed up Potentiation's Time Frame, or whether it might be accelerating on its own due to cosmic or evolutionary factors. Based on years of observation and experience, the simple answer here appears to be *no*.

Others have asked what is so special about the number 8—when the number 9 is sacred to many traditions, including Taoism, where it often signifies completion.

A helpful perspective here is that Potentiation establishes a personal infinity circuit of eight bioenergy centers that link to a ninth center. The Master Field represents the Creator and the ultimate completion that is a return to our Source's consciousness.

Because of the existence of the Fragmentary Body, an unpotentiated blueprint of nine bioenergy centers is imbalanced and connects in an unstable and awkward manner to a tenth center.

Certainly, if recalibrating to eight personal bioenergy centers were somehow unnatural, you would never know it from the enthusiastic response of so many whose health and lives have been reinvented by this work.

Keeping Track of the Time Frame

As bioenergy moves through your ecosystems during Potentiation, you often can feel it—physically, mentally, emotionally, and even spiritually. It is here that your ability to read your Electromagnetic Schematic can come in particularly handy.

A quick glance at the ecosystem the Potentiation energy is in when you experience detoxification, healing or other movement can speak volumes about what actually is happening.

A practical example for a member of Electromagnetic Group 1 might be a so-called healing crisis that kicks off as soon as you enter the seventh ecosystem that uncannily matches the categories for that bioenergy center.

Your bladder, kidneys and bones ache. Your Candida becomes energized. Old symptoms of fibromyalgia or chronic fatigue rear their ugly heads. And a tide of emotions such as disillusionment, frustration and helplessness washes over you.

Despite not feeling so hot, you are amazed that your Schematic and Time Frame are so accurate. And it is extraordinary to *experience* how closely interwoven are the various factors (physical, mental, emotional, etc.) surfacing together connected to your condition(s).

Before Potentiation, such a situation would have been deeply disturbing. But you take comfort in the fact that in all likelihood, based on your Schematic and Time Frame, you simply are purging toxins, pathogens, traumas and negative emotions associated with the seventh ecosystem.

Fortunately, *there is an enormous functional difference between a health crisis and a healing crisis.* Within days, sure enough, you notice that you are releasing a lot of funky stuff through your stools and urine that has no business in a human body.

Within a couple more days, right about the time the Potentiation energy is transitioning into the next ecosystem, you feel cleaner, stronger and happier than you can remember feeling.

Congratulations! You have just weathered a much-needed detoxification and, as a reward, entered a *window* of relative comfort and stability!

Can you see why it is an excellent idea to chart the Time Frame for your Potentiation in your calendar or planner as soon as you start this process?

The easiest way to chart your own Time Frame is to write "9 Down" beside the date of your Potentiation, "8 Down" beside the date that falls ten days later, "7 Down" ten days after that, and so on.

By doing this immediately after your session, you will know in which ecosystem the energy is working—as well as the direction of the energy— at any given moment.

When you reach "1 Down," beside the date that falls ten days later, write "1 Up." Beside the date for seven days further on, write "2 Up," followed by "3 Up" seven days after that, etc.

When the energy arrives at the ninth ecosystem again, write "Sealing Begins" and count eleven days before writing "Sealing Ends: Charging 8 Down."

This latter entry indicates that 1) your ninth and second ecosystems have become one in the second bioenergy center; and 2) the charging phase has begun with the eighth ecosystem.

Count seventeen days and write "Charging 7 Down," seventeen more days and note "Charging 6 Down," and so on. Seventeen days after the date for "Charging 1 Down," you will have completed your Potentiation!

The Fragmentary Body after Sealing

Detailed perspectives on the Fragmentary Body were provided in Parts I and II of this book.

Here, I simply wish to emphasize that after sealing, you no longer have a Fragmentary Body. Nor do you have a ninth bioenergy center (ignoring the Master Field).

In place of the Fragmentary Body and your old ninth bioenergy center, occupying your second bioenergy center from the bottom, is a completely new ecosystem.

For all Electromagnetic Groups, added to the elements listed for the former Fragmentary Body, this new ecosystem now controls DNA as well as the nervous system.

Additionally, this freshly sealed bioenergy center includes the emotions of atonement, deprivation, resentment, sense of being trapped, and unforgivingness.

Beyond these similarities, when it comes to glands, organs and conditions, the exact nature of this new ecosystem can differ significantly from one Electromagnetic Group to another.

When reading your sealed second bioenergy center, simply add all of the elements from your old ninth ecosystem, as listed in your Electromagnetic Schematic, to the elements indexed for the second ecosystem.

Intentionally Become the Creator

To conclude our exploration of Era II tools for promoting conscious personal mastery in tandem with the Regenetics Method, I will share a few thoughts relative to intention before outlining a series of consciousness-expanding exercises you can practice on a daily basis.

It is exceedingly important to respect the power of intention for healing and transformation. This is especially true in the context of Potentiation and the Regenetics Method—which by raising your personal frequency, magnify the power of your intention exponentially.

Intention is a cornerstone of manifestation, a vibration that bridges realities and attracts like energies. Intention links internal experience with external creation and is a driving force behind healing and transformation.

Every intention is an assertion of personal power and potentially an expression of our real reason for being here.

Focusing on what you truly want to achieve in life, on what does or would fulfill you, rather than fixating on problems or obstacles, is the best way to maintain intention for healing and transformation.

Of course, it is appropriate to acknowledge problems and obstacles, as well as the need to transcend them in order to heed your higher calling.

But know that *positive intentional energy moves mountains, whereas continuous focus on negatives makes mountains.*

Greatly exceeding the reach of any purely mental wish, *genuine intention is imbued with the power of positive feeling.* Living in the present as you want to live, emotionally speaking, is so potent an act that it draws into itself the very future you are energizing.

If you do not in some sense *feel* what you long to achieve, you are not putting your heart behind your intention—and your results will diminish accordingly.

The most effective way to create what our heart desires is simply to become the Creator. We *are* the Creator at our core, so why not drop false beliefs about who we are and the resultant emotive distortions (re: the emotions tied to our individual ecosystems) and live this metamorphic truth?

In the stirring words of Marianne Williamson, "You are a child of God. Your playing small doesn't serve the world. There's nothing enlightened about shrinking so that other people won't feel insecure around you ... We were born to make manifest the glory of God that is within us."

So how *do* we become the Creator? Quite simply, we feel what the Creator feels. And what *does* the Creator feel?

The Creator feels the emotions—and many more that are similarly expansive and uplifting—listed for the Master Field in all Electromagnetic Schematics: creativity, empathy, gratitude, faith, inspiration, joy, love, trust, and unity.

The more time we spend experiencing these and related positive feelings, the more we move forward on our path of conscious personal mastery toward embodying the Creator.

"Embodying the Creator" is just another phrase for becoming whole—which means healing, and ultimately transforming, our lives.

With the above thoughts on intention and conscious personal mastery in mind, I suggest that the following series of exercises quoted from the unparalleled intuitive source known as *The Law of One*, practiced regularly, will help you like nothing else in integrating and maximizing the energies of Potentiation:

Exercise One. This is the most nearly centered and useable within your illusion ... The moment contains love. That is the lesson/goal of this illusion ... The exercise is to consciously see that love in awareness and understanding distortions. The first attempt is the cornerstone. Upon this choosing rests the remainder of [your] life-experience. The second seeking of love within the moment begins the addition. The third seeking empowers the second, the fourth powering or doubling the third ... [T]here will be some loss of power due to flaws within the seeking in the distortion of insincerity. However, the conscious statement of self to self of the desire to seek love is so central an act of will that ... the loss of power due to this friction is inconsequential.

Exercise Two. The universe is one being. When a [person] views another [person], see the Creator ...

Exercise Three. Gaze within a mirror. See the Creator.

Exercise Four. Gaze at the creation which lies about ... each [person]. See the Creator.

The foundation or prerequisite of these exercises is a predilection towards what may be called meditation, contemplation, or prayer. With this attitude, these exercises can be processed. Without it, the data will not sink down into the roots of the tree of mind, thus enabling and ennobling the body and touching the spirit.

The mention of the importance of a "predilection towards ... meditation, contemplation, or prayer" speaks to a way of being, an internal intention to be present in the Now, not a rote activity.

Eventually, if you are performing them correctly, meditation, contemplation and prayer should cease to be isolated events and, instead, inform every moment as you go about activating your potential and living to the fullest.

When I shared these exercises with members of the Regenetics Method Forum, someone recommended a fifth exercise that seemed to encapsulate the other four and round them off beautifully:

Exercise Five. While doing the four exercises above, think or say, "I love you. I am you."

CHAPTER 14
Era III Tools

Era I tools for promoting conscious personal mastery center on nurturing the body during the phenomenal ener-genetic upgrades made possible by Potentiation and the Regenetics Method.

Going beyond the body and genetics, Era II tools are inspired by an epigenetic (mind-body) approach to integrating the uniquely potent energies of this work.

In order to complete our discussion of ways to maximize healing and transformation through DNA activation, it is necessary to touch on Era III, or meta-genetic, tools for conscious personal mastery.

Era III tools are capable of benefiting both the body and mind in extraordinary ways—yet *the primary characteristic of genuine meta-genetic medicine is that it is decidedly spiritual in nature.*

As explained in Part I, Era III techniques bypass our individual bodies and minds and go directly to the root of problems by changing the spiritual blueprint in the collective consciousness field responsible for creating them (Figures 8 and 9).

This final chapter serves as a brief introduction to the other three primary DNA activations in the Regenetics Method: Articulation Bioenergy Enhancement, Elucidation Triune Activation, and Transcension Bioenergy Crystallization.

Meta-genetic to their core in both theory and practice, these three modalities transcend even Potentiation in their ability to increase your consciousness, raise your personal frequency, and heal and transform areas still in need of attention.

We will begin with a description of each phase, before exploring the Regenetics Method Timeline (Figure 19), and concluding with a brief discussion of the "archeological" progression through the subtle bodies represented by the four-part Regenetics Method.

The second, third and fourth phases of this work, being somewhat more complex to perform than Potentiation, are meant to be facilitated—either remotely or in person—by someone with specialized training in the Regenetics Method.

If you would like to continue your healing and transformational journey with Regenetics beyond Potentiation, a regularly updated list of certified Facilitators grouped by country is available at **www.phoenixregenetics.org** and **www.potentiation.net**.

Make sure the Facilitator you choose for any of the DNA activations outlined below 1) is listed in our official database of certified Facilitators and 2) has training in the particular level(s) of this work you wish to experience.

At both of the websites above, you also can read about how to become a certified Regenetics Method Facilitator yourself.

Additionally, you will find more detailed information on all phases of the Regenetics Method online—including several pages of client Testimonials, a description of our supplemental series of ener-genetic fortifications (Songs of Distinction), and instructions for accessing the Regenetics Method Forum.

Individuals interested in the more esoteric aspects of Regenetics— such as luminous embodiment—are encouraged to read *Conscious Healing* (also available through the above websites), where conscious evolution and human potential are examined from a truly broad and pioneering perspective.

Articulation Bioenergy Enhancement

Focus: mental subtle body

Minimum Eligibility: five-month mark following the Potentiation session

Duration: ongoing

Some Reported Benefits: youthful energy; mental sharpness; improved memory; clearer communication; increased creativity; heightened sexuality; easier periods; less PMS; less intellectualizing; enhanced intuition; meditative mindfulness; decreased acne; better exercise; greater flexibility; allergy elimination; increased abundance

Potentiation can be life-altering in itself—and certainly was in my case. Not only did it save my life; it also gave me back my life after years of debilitating allergies and chronic autoimmune illness.

But Leigh and I knew from the outset it was possible to reinforce the process of DNA activation through other meta-genetic intercessions employing different vowel codes of sound and light.

Initiated by a one-time, half-hour session similar to Potentiation, Articulation is appropriate as of the five-month mark after the Potentiation session.

This second phase of the Regenetics Method is designed to enhance the enormous creative potential of the second bioenergy field and corresponding chakra.

As explained, the Regenetics Method grew out of the discovery that the human bioenergy centers are ecosystems where a number of factors spanning the body-mind-spirit spectrum function either harmoniously to create wellness or disharmoniously to produce illness.

Regenetics further recognizes that the second ecosystem, the Fragmentary Body, exists in most people as a bioenergy vacuum that to a large degree separates spirit and matter—keeping torsion energy from naturally healing and transforming our lives.

In Potentiation the bioenergy centers recalibrate from an imbalanced and unstable nine to an infinite and harmonious eight in number as the Fragmentary Body is repatterned out of existence. This creates an infinity circuit in the bioenergy blueprint (Figures 10 and 18).

In this process, the ninth ecosystem merges with and seals the second ecosystem. Sealing occurs at approximately the five-month mark of Potentiation—at which point the second bioenergy center transforms from an energetic liability to an important ener-genetic switchboard governing DNA function.

Articulation "potentiates" this newly established ecosystem, facilitating the integration of novel bioenergetic potentials that begin unfolding from the ninety-seven percent of potential DNA now ready to be accessed.

Many of these new potentials are related directly to the potent life energy of the second bioenergy field, the corresponding chakra, and the associated organs: the oral and reproductive systems (Figure 5). This life force, which is a concentrated form of bioenergy, has been called "kundalini."

Kundalini is the individual's own life-wave of torsion energy. This energy is pure universal creative consciousness placed in the individual at conception.

In Vedic teachings, kundalini is considered the highest evolutionary force humans possess with the power to unfold our full bio-spiritual potential when awakened.

To clarify a point for those familiar with the metaphysical tradition of India, kundalini is a primal energy that sits atop the first chakra, serpentlike and mostly dormant because of the energy disruption constituted by the Fragmentary Body just above it.

The key to raising your kundalini without forcing things and hurting yourself lies in the second chakra—which when sealed, naturally begins to bridge kundalini at its font with the higher bioenergy centers.

Articulation activates this life-wave at the genetic and cellular levels, providing a constant bioenergy supply for creativity in all areas—including artistic expression, interpersonal communication, healthy sexuality, and rebuilding through diet and exercise.

Many people who feel they have become "stuck" in some aspect of their Potentiation report being propelled forward again in their healing and transformation following Articulation.

This makes sense because with a new bioenergy matrix (with no energy disruption or leakage in the form of the Fragmentary Body) in place after sealing, the body, mind and spirit begin to crave the evolutionary energy that Articulation activates.

Since the Fragmentary Body has been sealed through Potentiation, the stimulation of kundalini through Articulation is safe, gentle, and continuous.

Sealing the Fragmentary Body during Potentiation, followed by activation of the former Fragmentary Body in Articulation, makes possible further healing—including the profound level of emotional transformation that often occurs during Elucidation.

Elucidation Triune Activation

Focus: emotional subtle body

Minimum Eligibility: 42-week mark following Potentiation session and at least one month after Articulation

Duration: 42 weeks (9+ months)

Some Reported Benefits: increased self-love; more joy; trauma release; forgiveness; acceptance; authentic relationships; clearer life purpose; self-empowerment; hormonal regulation; fewer hot flashes; healthier joints; greater stamina; body wisdom

As noted already, one intriguing aspect of DNA is that most people use less than ten (some say as little as three) percent of it. The rest has been dismissed by mainstream science as "junk."

The fact that we use less than ten percent of our DNA correlates to the fact that we use at best ten percent of our brain. Still more fascinating is that less than ten percent of the matter in the universe may be visible. The other ninety percent has been called "dark matter" and may reside in other dimensions.

Could there be an evolutionary purpose to "junk" DNA? Could it have hidden potential awaiting activation? Could it somehow activate the unused portion of our brain? Could this activation open up our perceptual faculties and allow us to see the invisible ninety percent of the universe?

Many researchers believe the answer to all these questions is an emphatic *yes*.

The Regenetics Method initially was designed to heal my chronic illness, but it turned out to be much more. At its heart, Regenetics encourages not just healing, but profound bio-spiritual transformation through conscious personal mastery.

Following Potentiation and Articulation, Elucidation—also initiated by a thirty-minute session—is designed to activate, via the neocortex and triune brain, the prefrontal cortex, sometimes called the "bird brain" to distinguish it from the new mammalian, mammalian and reptilian cortices.

Within the brain's triune nature, to use a phrase coined by neuroscientist Paul MacLean, we can chart the cognitive evolution of our species from the dominance of the reptilian brain; to the development of the limbic, old mammalian or emotional-cognitive brain; to the ascendancy of the neocortex, verbal-intellectual or new mammalian brain.

Today, in addition to this nested tripartite structure that reads like a three-stop roadmap through human history, we are beginning to see activity in our "fourth brain," the prefrontal lobes.

"Neuroscientists have a variety of viewpoints on this comparatively new portion of our neural system, which was once called 'the silent area' of the brain because its function was largely unknown and no activity was indicated there," explains Joseph Chilton Pearce.

"Paul MacLean considered the prefrontals a fourth evolutionary system, however, and called them the 'angel lobes,' attributing to them our 'higher human virtues' of love, compassion, empathy, and understanding."

I offer that MacLean was essentially correct, and that our evolution into a more highly evolved human involves activation—to some degree—of the prefrontal cortex.

In an article entitled "Enlightenment and the Brain" republished in *DNA Monthly*, neurophysicist Christian Opitz reports that Sri Bhagavan, developer of a popular energy healing technique known as *deeksha*, insists that

> activation of the Frontal Lobes is involved in God-realization. The experience of enlightenment, of non-separation, does not necessarily coincide with the experience of a living God-presence. In Sri Bhagavan's teaching more than the deactivation of the overactivity in the parietal lobes is necessary to move from enlightenment to God-realization. He speaks about the activation of the frontal lobes as a necessary neurological change for God to come alive in the consciousness of a person. The frontal lobes are associated with the individual will. Many mystical traditions speak about the merging of the individual will with the will of God as both a doorway to and result of God-realization. This cannot happen, however, if the frontal lobes are underactive.

Sri Bhagavan is making an important, often overlooked distinction between the meditative calming of the parietal lobes during the so-called enlightenment of many Eastern mindfulness practices, and genuine bio-spiritual conscious personal mastery.

Unlike mental "enlightenment," conscious personal mastery culminates not just in perceptual oneness (transformative as that may be), but *physical illumination*—what Sri Bhagavan calls God-realization. Moreover, such divine embodiment clearly is stated to involve activation of certain regions of the brain.

Elucidation stimulates the prefrontal cortex by way of the neocortex, owing to what I describe in *Conscious Healing* as a "cortical resonance" in the brain's triune structure that harmonically activates the fourth brain. It is for this reason that Leigh and I chose "Triune Activation" to characterize Elucidation.

In my own case, I felt decidedly "otherworldly" for months following Elucidation—as if my brain chemistry had been shifted fundamentally and permanently.

I was and am reminded of Opitz's line in the aforementioned article that "[d]opamine, the essential neurotransmitter for frontal lobe activity, is necessary for feelings of enchantment with life and bliss, often described as accompanying mystical union with God."

Elucidation greatly facilitates conscious personal mastery by assisting the individual to replace limiting and/or harmful beliefs—including associated emotions and attitudes—with life-affirming ones.

Restructuring the belief system and matching emotional states can change one's experience of reality dramatically. The movement here is toward embodiment of a radical new way of being based no longer on duality and separation, but on unity consciousness and unconditional love.

This third phase of the Regenetics Method prompts potential DNA to reconfigure the individual's infinity circuit, established through Potentiation, to a new unified frequency throughout the bioenergy blueprint called the "Unified Consciousness Field."

Creation of the Unified Consciousness Field occurs through a process of torsion energy repatterning similar to what happens during Potentiation.

The Unified Consciousness Field establishes and helps maintain a heightened unity consciousness by and through which, over time, our new bio-spiritual identity comes into being.

While the Unified Consciousness Field is experienced as a single torsion gestalt, like a bubble of universal creative consciousness surrounding the body, this Field remains a composite of eight bioenergy fields and chakras that constantly balance themselves.

In other words, the Unified Consciousness Field is a result of a continuously running "ener-genetic program," uploaded through Elucidation, designed to keep the bioenergy centers in a harmonious state of heightened energy.

Only when the ecosystems are sufficiently balanced and energized can further bio-spiritual evolution, such as that encouraged by Transcension, occur.

Transcension Bioenergy Crystallization

Focus: spiritual subtle body

Minimum Eligibility: 42-week mark following Elucidation session

Duration: 42 weeks (9+ months)

Some Reported Benefits: oneness; unity consciousness; unconditional love (of self and others); heightened faith; inner knowing; higher guidance; greater patience; peace and tranquility; youthing; professional transformation; dramatic abundance; daily miracles

Emerging from the same torsion energy principles applied to genetics as Potentiation, Articulation and Elucidation, Transcension is designed for the spiritual seeker—and is appropriate after the nine-month (42-week) Elucidation phase is complete.

Both Articulation and Transcension increase the activity of kundalini. But the degree of kundalini stimulation in Transcension, while still safe and manageable, far exceeds that of Articulation.

Indeed, *Transcension "supercharges" the bioenergy blueprint.*

Another important difference between these two DNA activations is that Transcension energizes a cyclical movement of torsion energy through the bioenergy centers similar to that experienced during Potentiation and Elucidation—whereas Articulation radiates kundalini from a fixed position in the second bioenergy center.

In discussing the unifying effects of Elucidation in the previous section, we were touching on an understanding of the Unified Consciousness Field as an example of divine paradox: of the One simultaneously being the many, and vice versa.

It was stated that while the Unified Consciousness Field is experienced as a gestalt, so much so that it often is seen by clairvoyants as pure white light, this Field remains a composite of eight bioenergy fields and chakras.

The bio-spiritually balanced structure of the Unified Consciousness Field can be understood even better using the analogy of the rainbow, which serves as a model of creation.

Each bioenergy center has a native harmonic frequency whose visible equivalent manifests as a true color of the rainbow. Many esoteric traditions refer to these colors as *rays*.

Starting with the first bioenergy center, these colors/rays are always the classic ROYGBIV of high school science: red, orange, yellow, green, blue, indigo, and violet.

Crucially, the eighth "color" in this model is the amalgam of all true colors—white—and corresponds to the eighth ecosystem.

In a potentiated person, the all-important eighth ecosystem subsumes all other ecosystems and links directly to the Master Field—which *is* the Unified Consciousness Field.

As a microcosmic representation of the greater consciousness field of the Creator, the eighth bioenergy center, when "elucidated," becomes capable of maintaining the individual's own Unified Conscious Field, which permeates all of one's lower ecosystems with the Consciousness of Love (Figures 1 and 4).

As we connect more fully to our Source and experience further healing and transformation by its unifying influx into our own bioenergy centers, conscious personal mastery can be understood as a very real phenomenon—encouraging a more self-actualized way of being—experienced by a relatively evolved individual (Figure 9).

As in Potentiation, Articulation and Elucidation, Transcension employs specific vowel combinations of sound and light to stimulate a metamorphic potential in human genetics.

The main difference (other than the time it takes to perform Transcension, forty-five as opposed to thirty minutes) is that the sound and light codes used in Transcension are even more ordered and harmonious than in previous activations.

By focusing on the spiritual subtle body, which acts as a "consciousness shuttle" between our Source and ourselves, Transcension establishes the possibility of a thoroughgoing transmutation of the emotional, mental and physical subtle bodies.

This fourth and final DNA activation draws in torsion energy directly from Source to transfigure the individual's bioenergy centers.

Conscious evolution accelerates exponentially as the bioenergy centers—which are maintained in balance through the Unified Consciousness Field established via Elucidation—are "crystallized," or activated to an even higher order of consciousness.

This level of conscious personal mastery—when fully integrated throughout our body-mind-spirit—allows us to live the fundamental truth that there is no difference between self and other since, in the grand scheme of creation, there is only the One.

The reality-restructuring concept behind Transcension is that it is only by knowing and experiencing who we truly are, and then allowing the Creator in us to express its wholeness through our individual lives, that we heal the world.

269

Timeline for Regenetics Activations

Figure 19 shows the Timeline on which the various DNA activations that make up the Regenetics Method are designed to be experienced.

When you have spent five months potentiating, you are ready for Articulation. Slightly over four months later, at forty-two weeks after your Potentiation session, you can receive Elucidation. Forty-two weeks later, you become eligible for Transcension.

The Regenetics Method Timeline

Potentiation	Articulation	Elucidation	Transcension
Start	5 months	9+ months	18+ months	27+ months

Songs of Distinction

New research shows self-healing can occur by "ener-genetically" activating DNA.

The **Regenetics Method** uses **sound** and **intention** to stimulate DNA to repattern the body's electromagnetic (EM) fields. This, in turn, encourages healing on the cellular level.

Regenetics activates a genetic potential that already exists in us, by "potentiating" so-called "junk" DNA.

Potentiation focuses on the physical body and "seals" the Fragmentary Body, establishing a basic unity consciousness that greatly promotes healing.

The Fragmentary Body is sealed at around 5 months following **Potentiation**. The EM fields have recalibrated from an imbalanced 9 to a harmonious 8. The "infinity circuit" in the body's energetics is complete.

Designed to harmonize the mental body, **Articulation** "switches on" healing bioenergy in the body's second energy center.

Articulation enhances creativity in all areas while facilitating the transformation of limiting thought-forms and behaviors.

Elucidation activates a mostly dormant portion of the prefrontal lobes via the neocortex, facilitating creation of a higher energy body to assist in our "ascension" to a higher organic expression of unity consciousness.

Elucidation works through the emotional body to assist the individual to replace limiting and/or harmful beliefs with life-affirming ones.

The Unified Consciousness Field is the result of a continuously running ener-genetic "program" that is "uploaded" out of DNA through **Elucidation**. This program is designed to keep the individual's bioenergy centers in a state of balance during further evolution of consciousness having to do with the spiritual body.

Transcension focuses on healing the spiritual body, which links conscious Source energy with our physical, mental and emotional bodies.

Transcension energizes a cyclical movement of this "torsion" energy, further activating and harmonizing the EM fields and related *chakras*.

Transcension thus promotes bioenergy "crystallization" (stability, order, creativity, and harmony).

By instituting a higher degree of systemic order at the ener-genetic level, **Transcension** encourages an advanced level of conscious personal mastery.

This is as it should be, since the **Regenetics Method** progressively stimulates consciousness and healing in a safe, integrated and integratable manner.

Songs of Distinction work on specific glands and related organs to stimulate further release of toxins and rebuilding, as well as additional mental, emotional and spiritual growth.

Songs work synergistically to cross-fortify each other.

Songs of Distinction can be experienced 42 weeks after **Potentiation** at a rate of one Song per month.

For more information on the Regenetics Method, visit us online at http://www.phoenixregenetics.org.

Figure 19: Regenetics Method Timeline

The above chart delineates the minimum Timeline for experiencing the four primary DNA activations in the Regenetics Method, as well as Songs of Distinction.

While these activations can occur later than this minimum Timeline, without diminishing their effectiveness, note that they cannot be experienced earlier.

The rationale for having a minimum Timeline is simple and practical. Regenetics activations can be very powerful, and typically require a certain amount of integration time to unfold to a point where even deeper levels of healing and transformation can occur.

Any tendency to want to go faster is most likely the ego talking. Wanting to speed up the process also means you probably are not being as present as you could be with—and thus maximizing—the changes that may be happening in the Now.

Raising Your Personal Frequency

Three interrelated aspects of Regenetics worth emphasizing are that by raising your personal frequency, this Method:

1. Strengthens your natural immunity to lower-vibrating toxins, energies, pathogens, situations, and even people;

2. Increases the power of your attractor fields to pull higher-vibrating individuals and outcomes into your life; and

3. Provides an unprecedented level of spiritual guidance and protection as you come into ever greater resonance with the vibration of your Higher Self.

The benefits of increasing your individual vibration can range from coming down with fewer colds and flus, to having more friends and greater financial support, to being able to safely and gracefully navigate even the most difficult challenges.

Raising your personal frequency also encourages detoxification of physical, mental, emotional and spiritual hindrances that are no longer a fit for your evolving consciousness.

Archeological Approach to Healing & Transformation

The process of raising one's personal frequency over the course of Regenetics is related closely to the way this Method progresses through the subtle bodies.

In *Psychoenergetic Science: A Second Copernican-scale Revolution*, physicist William Tiller describes humans as composed of a seemingly individual identity informed by a "rich infrastructure [of] subtle bodies" that represent the true key to "greater human performance and expanded capabilities."

The subtle bodies are multidimensional templates for human beings which, in complex ways that transcend the parameters of this book, govern the bioenergy blueprint itself.

These subtle bodies—which form ener-genetic templates for our bio-spiritual incarnation and are not to be confused with the actual physical body—are arranged in a specific order, from the lowest to the highest frequency, thus: physical, mental, emotional, spiritual.

Some metaphysical traditions place the mental body higher than the emotional body. But based on kinesiology, experience and observation, the order above represents the true functional arrangement of the subtle bodies.

Potential DNA interfaces not only with the bioenergy fields, but also—and even more crucially—with the physical, mental, emotional and spiritual subtle bodies.

In order to correct distortions in the bioenergy blueprint as detailed in Part I, Regenetics activations technically first activate the subtle bodies, which in turn heal and transform the aspects of the bioenergy fields to which they relate.

The four primary DNA activations in the Regenetics Method—which promote spiritual mastery, first and foremost—are overseen individually by a subtle body that is actually an extension of our Higher Self.

Potentiation activates the physical subtle body. Articulation centers on the mental subtle body. Elucidation is keyed to the emotional subtle body. And Transcension stimulates the spiritual subtle body.

In discussing the subtle bodies, we are entering a realm of inverse relationships that turn the perceived primacy of physicality within the holographic matrix of our world on its head.

In other words, the higher the subtle body, the more powerful it is than—and the more responsible it is for creating—our manifest experience of reality.

Because an increase in subtlety of energy indicates that the energy is becoming more potent by harmonically approximating pure Source energy, *the mental body is more fundamental than the physical body, the emotional body is more elemental than the mental body, and the spiritual body is the primary subtle body.*

By respecting this inherent progression, the Regenetics Method takes what might be described as an *archeological* approach to healing and transformation.

This approach starts with a focus on the top, surface or physical level of the subtle bodies with Potentiation; goes deeper into the mental realm with Articulation; then plumbs the even more important creational domains of the emotional body in Elucidation and the spiritual body in Transcension.

A practical example may aid in understanding how this archeological approach facilitates healing and transformation by assisting the individual in releasing energy distortions in the area of the subtle anatomy where such distortions exist.

Let us imagine that an individual chooses to experience the Regenetics Method mainly because she suffers from severe allergies to certain foods.

It is very common for clients to report lessening or disappearance of allergies following Potentiation, especially when the allergies have been induced physically by an adverse reaction to vaccines or other external factors.

But in the case of our theoretical client, after several months of potentiating, it becomes obvious that her allergies, which have not abated, are rooted at a deeper level.

So at the five-month mark following the Potentiation session, when she becomes eligible to experience Articulation, she decides to move forward with this activation focused on the mental subtle body.

On numerous occasions, clients have reported that their allergies completely went away after Articulation—and such, thankfully, is the case for our theoretical client.

If, however, her allergies persisted, we would assume they stem from a distortion either at the emotional level, addressed through Elucidation, or at the spiritual level, the focus of Transcension.

As a final clarification, just because a particular DNA activation focuses on a specific subtle body—such as Potentiation centering on the physical subtle body—does not mean that healing and transformation cannot occur simultaneously on mental, emotional and spiritual levels.

To the contrary, since the subtle bodies are interconnected like an intricate tapestry forming part of the Higher Self, it is normal for Potentiation to produce far more than physical results, Articulation to create numerous breakthroughs that are not just mental, and so on.

Final Thoughts on Conscious Personal Mastery

Integral to the notion of conscious personal mastery are the words "conscious" and "personal."

Insofar as we fail to use our daily experiences to learn to love ourselves and others *consciously* as one, we are not maximizing our level of mastery.

The journey to conscious personal mastery, which charts a life-changing trajectory from healing to transformation, requires both our regular intention and *attention*.

In addition, the life-changing journey to wholeness is in all instances decidedly *personal*.

While it is true that each of us is moving toward the inevitable center that is the Creator, like spokes of a wheel we come from all directions. In the end, you must walk your own path back to the One.

If you deem that Potentiation and the Regenetics Method can assist you in activating your potential for conscious personal mastery, the only thing to do is proceed confidently by placing one foot in front of another.

If you choose a different path, the only thing to do is proceed confidently by placing one foot in front of another. We all eventually will meet in the middle, anyway.

As in the Irish blessing, may the road rise up to meet you, and may the wind be always at your back!

APPENDIX A: FREQUENTLY ASKED QUESTIONS

Q: Is it possible for me to "mess up" my Potentiation?

A: As long as your session is performed more or less as taught and you approach your Potentiation with an open mind and especially heart, there is practically no way you can botch your DNA activation and bioenergy repatterning. Note that this includes previous, simultaneous or subsequent exposure to other forms of DNA activation, other types of energy work, and even environmental radiation sources such as computers and cell phones.

Q: Is there ever a reason to redo Potentiation?

A: Not really. Even in the case where you flub a line or two of Potentiation, or a distance recipient forgets the appointment, the energies of this DNA activation—once set in motion—remain available for access by yourself or another "morphogenetically." Simply use your intention to tap into the healing and transformational potential of this work that already exists.

Q: Can a person who already has been potentiated by someone else benefit from potentiating him or herself?

A: Benefit, yes, in a meditative way. Please be aware, however, that repeated Potentiation does not change or improve the bioenergy repatterning process.

Q: So Potentiation can be used as a daily meditation?

A: Absolutely. But here again, Potentiation does not require repeating in order to be one hundred percent effective. The vast majority of individuals—including most who have contributed Testimonials—experience Potentiation one time only.

Q: Will Potentiation interfere with any other energetic methods I might be trying?

A: To the contrary, Potentiation may make other modalities more effective—and even too powerful. This applies not only to energetic therapies, but to any modality. Whether to try other modalities following Potentiation is entirely up to you. Always trust your intuition. You, and only you, know what is right for your body, mind, and spirit. Remember to ask other practitioners to treat you gingerly, as repatterning your bioenergy blueprint and raising your personal frequency through Potentiation allow your system to accomplish more with less external energy input.

Q: Are there any things I might do that can interfere with my Potentiation?

A: Nothing except an individual's free will can impede the proper unfoldment of Potentiation. That said, there are some basic considerations for people passing through deeper periods of healing during Regenetics. Always trust your intuition in supporting the unblocking of distortions in—and detoxification of—your physical, mental, emotional and spiritual bodies. If something feels as if it is pushing you too hard, it probably is. Sometimes, supplemental healing activities are appropriate. But often, especially for those learning to trust the wisdom of their body-mind-spirit as it self-corrects its imbalances, more is less and less is more.

Q: Does everyone experience physical detoxification after Potentiation?

A: No. This work is highly individualized. But keep in mind that since detoxification can include not just physical, but also mental, emotional and even spiritual elements, some form of beneficial release often occurs during Potentiation.

Q: Does Potentiation transform my basic DNA?

A: As applied to the three percent of protein-building DNA that makes you yourself, the answer is no. Wave-genetics reveals that DNA activation is capable of shifting potential DNA and regulating the activity of specific genes, however, as bioenergy flows from the consciousness field through noncoding into coding DNA to promote healing and transformation.

Q: Are there any contraindications involved with Potentiation?

A: As for contraindications, there are no "indications." Potentiation is not a therapy, but the first phase of an integrated Method for facilitating conscious personal mastery as a bio-spiritual healing path, or way of becoming whole. While making no medical claims, there is every reason to believe—based on hard science—that a successful reset of the bioenergetic disharmonies that have created problems can be profoundly restorative.

Q: I've read online that DNA activation is dangerous. How do you respond to this?

A: Such thinking reflects programmed victim consciousness and the propagandistic view that the world is a "dangerous" place. The simple fact is that listening to beautiful music or making love stimulates DNA. Our genetic structure also is stimulated continuously by cosmic gamma rays. DNA activation has been a great blessing for thousands of people—many of whom had given up hope of ever being well again prior to discovering Potentiation and the Regenetics Method.

Q: Does everyone benefit from Potentiation?

A: While some people have more profound results than others, it seems that anyone approaching Potentiation with a truly open mind and heart experiences a positive shift—even if it was not what was expected. Make sure to set your intention specifically yet flexibly on what you want to achieve, then trust the wisdom of your DNA as you go about living with joy. A good way to maintain intention is to journal on your own conscious personal mastery as it expresses itself in your individualized evolutionary path. Also, the importance of inviting more and more love into all levels of your being cannot be overemphasized, as "exercising the heart" ultimately is what makes your DNA available for activation.

Q: Can someone who is already healthy benefit from Potentiation?

A: How do you define "healthy"? *Healthy* describes someone who is whole in every way: physically, mentally, emotionally, and spiritually. From this perspective, few people are entirely healthy. Clients with no physical problems often report substantial healing on mental, emotional and/or spiritual levels. Others experience Potentiation more palpably. No two individuals are alike, but most people (even those who consider themselves healthy) report positive shifts in one or more areas.

Q: How do I know if Potentiation is right for me?

A: Trust your intuition. We live in a world based largely on denying our own power. The Regenetics Method involves experiencing firsthand that real power exists in and through you. If you are afraid to change; feel locked in victim consciousness; believe that only someone or something outside yourself can cure you; or are addicted to old illness or relational patterns, Potentiation probably is not for you—at this time. If, however, the concept of conscious personal mastery excites you; you are committed to your own empowerment; you believe it is possible to transcend limitation; and Potentiation resonates with you—go for it!

Q: Is there any required avoidance period of foods or other substances following Potentiation as there is with NAET and its derivatives?

A: None.

Q: Can someone who is deaf or hard of hearing be potentiated in person?

A: Yes. The person's DNA will feel and be activated by the vibration and energy of the in-person Potentiation codes.

Q: Can I potentiate someone else without potentiating myself, either beforehand or simultaneously?

A: This does not appear to be possible. Nor should it be desirable.

Q: Is it possible for two or more people to facilitate their own or another's Potentiation together?

A: Yes. Leigh and I performed the very first Potentiation this way.

Q: Can I do Potentiation without the Mi tuning fork?

A: Not if you want to do it properly and still call it Potentiation.

Q: Can nonphysical things be potentiated?

A: Definitely. People have observed positive outcomes by potentiating businesses, homes, physical locations, and even abstract situations. Note that potentiating a relationship, for example, does not mean necessarily that you are potentiating another person in the relationship.

Q: Is there any difference, in terms of effectiveness, between a remote and in-person Potentiation?

A: None whatsoever.

Q: Given that this work is nonlocal at its base, why are there two sets of Potentiation codes—one for in-person sessions, the other for distance recipients?

A: The simple answer is that this work came through this way. Both sets of Potentiation codes activate exactly the same bioenergetic repatterning process. Theoretically, one could use the distance codes exclusively for all sessions. In fact, subsequent phases of the Regenetics Method require only one set of codes. In this book, a conscious decision was made to teach Potentiation exactly as it was communicated.

Q: Can I perform Potentiation for someone who doesn't know it?

A: Typically, for ethical reasons having to do with free will, you are strongly discouraged from doing so. There are three—and only three—exceptions to the permission rule when it comes to in-person or distance Potentiation for people: embryos/fetuses, young children (under twelve), and communication-impaired adults. And obviously, you do not need permission to potentiate a pet.

Q: Before offering this work to family and friends, should I muscle test to make sure they're ready for it?

A: Except in the aforementioned three exceptions to the permission rule, where it is acceptable to muscle test this way, you should empower others by letting them decide for themselves whether they are ready to be potentiated. To help them decide, you can share your own perspective on Potentiation, refer them to **www.phoenixregenetics.org** or **www.potentiation.net**, or provide them with a copy of this book. Whenever possible, it is important to honor other people's free will in making their own decisions.

Q: Can I charge money for this work?

A: It is recommended that you receive certification in the appropriate level(s) of the Regenetics Method before charging money to facilitate this work. For information on training seminars, visit **www.phoenixregenetics.org** or **www.potentiation.net**.

Q: What is the protocol for moving forward with Articulation?

A: As of the five-month mark following your Potentiation session, you become eligible to receive Articulation from a certified Regenetics Method Facilitator. Like Elucidation and Transcension, Articulation can be done in person, but usually is performed at a distance. Visit **www.phoenixregenetics.org** or **www.potentiation.net** for an updated list of certified Facilitators grouped by country.

APPENDIX B: POTENTIATION CONSENT FORM

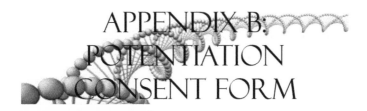

Potentiation Recipient's Name

_____

Last   First

Potentiation Facilitator's Name

_____

Last   First

Waiver: With respect to my Potentiation Electromagnetic Repatterning session, also called "Potentiation," I, for myself, my heirs, personal representatives or assigns, do hereby release, waive and discharge (with covenant not to sue) my Potentiation Facilitator, the author of _Potentiate Your DNA: A Practical Guide to Healing and Transformation with the Regenetics Method_ or the Developers of Potentiation and the Regenetics Method from liability from any and all claims, including practicing medicine without a license, resulting in any loss, damage or injury caused, or alleged to be caused, directly or indirectly, from receiving Potentiation.

Assumption of Risks: Participation in Potentiation carries with it certain inherent risks that cannot be eliminated regardless of the care taken. The specific risks vary, but range from 1) physical, mental and/or emotional detoxification and release to 2) "healing crises" requiring days or weeks of rest to move through. I know, understand and appreciate any and all risks inherent in Potentiation. I hereby assert that my participation is voluntary and that I knowingly assume all such risks.

Indemnification and Agreement to Hold Harmless: I agree to indemnify and hold harmless my Potentiation Facilitator, the author of _Potentiate Your DNA: A Practical Guide to Healing and Transformation with the Regenetics Method_ and the

Developers of Potentiation and the Regenetics Method from any and all claims, actions, suits, procedures, costs, expenses, damages and liabilities, including attorney's fees, brought as a result of my receiving Potentiation, and to reimburse them for any such expenses incurred.

Severability: I expressly acknowledge that this agreement is intended to be as broad and inclusive as is permitted by the law of the state or country in which Potentiation is performed or received, and that if any portion thereof is held invalid, it is agreed that the balance shall, notwithstanding, continue in full legal force and effect.

Acknowledgment of Understanding: I have read in its entirety this waiver of liability, assumption of risk, indemnity and severability agreement, fully understand its terms, and acknowledge that I am giving up substantial rights, including my right to sue. I acknowledge that I am signing this agreement freely and voluntarily, and intend by my signature to effect a complete and unconditional release of all liability to the greatest extent allowed by law.

_____

Signature of Recipient   Date

-or-

_____

Signature of Parent/Guardian/Caregiver   Date

Recipient's Name (if a minor or communication-impaired):

BIBLIOGRAPHY
& WEBOGRAPHY

NOTE: Back issues of *DNA Monthly*, where a number of articles listed below appear, can be read online at **www.potentiation.net**.

Adams, Mike, personal website (www.naturalnews.com)

Berendt, Joachim-Ernst, *The World Is Sound—Nada Brahma: Music and the Landscape of Consciousness* (Inner Traditions International, 1991)

Bohm, David, *Wholeness and the Implicate Order* (Routledge, 2002)

—*On Creativity* (Routledge, 2004)

Booth, Robert, "Dust 'Comes Alive' in Space" (*UK Times Online* at www.timesonline.co.uk, August 2007)

Braden, Gregg, *The God Code: The Secret of Our Past, the Promise of Our Future* (Hay House, 2004)

Bryce, Sheradon, *Joy Riding the Universe: Snapshots of the Journey* (HomeWords Publishing, 1993)

Carey, Ken, *The Starseed Transmissions* (HarperSanFrancisco, 1982)

—*Terra Christa* (Uni-Sun, 1985)

—*Return of the Bird Tribes* (Uni-Sun, 1988)

—*Starseed—The Third Millennium: Living in the Posthistoric World* (HarperSanFrancisco, 1991)

—*Vision: A Personal Call to Create a New World* (HarperCollins, 1992)

Castaneda, Carlos, *The Teachings of Don Juan: A Yaqui Way of Knowledge* (University of California Press, 2008)

Cutler, Ellen, *Winning the War against Immune Disorders and Allergies: A Drug Free Cure for Allergies* (Delmar Thomson Learning, 1998)

Darwin, Charles, *The Origin of Species* (Signet Classics, 2003)

Dossey, Larry, *Healing Words: The Power of Prayer and the Practice of Medicine* (HarperSanFrancisco, 1997)

—*Reinventing Medicine: Beyond Mind-body to a New Era of Healing* (HarperSanFrancisco, 1999)

Elkins, Don, Rueckert, Carla and McCarty, James Allen, *The Law of One: Books I-V* (Whitford Press, 1984-98)

Fisher, M. F. K., *The Art of Eating* (Wiley, 2004)

Flournoy, Bryan, "Have You Helped Your DNA Today?" (*DNA Monthly*, January 2008)

Fosar, Grazyna and Bludorf, Franz, *Vernetzte Intelligenz* ("Networked Intelligence") (Omega Verlag Bongart-Meier, 2001) (Currently unavailable in English. Visit the authors' website at www.fosar-bludorf.com.)

Free, Wynn with Wilcock, D., *The Reincarnation of Edgar Cayce?: Interdimensional Communication and Global Transformation* (Frog, Ltd., 2004)

Gariaev, Peter, "An Open Letter from Dr. Peter Gariaev, the Father of Wave-genetics" (*DNA Monthly*, September 2005)

—"A Brief Introduction to Wave-genetics: Scope and Possibilities" (*DNA Monthly*, April 2009)

—"Crisis in Life Sciences" (*DNA Monthly*, August 2009)

Gerber, Richard, *Vibrational Medicine: New Choices for Healing Ourselves* (Bear & Co., 1988)

Gibbs, W. Wayt, "The Unseen Genome: Gems among the Junk" (*Scientific American*, November 2003)

Goettemoeller, Jeffrey, *Stevia Sweet Recipes: Sugar-free-naturally* (Vital Health Publishing, 1999)

Gray, William, *The Talking Tree* (Weiser, 1977)

Hahnemann, Samuel, *Organon of Medicine* (Nabu Press, 2010)

Hancock, Graham, *Supernatural: Meetings with the Ancient Teachers of Mankind* (The Disinformation Company, 2007)

Hawks, John, personal weblog (www.johnhawks.net)

Hay, Louise, *You Can Heal Your Life* (Hay House, 1984)

Heinemann, Klaus and Ledwith, Miceal, *The Orb Project* (Atria Books/Beyond Words, 2007)

Hoagland, Richard C., personal website (www.enterprisemission.com)

Holtje, Dennis, *From Light to Sound: The Spiritual Progression* (Blue Star, 1995)

Horowitz, Leonard G., *Emerging Viruses: AIDS and Ebola—Nature, Accident or Intentional?* (Tetrahedron, 1996)

—*DNA: Pirates of the Sacred Spiral* (Tetrahedron, 2004)

Horowitz, Leonard G. and Puleo, Joseph S., *Healing Codes for the Biological Apocalypse* (Tetrahedron, 1999)

Houston, Jean, Foreword to Ken Carey's *The Starseed Transmissions* (HarperCollins, 1991)

Huggins, Hal, *It's All in Your Head: The Link between Mercury Amalgams and Illness* (Avery Publishing Group, 1993)

Hulse, David, *A Fork in the Road* (AuthorHouse, 2009)

Hunt, Valerie, *Infinite Mind: Science of the Human Vibrations of Consciousness* (Malibu Publishing Co., 1989)

Institute of Heartmath (www.heartmath.org)

Judd, Gerard, *Good Teeth Birth to Death* (Research Publications Co., 1996)

Klinghardt, Dietrich, personal website (www.neuraltherapy.com)

Larson, Dewey, website devoted to Reciprocal System of physical theory (www.rstheory.org)

Liedloff, Jean, *The Continuum Concept: In Search of Happiness Lost* (Da Capo Press, 1986)

Lipton, Bruce, *The Biology of Belief: Unleashing the Power of Consciousness, Matter, and Miracles* (Mountain of Love/Elite Books, 2005)

—"Embracing the Immaterial Universe" (*Shift: At the Frontiers of Consciousness*, December 2005-February 2006; reprinted in *DNA Monthly*, October 2009)

Lipton, Bruce and Bhaerman, Steve, *Spontaneous Evolution: Our Positive Future (and a Way to Get There from Here)* (Hay House, 2009)

Luckman, Sol, *Beginner's Luke: Book I of the Beginner's Luke Series* (Crow Rising Transformational Media, 2007)

—*Conscious Healing: Book One on the Regenetics Method* (Crow Rising Transformational Media, 2009)

Lupu, Alexandra, "Coffee: A Handy Natural Remedy" (www.news.softpedia.com)

Medical Voices Vaccine Information Center (www.imcv.info)

Mercola, Joseph, personal website (www.mercola.com)

Miller, Neil Z., *Immunization: Theory vs. Reality* (New Atlantean Press, 1996)

Miller, Iona and Miller, Richard A., "From Helix to Hologram: An Ode on the Human Genome" (*Nexus*, September-October 2003; reprinted in *DNA Monthly*, October 2005)

Miller, Richard A., Webb, Burt and Dickson, Darden, "A Holographic Concept of Reality" (*Psychoenergetic Systems*, Vol. 1, 1975; reprinted in *DNA Monthly*, May 2007)

Mindell, Arnold, *Dreambody: The Body's Role in Revealing the Self* (Lao Tse Press, 1998)

Mohr, Bärbel, "DNA's Hypercommunication: The 'Living Internet' inside of Us" (2002) (Summary of the German book *Vernetzte Intelligenz* ["Networked Intelligence"] by Grazyna Fosar and Franz Bludorf) (http://www.bibliotecapleyades.net/ciencia/ciencia_genetica02.htm)

Motoyama, Hiroshi, *Theories of Chakras: Bridge to Higher Consciousness* (Quest, 1981)

Myss, Caroline, *Anatomy of the Spirit: The Seven Stages of Power and Healing* (Three Rivers Press, 1997)

—*Sacred Contracts: Awakening Your Divine Potential* (Three Rivers Press, 2003)

Nambudripad, Devi, *Say Goodbye to Illness* (Delta Publishing Co., 1999)

Narby, Jeremy, *The Cosmic Serpent: DNA and the Origins of Knowledge* (Jeremy P. Tarcher/Putnam, 1998)

Opitz, Christian, "Enlightenment and the Brain" (*DNA Monthly*, May 2006)

Peale, Norman Vincent, *The Power of Positive Thinking* (Fireside, 2007)

Pearce, Joseph C., *The Biology of Transcendence: A Blueprint of the Human Spirit* (Inner Traditions, 2001)

Peirce, Penney, *Frequency: The Power of Personal Vibration* (Atria Books/Beyond Words, 2009)

"Phoenix (mythology)" (Webpage on the history of the legendary phoenix bird) (en.metapedia.org/wiki/Phoenix_(mythology))

Price, Weston A., *Nutrition and Physical Degeneration* (Price Pottenger Nutrition, 2008)

—The Weston A. Price Foundation (www.westonaprice.org)

Rein, Glen, "Effect of Conscious Intention on Human DNA" (Proc.Internat.Forum on New Science, 1996)

Roshoniel, "Activating DNA's Higher Potentials" (*DNA Monthly*, June-July 2006)

Ruiz, Miguel, *Beyond Fear: A Toltec Guide to Freedom and Joy* (Council Oak Books, 1997)

Sahelian, Ray and Gates, Donna, *The Stevia Cookbook: Cooking with Nature's Calorie-free Sweetener* (Avery Trade, 2004)

Sahtouris, Elisabet, "Living Systems in Evolution" (*DNA Monthly*, April 2007)

Sams, Jamie and Carson, David, *Medicine Cards: The Discovery of Power through the Ways of Animals* (St. Martin's Press, 1999)

Sanderson, Ivan, "The Twelve Devil's Graveyards around the World" (*Saga*, 1972)

Sheldrake, Rupert, *The Presence of the Past: Morphic Resonance and the Habits of Nature* (Inner Traditions, 1995)

Schucman, Helen (Editor), *A Course in Miracles: Combined Volume* (Foundation for Inner Peace, 2007)

Stein, Rob, "Reports Accuse WHO of Exaggerating H1N1 Threat, Possible Ties to Drug Makers" (*Washington Post Online* at www.washingtonpost.com, June 2010)

St. John of the Cross, *The Dark Night of the Soul* (Hodder & Stoughton, 2010)

Talbot, Michael, *The Holographic Universe* (HarperPerennial, 1992)

Tiller, William A., *Psychoenergetic Science: A Second Copernican-scale Revolution* (Pavior, 2007)

Tolle, Eckhart, *The Power of Now: A Guide to Spiritual Enlightenment* (New World Library, 1999)

"Vision Quest" (Webpage describing Native American rites of passage) (www.crystalinks.com/visionquest.html)

Vonderplanitz, Aajonus, *We Want To Live* (Carnelian Bay Castle Press, 1997)

Wade, Nicholas, "A Decade Later, Genetic Map Yields Few New Cures" (*New York Times Online* at www.nytimes.com, June 2010)

Wilcock, David, personal website and weblog (www.divinecosmos.com)

—"Kozyrev: Aether, Time and Torsion" (www.divinecosmos.com; reprinted in *DNA Monthly*, May 2008)

Williamson, Marianne, *A Return to Love: Reflections on the Principles of "A Course in Miracles"* (Harper, 1992)

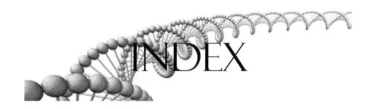

INDEX

Sol Luckman is an acclaimed author of fiction and nonfiction and pioneering ink painter whose work has appeared on mainstream book covers. His books include the international bestselling *Conscious Healing: Book One on the Regenetics Method* and its popular sequel, *Potentiate Your DNA: A Practical Guide to Healing & Transformation with the Regenetics Method*. His visionary novel, *Snooze: A Story of Awakening*, won the 2015 National Indie Excellence Award for New Age Fiction. *Snooze* further proved its literary merit by being selected as a 2016 Readers' Favorite International Book Award Finalist in the Young Adult-Coming of Age category and receiving an Honorable Mention in the 2014 Beach Book Festival Prize Competition in the General Fiction category. Sol's latest book, *The Angel's Dictionary: A Spirited Glossary for the Little Devil in You*, winner of the 2017 National Indie Excellence Award for Humor, reinvigorates satire to prove that—though we might not be able to change the world—we can at least have a good laugh at it. Then again, maybe laughter can transform the world! View Sol's paintings, read his blog and learn more about his work at **www.CrowRising.com**.

If you would like to help spread the word about the Regenetics Method, please submit a personal Testimonial and/or Book Review of *Potentiate Your DNA* through either of the websites below.

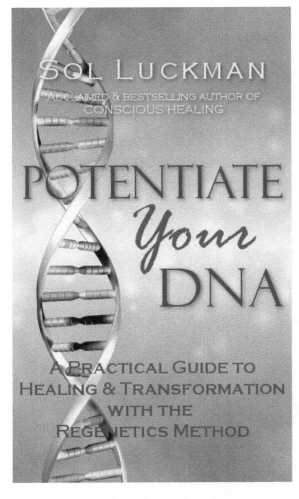

Those desirous to share *Potentiate Your DNA* with family and friends may be interested in our "Pay It Forward" program— which provides substantial discounts on orders of ten or more paperback copies.

For more information, visit
www.phoenixregenetics.org or
www.potentiation.net.

The classic, definitive book on DNA activation, *Conscious Healing*, now updated and expanded with a wealth of empowering new information, is far more than the inspiring story of the development of a "revolutionary healing science" (*Nexus*).

An unparalleled synthesis of modern and ancient healing wisdom, this leading-edge text is essential reading for anyone interested in alternative medicine, energy healing, consciousness research, quantum biology, human evolution, or personal enlightenment.

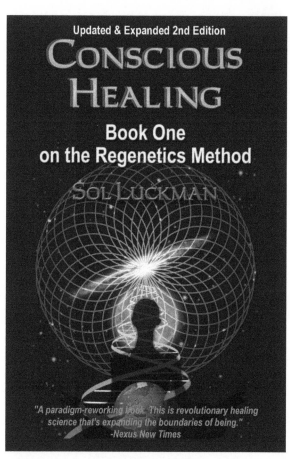

Updated & Expanded 2nd Edition

CONSCIOUS HEALING

Book One
on the Regenetics Method

SOL LUCKMAN

"A paradigm-reworking book. This is revolutionary healing science that's expanding the boundaries of being."
-Nexus New Times

Order your paperback or ebook copy today at
www.phoenixregenetics.org or
www.potentiation.net.

All DNA activations in the Regenetics Method employ notes from the ancient Solfeggio scale.

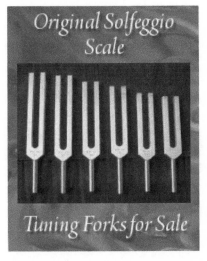

The Phoenix Center for Regenetics is proud to offer the six original Solfeggio frequencies in tuning forks made of the highest quality alum for excellent overtone production.

Purchase your Solfeggio scale tuning forks today at **www.phoenixregenetics.org** or **www.potentiation.net**.

The Regenetics Method of DNA activation can be life-changing not only for those who experience it, but equally for those who facilitate it.

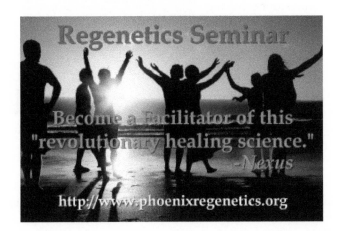

Learn more about Facilitator certification at **www.phoenixregenetics.org** or **www.potentiation.net**.

Could it be there's no such thing as the paranormal ... only infinite varieties of normal we've yet to understand?

From acclaimed author Sol Luckman comes *Snooze*, the riveting tale of one extraordinary boy's awakening to the world-changing reality of his dreams, winner of the 2015 National Indie Excellence Award for New Age Fiction and 2016 Readers' Favorite International Book Award Finalist in the Young Adult-Coming of Age category.

Join Max Diver, aka "Snooze," along the razor's edge of a quest to rescue his astronaut father from a fate stranger than death in the exotic, perilous Otherworld of sleep.

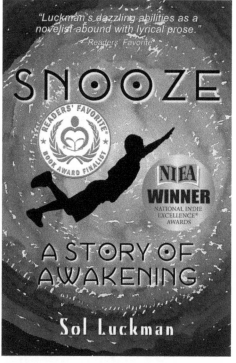

An insightful look at a plethora of paranormal subjects, from Sasquatch and lucid dreaming to time travel via the Bermuda Triangle, *Snooze* also shines as a work of literature featuring iconic characters, intense drama and breathless pacing to stir you wide awake!

"Luckman's dazzling abilities as a novelist abound with lyrical prose ... If you enjoy colorful characters, a fast-paced plot and stories that tug at your heart, this novel in eighty-four chapters is anything but a yawn."
—Readers' Favorite

Snooze is "a multi-dimensional, many-faceted gem of a read. From mysteries to metaphysics, entering the dream world, Bigfoot, high magic and daring feats of courage, this book has it all."
—Lance White, author of *Tales of a Zany Mystic*

"*Snooze* is a book for readers ready to awaken from our mass cultural illusion before we self-destruct. *Snooze* calls out for readers open to the challenging adventure of opening their minds." —Merry Hall, Co-Host of *Envision This*

Learn more at **www.CrowRising.com**.

Denis Johnson is the author of eight previous novels, one collection of short stories, three collections of poetry and one book of reportage. His novel *Tree of Smoke* won the 2007 National Book Award, and *Train Dreams* was a finalist for the 2012 Pulitzer Prize.

THE LAUGHING MONSTERS

Freetown, Sierra Leone. A city of heat and dirt, of guns and militia, where suspicion has become the law. Alone in its crowded streets, Captain Roland Nair has been given a single assignment. He must find Michael Adriko, maverick and warrior — also the man who has saved Nair's life three times, but risked it many more . . . The two have schemed, fought and profited together in the most hostile regions of the world. But on this new level — that of espionage, state secrets and treason — their loyalties will be tested to the limit.

Books by Denis Johnson
Published by Ulverscroft:

NOBODY MOVE

DENIS JOHNSON

THE LAUGHING
MONSTERS

Complete and Unabridged

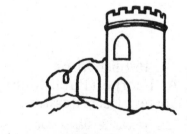

ULVERSCROFT
Leicester

First published in Great Britain in 2015 by
Harvill Secker
London

First Large Print Edition
published 2017
by arrangement with
Penguin Random House
London

A catalogue record for this book is available
from the British Library.

ISBN 978–1–4448–3120–7

Published by
F. A. Thorpe (Publishing)
Anstey, Leicestershire

Set by Words & Graphics Ltd.
Anstey, Leicestershire
Printed and bound in Great Britain by
T. J. International Ltd., Padstow, Cornwall

This book is printed on acid-free paper

For Charlie and Scout

For Charlie and Oscar

Acknowledgements

For assistance way beyond the call
of duty, the author thanks
Michele Thompson

ONE

Eleven years since my last visit and the Freetown airport still a shambles, one of those places where they wheel a staircase to the side of the plane and you step from European climate control immediately into the steam heat of West Africa. The shuttle to the terminal wasn't bad, but not air-conditioned.

Inside the building, the usual throng of fools. I studied the shining black faces, but I didn't see Michael's.

The PA spoke. Only the vowels came through. I called over the heads of the queue at the desk — 'Did I hear a page for Mr. Nair?'

'No, sir. No,' the man called back.

'Mr. Nair?'

'Nothing for such a name.'

A man in a dark suit and necktie said, 'Welcome, Mr. Naylor, to Sierra Leone,' and helped me through the mess and chatted with me all through customs, which didn't take long, because I'm all carry-on. He helped me outside to a clean white car, a Honda Prelude. 'And for me,' he said, with a

queasy-looking smile, 'two hundred dollars.' I gave him a couple of one-euro coins. 'But, sir,' he said, 'it's not enough today, sir,' and I told him to shut up.

The driver of the Honda wanted in the area of a million dollars. I said, 'Spensy mohnee!' and his face fell when he saw I knew some Krio. We reached an arrangement in the dozens. He couldn't go any lower because his heart was broken, he told me, by the criminal cost of fuel.

At the ferry there was trouble — a woman with a fruit cart, policemen in sky-blue uniforms throwing her goods into the bay while she screamed as if they were drowning her children. It took three cops to drag her aside as our car thumped over the gangway. I got out and went to the rail to catch the wet breeze. On the shore the uniforms crossed their arms over their chests. One of them kicked over the woman's cart, now empty. Back and forth she marched, screaming. The scene grew smaller and smaller as the ferry pulled out into the bay, and I crossed the deck to watch Freetown coming at us, a mass of buildings, many of them crumbling, and all around them a multitude of shadows and muddy rags trudging God knows where, hunched forward over their empty bellies.

At the Freetown dock I recognized a man, a skinny old Euro named Horst, standing beside a hired car with his hand shading his eyes against the sunset, taking note of the new arrivals. As our vehicle passed him I slumped in my seat and turned my face away. After we'd passed, I kept an eye on him. He got back in his car without taking on any riders.

Horst . . . His first name was something like Cosmo but not Cosmo. Leo, Rollo. I couldn't remember.

I directed Emil, my driver, to the Papa Leone, as far as I knew the only place to go for steady electric power and a swimming pool. As we pulled under the hotel's awning another car came at us, swerved, recovered, sped past with a sign in its window — SPLENDID DRIVING SCHOOL. This resembled commerce, but I wasn't feeling the New Africa. I locked eyes with a young girl loitering right across the street, selling herself. Poor and dirty, and very pretty. And very young. I asked Emil how many kids he had. He said there were ten, but six of them died.

Emil tried to change my mind about the hotel, saying the place had become 'very demoted.' But inside the electric lights burned, and the spacious lobby smelled clean, or poisonous, depending on your

5

opinion of certain chemicals, and everything looked fine. I'd heard the rebels had shot it out with the authorities in the hallways, but that had been a decade before, just after I'd run away, and I could see they'd patched it all up.

The clerk checked me in without a reservation, and then surprised me:

'Mr. Nair, a message.'

Not from Michael — from the management, in purple ink, welcoming me to 'the solution to all your problems,' and crafted in a very fine hand. It was addressed 'To Whom It May Concern.' Clipped to it was a slip of paper, instructions for getting online. The desk clerk said the internet was down but not always. Maybe tonight.

I had a Nokia phone, and I assumed I could get a local SIM card somewhere, but — the clerk said — not at this hotel. For the moment, I was pretty well cut off.

Good enough. I didn't feel ready for Michael Adriko. He was probably here at the Papa in a room right above my head, but for all I knew he hadn't come back to the African continent and he wouldn't, he'd only lured me here in one of his incomprehensible efforts to be funny.

★ ★ ★

The room was small and held that same aroma saying, 'All that you fear, we have killed.' The bed was all right. On the nightstand, on a saucer, a white candle stood beside a red-and-blue box of matches.

I'd flown down from Amsterdam through London Heathrow. I'd lost only an hour and I felt no jet lag, only the need of a little repair. I splashed my face and hung a few things and took my computer gear, in its yellow canvas carrier-kit, downstairs to the poolside.

On the way I stopped to make an arrangement with the barman about a double whiskey. Then at a poolside table in an environment of artful plants and rocks, I ordered a sandwich and another drink.

A woman alone a couple of tables away pressed her hands together and bowed her face toward her fingertips and smiled. I greeted her:

'How d'body?'

'D'body no well,' she said. 'D'body need you.'

I cracked my laptop and lit the screen. 'Not tonight.'

She didn't look in the least like a whore. She was probably just some woman who'd stopped in here to ease her feet and might as well seize a chance to sell her flesh. Right by the pool, meanwhile, a dance ensemble and

7

percussionist had all found their spots, and the patrons got quiet. Suddenly I could smell the sea. The night sky was black, not a star visible. A crazy drumming started up.

Off-line, I wrote to Tina:

I'm at the Papa Leone Hotel in Freetown. No sign of our old friend Michael.

I'm at the poolside restaurant at night, where there's an African dance group, I think they're from the Kissi Chiefdom (they look like street people), doing a number that involves falling down, lighting things on fire, and banging on wild conga drums. Now one guy's sort of raping a pile of burning sticks with his clothes on and people at nearby tables are throwing money. Now he's rolling all around beside the swimming pool, embracing this sheaf of burning sticks, rolling over and over with it against his chest. It's a bunch of kindling about half his size, all ablaze. I'm only looking for food and drink, I had no idea we'd be entertained by a masochistic pyromaniac. Good Lord, Dear Baby Girl, I'm at an African hotel watching a guy in flames, and I'm a little drunk because I think in West Africa it's best always to be

just a tiny bit that way, and the world is soft, and the night is soft, and I'm watching a guy

Across the large patio, Horst appeared and threaded himself toward me through the fire and haze. He was a tanned, dapper white-haired white man in a fishing vest with a thousand pockets and usually, I now remembered, tan walking shoes with white shoelaces, but I couldn't tell at the moment.

'Roland! It's you! I like the beard.'

'C'est moi,' I admitted.

'Did you see me at the quay? I saw you!' He sat down. 'The beard gives you gravitas.'

We bought each other a round. I told the barman, 'You're quick,' and tipped him a couple of euros. 'The staff are efficient enough. Who says this place has gone downhill?'

'It's no longer a Sofitel.'

'Who owns it?'

'The president, or one of his close companions.'

'What's wrong with it?'

He pointed at my machine. 'You won't get online.'

I raised my glass to him. 'So Horst is still coming around.'

'I'm still a regular. About six months per

year. But this time I've been kept home almost one full year, since last November. Eleven months.'

The entertainment got too loud. I adjusted my screen and put my fingers on the keyboard. Rude of me. But I hadn't asked him to sit down.

'My wife is quite ill,' he said, and he paused one second, and added, 'terminal,' with a sort of pride.

Meanwhile, two meters off, by the pool, the performer had set his shirt and pants on fire.

To Tina:

I saw a couple of US soldiers in weird uniforms at the desk when I checked in. This place is the only one in town that has electricity at night. It costs $145 a day to stay here.

Hey — the beard's coming off. It's no camouflage at all. I've already been recognized.

With the drumming and the whooping, who could talk? Still, Horst wouldn't let me off. He'd bought a couple of rounds, discussed his wife's disease . . . Time for questions. Beginning with Michael.

'What? Sorry. What?'

10

'I said to you: Michael is here.'

'Michael who?'

'Come on!'

'Michael Adriko?'

'Come on!'

'Have you seen him? Where?'

'He's about.'

'About where? Shit. Look. Horst. In a land of rumors, how many more do we need?'

'I haven't seen him personally.'

'What would Michael be here for?'

'Diamonds. It's that simple.'

'Diamonds aren't so simple anymore.'

'Okay, but we're not after simplicity, Roland. We're after adventure. It's good for the soul and the mind and the bank balance.'

'Diamonds are too risky these days.'

'You want to smuggle heroin? The drugs racket is terrible. It destroys the youth of a nation. And it's too cheap. A kilo of heroin nets you six thousand dollars US. A kilo of diamonds makes you a king.'

To Tina I wrote: Show's over now. Everyone appears uninjured. The whole area smells like gasoline.

'What do you think?' Horst said.

'What I think is, Horst — I think they'll snitch you. They'll sell you diamonds and then they'll snitch you, you know that,

11

because around here it's nothing but snitches.'

Maybe he took my point, because he stopped his stuff while I wrote to Tina:

I'm getting drunk with this asshole who used to be undercover Interpol. He looks far too old now to get paid for anything, but he still sounds like a cop. He calls me Roland like a cop.

At any point I might have asked his first name. Elmo?

Horst gave up, and we just drank. 'Israel,' he told me, 'has six nuclear-tipped missiles raised from the silos and pointing at Iran. Sometime during the next US election period — boom-boom Teheran. And then it's tit for tat, that's the Muslim way, my friend. Radiation all around.'

'They were saying that years ago.'

'You don't want to go home. Within ten years it will be just like here, a bunch of rubble. But our rubble here isn't radioactive. But you won't believe me until you check it with a Geiger counter.' The whiskey had washed away his European manner. He was a white-haired, red-faced, jolly elfin cannibal.

In the lobby we shook hands and said good night. 'Of course they'd *like* to snitch you,' he

said. He stood on his toes to get close to my left ear and whisper: 'That's why you don't go back the way you came.'

∗ ∗ ∗

Later I lay in the dark holding my pocket radio against the very same ear, listening with the other for any sound of the hotel's generator starting. A headache attacked me. I struck a stinky match, lit the candle, opened the window. The batting of insects against the screen got so insistent I had to blow out the flame. The BBC reported that a big storm with 120-kilometer-per-hour winds had torn through the American states of Virginia, West Virginia, and Ohio, and three million homes had suffered an interruption in the flow of their electricity.

Here at the Papa Leone, the power came up. The television worked. CCTV, the Chinese cable network, broadcasting in English. I went back to the radio.

The phones in Freetown emit that English ring-ring! ring-ring! The caller speaks from the bottom of a well:

'Internet working!'

Working! — always a bit of a thrill. My machine lay beside me on the bed. I played with the buttons, added a PS to Tina:

I drew cash on the travel account — 5K US. Credit cards still aren't trusted. Exchange rate in 02 was 250 leones per euro, and the largest bill was 100 leones. You had to carry your cash in a shopping bag, and some used shoeboxes. Now they want dollars. They'll settle for euros. They hate their own money.

I sent my e-mails, and then waited, and then lost the internet connection.

The BBC show was *World Have Your Say*, and the subject was boring.

The walls ceased humming and all went black as the building's generator powered down, but not before I had a short reply from Tina:

Don't go back the way you came.

Suddenly I had it. Bruno. Bruno Horst.

★ ★ ★

Around three that morning I woke and dressed in slacks, shirt, and slippers, and followed my Nokia's flashlight down eight flights to the flickering lobby. Nobody around. While I stood in the candle glow among large shadows, the lights came on and

the doors to both elevators opened and closed, opened and closed once more.

I found the night man asleep behind the desk and sent him out to find the girl I'd seen earlier. I watched while he crossed the street to where she slept on the warm tarmac. He looked one way, then the other, and waited, and finally nudged her with his toe.

I took an elevator upstairs, and in a few minutes he brought her up to my room and left her.

'You're welcome to use the shower,' I said, and her face looked blank.

Fifteen years old, Ivoirian, not a word of English, spoke only French. Born in the bush, a navel the size of a walnut, tied by some aunt or older sister in a hut of twigs and mud.

She took a shower and came to me naked and wet.

I was glad she didn't know English. I could say whatever I wanted to her, and I did. Terrible things. All the things you can't say. Afterward I took her downstairs and got her a taxi, as if she had somewhere to go. I shut the car's door for her and heard the old driver saying even before he put it in gear: 'You are a bad woman, you are a whore and a disgrace . . . ' but she couldn't understand any of it.

15

I woke to the sound of a groundskeeper whisking dead mayflies from the walk below my balcony with a small broom. Around six it had rained hard for fifteen minutes, knocking insects out of the sky, and I call these mayflies for convenience, but they seemed half cockroach as well. Later, in the lobby, when I asked the concierge what sort of creature this was, he said, 'In-seck.'

Michael had called and left a message at the front desk. I asked the clerk, 'Why didn't you put him through to the phone in my room?' and the young man scratched at the desk with his fingernail and examined his mark and seemed to forget the question until he said, 'I don't know.'

Michael wanted to meet me at 1600. At the Scanlon. That said a lot about his circumstances.

I wandered into the Papa's restaurant twenty minutes before the ten o'clock conclusion of the free buffet, the last person down to breakfast, and I found the staff thronging the metal warming pans, forking stuff onto plates for themselves. So this is what they eat, I thought, and by turning up with my own plate here I'm sort of fishing this fat banger sausage right out of

16

somebody's mouth. You half-American pig. I took some fried potatoes too — the word for them is 'Irish' — and then I couldn't eat, but I ate anyway, because they were watching me. Under their compassionate gazes I ate every crumb.

It was October, with temperatures around thirty Celsius most of the daytime, not unbearable in the shade, as always very humid. Right now we had a cool sea breeze, a few bright clouds in a blue sky, and a white sunshine that by noon would crash down like a hot anvil. The only other patron was a young American-looking guy in civilian clothing with a tattoo of a Viking's head on his forearm.

The power was up. American country music flowed through the PA speakers. I took the latter half of my coffee to a table near the television to catch the news on Chinese cable, but the local network was playing, and all I got was a commercial message from Guinness. In this advertisement, an older brother returns home to the African bush from his successful life in the city. He's drinking Guinness Draught with his younger brother in the sentimental glow of lamps they don't actually possess in the bush. Big-city brother hands little bush brother a bus ticket: 'Are you ready to drink at the table of men?' The

young one takes it with gratitude and determination, saying, 'Yes!' The announcer speaks like God:

'Guinness. Reach for greatness.'

⋆ ⋆ ⋆

After breakfast I went out front with my computer kit belted to my chest like a baby carrier. Sweat pressed through my shirt, but the kit was waterproof.

The only car out front had its bonnet raised. A few young men waited astride their okadas, that is, motorcycles of the smallest kind, 90cc jobs, for the most part. I chose one called Boxer, a Chinese brand. 'Boxer-man. Do you know the Indian market? Elephant market?'

'Elephant!' he cried. 'Let's go!' He slapped the seat behind him, and I got on, and we zoomed toward the Indian market over streets still muddy and slick from last night's downpour, lurching and dodging, missing the rut, missing the pothole, missing the pedestrian, the bicycle, the huge devouring face of the oncoming truck — missing them all at once, and over and over. On arrival at the market with its mural depicting Ganesha, Hindu lord of knowledge and fire, I felt more alive but also murdered.

The elephant-faced god remained, but Ganesha Market had a new title — Y2K Supermarket.

'I'm waiting for you,' my pilot told me.

'No. Finish,' I said, but I knew he'd wait.

I left the Boxer at the front entrance and went out by the side. I believe in the underworld they call this maneuver the double-door.

Outside again I found a small lane full of shops, but I didn't know where I was. I made for the bigger street to my left, walked into it, was almost struck down, whirled this way by an okada rider, that way by a bicycle. I'd lost my rhythm for this environment, and now I was miffed with the traffic as well as hot from walking, and I was lost. For forty-five minutes I blundered among nameless mud-splashed avenues before I found the one I wanted and the little establishment with its hoarding: ELVIS DOCUMENTS.

Three solar panels lay on straw mats in the dirt walkway where people had to step around them. The hoarding read, 'Offers: photocopying, binding, typing, sealing, receipt/invoice books, computer training.'

Inside, a man sat at his desk amid the tools of his livelihood — a camera on a tripod, a bulky photocopier, a couple of computers — all tangled in power cords.

He rose from his office chair, a leather swivel model missing its casters, and said, 'Welcome. How can I be of service?' And then he said, 'Ach!' as if he'd swallowed a seed. 'It's Roland Nair.'

And it was Mohammed Kallon. It didn't seem possible. I had to look twice.

'Where's Elvis?'

'Elvis? I forget.'

'But you remember me. And I remember you.'

He looked sad, also frightened, and made his face smile. White teeth, black skin, unhealthy yellow eyeballs. He wore a white shirt, brown slacks cinched with a shiny black plastic belt. Plastic house slippers instead of shoes.

'What's the problem here, Mohammed? Your store smells like a toilet.'

'Are we going to quarrel?'

I didn't answer.

Everything was visible in his face — in the smile, the teary eyes. 'We're on the same side now, Roland, because in the time of peace, you know, there can be only one side.' He opened for me a folding chair beside his desk while he resumed his swivel. 'I might have known you were in Freetown.'

I didn't sit. 'Why?'

'Because Michael Adriko is here. I saw

20

him. The deserter.'

'You call Michael a deserter?'

'Hah!'

'If he's a deserter, then call me a deserter too.'

'Hah!'

I felt irritated, ready to argue. Mohammed was still a good interrogator. 'Listen,' I said, 'Michael's not from any of these Leonean clans, any of the chiefdoms. I think he's originally from Uganda. So — if he left here suddenly back then, he didn't desert.'

'Can't you sit down to talk?'

'Bruno Horst is around.'

'I do believe it. So are you.'

'Is he working for one of the outfits?'

'How would I know?'

'I don't know how you'd know. But you'd know.'

'And who does Roland Nair work for?'

'Just call me Nair. Nair is in Freetown strictly on personal business. And it really does stink in here.'

'Who do you work for?'

I shrugged.

'Anyone. As usual,' he said.

I wasn't a torturer. I'd never stood ankle-deep in the fluids of my victims . . . 'I can't imagine how you ended up here,' I told him. 'You're all wrong for this.'

'Holy cow! All wrong for what?'

'You're a dirty player.'

Mohammed had lost his smile. 'I hear the pot saying to the kettle, 'You are black.' Do you know that expression?'

He had a point. 'All right,' I said, 'we're both black,' and it struck me as funny.

Mohammed found his smile again. 'Nair, I don't want to get off on the wrong foot after so long a time, honestly — because it's almost the moment when you take me to lunch!'

'Lunch isn't out of the question,' I said. 'But first give me a few minutes with your computers.'

'None of them are working.'

'The computers downstairs.'

'There's no downstairs.' He was a terrible liar. I stared until he understood. 'Bloody hell!'

'Let's have a look inside your closet.'

'Every day brings new surprises!' He looked as if he'd eaten something evil and delicious. 'You're with NIIA?'

'Let's follow the protocol.' The protocol called for his getting out of my way.

He sat back down and busied himself with a pile of receipts, bursting with a silly, private glee, while I went across the space to his mop closet, which stood open and which also served as a toilet, with a slop-bucket covered

by a wooden board and a roll of brownish paper on the floor beside it. That accounted for the stench in the place.

I consulted the readout on my coder, a unit that fits on a key chain. The eight-digit code changes every ninety seconds. I entered the closet and shut the door behind me, and by the glow of my Nokia I moved aside a patch on the rear wall and keyed the digits into the interlock and pushed the wall open and went down the metal stairs as the panel clicked shut behind me without my assistance.

Here the four lights were burning.

I'd entered this sunken place more than once, long ago. It had been built to American standards, not in meters, but in feet: ten by sixteen in area, with concrete walls eight feet in height, and one dozen metal stair steps leading down. A battery bank in a wire cage bolted to the concrete floor, an electric bulb in another such cage in each of the concrete walls. A desk, a chair, both metal, both bolted down. On the desk, two machines — much smaller units than we'd used a dozen years before.

I sat down and took from my carrier-kit an accessory disguised as a cigarette lighter, a NATO-issued device similar to a USB stick, with the algorithms built in. It actually makes a flame. I held it to my face and scanned my

iris and stuck it into the side of the machine in front of me and powered up and logged on. Through the NATO Intel proxy I sent a Nothing To Report — but I sent it twice, which warned Tina to expect a message at her personal e-address. For this exchange Tina would know to shelve the military algorithms. We used PGP encryption. As the name promised, it's pretty good protection.

I logged off of NIIA and attached my own keyboard to the console and went through the moves and established a Virtual Private Network and sent:

Get file 3TimothyA for me. Your NEMCO password will work.

Nothing now but the sound of my breath and the prayers of three small cooling fans. The fans cooled the units, not the user. I wiped my face and neck with my kerchief. It came away drenched. My breath came faster and faster. My Nokia's clock showed a bit after 1300 — noon in Amsterdam. I hadn't allowed time for getting lost. Tina might have gone to lunch. It irked me that I couldn't slow my breath.

But Tina was at her desk, and she was ready. I sent: 'I'm ready for those dirty pictures.'

Within two minutes it was done.

I believe that by making this transaction the two of us risked life sentences. But only one of us knew it. Like anyone in the field of intelligence, Tina asked no questions. Besides, she loved me.

I came up the stairs and into Elvis Documents with my kit clutched against my chest, as if it held the goods, but it didn't. A Cruzer device snugged in the waistline seam of my trousers held the goods.

Mohammed waited in his broken chair, his gaze fixed studiously in another direction.

'Let's eat,' I said.

★　★　★

We ate down the street at the Paradi. Decent Indian fare.

During the late nineties and for a few years after, when this place had drawn the interest of the media, Kallon had worked as a stringer for the AP and as a CIA informant, and then the CIA had levered him into the Leonean secret service to inform from down in the nasty heart of things, and he had hurt a lot of people. And now he'd got himself a job with NATO.

That the CIA once ran Mohammed Kallon was, I acknowledge, my own supposition,

prompted merely by my sharp nose for a certain perfume. Snitches stink.

I let Kallon order for both of us while I went to the men's lavatory. I slipped shut the lock and took my passport from my shirt pocket and the Cruzer from the seam in my trousers. I felt desperate to be rid of it. Cowardly — but the situation felt all too new.

Normally I carry my passport in a ziplock plastic bag. I removed the passport from the bag and replaced it with the Cruzer, wound the Cruzer tightly in the plastic, and looked for a hiding place.

The toilets, two of them, were set into the floor, each with a foot pedal for flushing. I examined the tiles on all four walls, fiddled with the mirror, ran my fingers around the windowsill. I tried lifting the posts of the divider between the two toilets — one came loose from the floor. With my finger I scratched a delve at the bottom of its hole, dropped the tiny package in, and replaced the post to cover it.

For the sake of realism, I pressed the pedal on one of the toilets. It didn't flush. The other one sprayed my shoe. I washed my hands at the sink and rejoined Mohammed Kallon.

Over lunch we talked about nothing really, except when I asked him outright, 'What's

going on?' and he said, 'Michael Adriko is going on.'

★ ★ ★

Having nowhere else to be, I arrived an hour early at the Scanlon, a hotel more central to Freetown than the better ones. When the region had drawn journalists, this was where many of them had lodged, a four-story place sunk in the diesel fumes and, when the weather was dry, in the hovering dust.

Inside the doors it was mute and dim — no power at the moment please sir — but crowded with souls. In the middle of the lobby stood a figure in a two-piece jogging suit of royal purple velour, a large man with a bald, chocolate, bullet-shaped head, which he wagged from side to side as he blew his nose loudly and violently into a white hand towel. People were either staring or making sure they didn't. This was Michael Adriko.

Michael folded his towel and draped it over his shoulder as I came to him. Though we had an appointment in an hour, he seemed to take my appearance here as some kind of setback, and his first word to me was, '*What*-what.' Michael often uses this expression. It serves in any number of ways. A blanket translation would be 'Bloody hell.'

27

'Thanks for meeting me at the airport.'

'I was there! Where were you? I watched everybody getting off the plane and I never saw you. I swear it!' He always lies.

He put out his monumental hand and gave mine a gentle shake, with a finger-snap.

'For goodness' sake, Nair, your beard is gray!'

'And my hair is still black as a raven's.'

'Do ravens have beards?' He had his feet under him now. 'I like it.' Before I could stop him, he reached out and touched it. 'How old are you?'

'Too close to forty to talk about.'

'Thirty-nine?'

'Thirty-eight.'

'Same as me! No. Wait. I'm thirty-seven.'

'You're thirty-six.'

'You're right,' he said. 'When did I stop counting?'

'Michael, you've got an American accent. I can't believe it.'

'And I can't believe you bring a lovely full beard to the tropics.'

'It's coming off right away.'

'So is my accent,' he said and turned to the waiter and spoke in thick Krio I couldn't follow, but I got the impression at least one of us was getting a chicken sandwich.

I asked the clerk if a barber was available,

and he shook his head and told me, 'Such a person does not exist.'

I asked Michael, 'Do you still carry your clippers?'

Smiling widely, he caressed his baldness. 'I'm always groomed. Send the sandwich to my room,' he told the clerk. 'Two three zero.'

'I know your room,' the clerk said.

'Come, Nair. Let's chop it down with the clippers. You'll feel younger. Come. Come.' Michael was moving off, calling over his shoulder to the desk clerk, 'Also bottled water!' Looking backward, he collided with a striking woman — African, light-skinned — who'd tacked a bit, it seemed to me, in order to arrange the collision. He looked down at her and said, '*What*-what,' and it was plain they were friends, and more.

It didn't surprise me she was beautiful, also young — not long out of university, I guessed. Such women succumbed to Michael quickly, and soon moved on.

She wore relief-worker or safari garb, the khaki cargo pants and fishing vest and light, sturdy hiking shoes. On this basis, I misjudged her. Really, that's all it was — I judged her according to her clothes, and the judgment was false. But the first impression was strong.

Michael looked put out with her. 'Every-body's here at once.'

'Not for long — I'm off exploring.' She sounded American.

'Exploring where?' He was smiling, but he didn't like it.

'I'm looking for postcards.'

I said, 'You'll have to go to the Papa for that.'

'Yes, the Papa Leone Hotel,' Michael explained, 'but it's too far.'

'All right, I'll take a car.'

Michael sighed.

'Don't pout,' she said. 'I'll be back in an hour.'

'Wait. Meet my friend Roland Nair. This is Davidia St. Claire.'

'Another friend? Everybody's his friend.' Davidia St. Claire was speaking to me. 'Did he say Olin?'

'My given name is Roland, but I never use it. Please call me Nair.'

'Nair is better,' Michael informed her. 'It's sharper. Look,' he went on, 'at the Papa, get your nails done or something, kill some time, and let's all meet at the Bawarchi for dinner — early dinner, six p.m. We all should know each other, because Nair is my closest friend.'

I said, 'He saved my life.'

'Oui?' Her eyebrows went up.

Michael said, 'C'est vrai.'

'More than once,' I said.

'Three times.'

'He kept me alive on a daily basis,' I said, and his woman looked me over — as if I explained something she'd wondered about, that kind of look, and I didn't understand it. I said, 'Are you Ivoirian?'

It made her laugh. 'Who, me?'

'I thought because of the French.'

'That's just for fun. I'm a Colorado girl.'

'I'm half American myself,' I said. I offered my hand. She laid two fingers on my wrist and seemed to watch my face as if to gauge the effect of her touch, which stirred me, in fact, like an anthem. She looked very directly into my eyes and said, 'Hello.'

And then, 'Goodbye.'

★　★　★

In room 230 I noticed a rollerbag I judged not quite in Michael's style, but nothing that clearly said the woman Davidia slept here.

Michael flipped the wall switch. 'Still no power!' He went to the dresser, opened a drawer, and turned to me gripping a braided leather whip about a meter in length, knotted at the narrow end. He grasped its handle and

31

pulled out a dagger. 'Nobody will know about my blade!'

'But, Michael — they'll know about your whip.'

'Well, let them know at least something. It's fair to be warned. Look how sharp. I could shave your beard with this.'

'Show me to the clippers, please.'

While I ran down the battery on his clippers at the sink, doing my best by the light through the small window, Michael cleaned his teeth, working away with a brush from whose other end a small spider dangled and swung.

There was another toothbrush sticking out of a water glass, and a tube of facial cream, and two kinds of deodorant. 'Tell me your friend's name again.'

He spat in the sink and said, 'I've got a million friends,' just like an American. 'Look!' he cried. 'It's Roland Nair emerging from the bush.' He resumed his brushing — still talking, foaming at the mouth. 'You have gray in the beard, but not on your head.'

'A couple of days with you should fix that.' I spoke to his reflection, side by side with my own.

I am Scandinavian but have black hair and gray eyes, or blue, according to the environment. If I wanted my appearance to

impress, I'd stay away from the sun and keep a very white complexion to go with my raven locks, that would be my look. But I like the sun on my face, even in the tropics.

Michael has handsome features, a brief, aquiline nose, high cheekbones, wide, inquiring eyes — like one of those Ethiopian models — and as for his lips, I can't say. You'd have to follow him for days to get a look at his mouth in repose. Always laughing, never finished talking. A hefty, muscular frame, but with an angular grace. You know what I mean: not a thug. Still — lethal. I'd never seen him being lethal, but in 2004 on the Kabul-Kandahar road somebody shot at us, and he told me to stay down and went over a hill, and there was more shooting, and soon — none. And then he came back over the hill and said, 'I just killed two people,' and we went on.

Once he showed me a photograph, a little boy with Michael Adriko's face, his hand in the hand of a man he said was his father. Michael's father had Arab blood apparent in his features, and so Michael — well, there's a dash of cream in the coffee, invisible to me, but obvious to his fellow Africans. Sometimes he introduced me to them as his brother. As far as I could tell, he was never disbelieved.

He stroked his teeth with vigor. The spider

whipped around on its strand. He rinsed his brush and the spider was gone.

Now he watched me comb my hair. I think it fascinated him because he was bald. He laughed. 'Your vanity doesn't make you look more lovely. It only makes you look more vain.' At that moment, the ceiling fixture flickered to life. 'Power's back. Let's see the news.'

He sat on the bed and punched buttons on the television's wand, pushing the device toward the screen as if to toss the signal at it. 'News. News. News.' Al Jazeera had sports. The soccer scores. He settled for Nigerian cable, some sort of amateur singing competition, and then he untied his very clean red jogging shoes and kicked them off and set about massaging both feet, each with one hand. Vivid yellow socks.

'Michael — '

Michael laughed at the television.

'Michael, it's time you told me something. You contact me, you get me down here — '

'You contacted me! You said, What's going on, I said, Come down to SL and I'll show you a plan.'

'Don't *show* me the plan. *Tell* me the plan.'

But I'd lost him. He watched the screen with his mouth half open, his hands clutching

his feet. The commercial ad from Guinness, the two black brothers, the bus ticket out of the bush . . . By the power brewed into this drink big-city brother frees his sibling from a curse that neither of them understands, and side by side they set out for the Kingdom of Civilization. Michael's eyes glistened and he smiled a wide, tight smile. I'd often seen him driven to tears — this was what it looked like. Something had caught him by the heart. Brother for brother, reaching for greatness. Michael was moved. Michael was weeping.

As quickly as the ad was over he leapt into the bathroom, splashed his face at the sink, blew his nose into the hand towel, loomed in the doorway.

'Here's the plan: I am a new man, and I plan to do what a new man does.'

Now he stood in the middle of the room, offering me tomorrow in his two outstretched hands. 'Do you want a plan? I'm just going to give you results. You'll live like a king. A compound by the beach. Fifty men with AKs to guard you. The villagers come to you for everything. They bring their daughters, twelve years old — virgins, Nair, no AIDS from these girls. You'll have a new one every night. Five hundred men in your militia. You know you want it. They dance at night, a big

bonfire, and the magic men come and stretch their arms to the length of a python, and change into all kinds of animals, and drums pounding, and naked dancers, all just for you, Nair! We want it. That's what we want. And you know it's here. There's no place else on earth where we can have it.'

'This land of chaos, despair — '

'And in the midst of it, we make ourselves unreachable. A man can choose a valley, one with narrow entrances — defensible entries — and claim it as his nation, like Rhodes in Rhodesia — '

'I can't believe I hear a black man talking like this.'

'We'll have the politicians kissing our feet. Every four years we'll assassinate the president.'

'The same president?'

'It's term limits! We'll be the ones controlling that.'

'How many men with AKs?'

'How many did I say? A thousand. Nair, I'll come around on my launch on Sundays. Run it up onto the sand of your protected beach. Our children will play together. Our wives will be fat. We'll play chess and plan campaigns.'

'You don't play chess.'

'You haven't seen me for seven years.'

'Man — you don't play chess.'

He looked at me, wounded. So naked in his face. 'That's why it has to be you. You're the one who knows those games.'

'And your games too, right?'

'It has to be you.'

I said, 'This better not be about diamonds.'

'Not diamonds. Not this time. This time we concern ourselves with metals and minerals.'

'And aren't diamonds actually minerals?'

'This is why I can never make a point,' Michael said, 'because you query the details like some kind of master interrogator.'

'Sorry. Is it gold, then?'

'I tell you now: Stay away from the gold here, unless I say otherwise. The gold around here is fake. You'd see that the minute you looked at a kilo bar of it — but by the time they give you a look, you're already in a dark place with bad people.'

'I'll wait for your signal.'

He sat beside me on the bed and placed a hand on my shoulder. 'I want you to understand me. I have this mapped from point A to point Z. And, Nair — point Z is going to be marvelous. Did I ever tell you about the time I saved the Ghanaian president's life?'

It made me uncomfortable when he sat so close, but it was just an African thing. I said,

'Michael, what about the girl? Who is she to you?'

'She's American.'

'She told me that herself.'

'I heard her telling you.'

'Who is she, Michael?'

'More will be revealed.'

This was his style, his tiresome, unchangeable way. Information was an onion, to be peeled back in layers.

'What about you? What's your passport?'

'Ghana,' he said, and he didn't look happy about it. 'Ghana will always welcome me.'

I shrugged away his heavy hand and got up. 'Enough of Michael's nonsense. Let's get a drink.'

'Prior to sixteen hundred,' he said, 'I drink only bottled water.'

'As they say, it's sixteen hundred somewhere.' I checked my phone. 'Here, as a matter of fact.'

'I stink! Get out while I shower.'

Looking down at him now — 'Final question: What about Congo gold?'

'Nair! — you're so far ahead of me.'

'If I was ahead of you, I'd know what I'm doing in Freetown instead of Congo, where all the gold is.'

'The important thing is that you came without knowing why.'

'I know why I came.'

'But not why I asked you. You came without an explanation.'

'You'd only lie to me, Michael.'

'For security purposes, perhaps. Yes. For your protection in transit. But we're friends. We don't lie to each other.' He believed it.

★   ★   ★

As I made for the elevator, the lights died in the hallway. I took the stairs. Candles at the front desk, in the lobby, the big dining room. In the bar, the smell of burning paraffin, the stench of cologne overlying human musk. Voices from the dark — laughter — candlelit smiles. I ordered a martini, and it tasted just like one.

Tina strayed into my mind. I drank quickly and ordered another.

Why hadn't I simply loaded the goods into my Cruzer in Amsterdam, and left Tina out of things? That seemed simple enough — now. But I'd been sent here to Freetown on an NIIA errand, and I had no idea what sort of last-minute scrutiny the powers might have authorized. Anything at all seemed possible, including my being called aside at airport security and confronted with a couple of NIIA comptrollers donning latex gloves.

Afraid of some kind of search, I'd made Tina some kind of patsy.

After I drained the second glass and ate the second olive — really, all would be well. Many people keep watch. Nobody sees. It takes a great deal to waken their curiosity. NATO, the UN, the UK, the US — poker-faced, soft-spoken bureaucratic pandemonium. They're mad, they're blind, they're heedless, and not one of them cares, not one of them.

I could have reasoned all this out from the start. But I'm a coward, and I couldn't bear living alone in the abyss. Therefore Tina, unaware, lived in it beside me.

Perhaps Tina and I would be married on my return, after I'd met my contact and sold the goods and made money enough for several honeymoons, and after I'd been relieved of my current duty, which was to report on the activities and, if possible, the intentions of Michael Adriko.

★ ★ ★

From half the distance down into my third martini, I heard Michael's voice in the lobby — 'What happened to my sandwich?'

The desk clerk followed him. 'It's coming to the room, sir.'

'Send it to the bar, will you?'

He took the vacant stool beside mine and ordered a Guinness. I said, 'Really? Guinness?'

'Guinness is good for you. Let's sit alone.'

I joined him at a table with my martini. Two more sips, and I was ready to take him on.

'Talk to me, Miguel. Talk, or I walk.'

'I'm here to talk,' he said. 'We're talking.' But all he did with his mouth was pull on his beer.

'This place is a dump. What's wrong with the Papa Leone?'

'Too many people know me there.'

'Right. You're broke.'

'I'm on a budget. Is that dishonorable?'

'It's troubling.'

'Why trouble yourself? Is it really your problem?'

'It is if I'm in business with you, because I'll end up living in this hovel. I can't run back and forth.'

'That's your choice, Nair. Don't blame me.'

'*Am* I in business with you?'

'That's also your choice.'

I took a breath and counted to five. I released a delirious sigh. 'What about the girl? Is she with us?'

'I met her in Colorado.'

'Congratulations.'

'Thanks. I'm a lucky man.'

'Who is she?'

'More will be revealed.' A lighter flared across the room, somebody starting a cigarette in a group of five white men. Michael cocked his head in that direction, not looking there, his face full of conspiracy. 'Now, who are these fellows?'

'Pilots. Russian. They work for the charter outfits.'

'They don't look like civilian pilots. They're all young, all fit. Why doesn't at least one of them have a beer belly? Look at the haircuts — regulation.'

'All right, very good. Who are they?'

Suddenly he stood up and strode over to their table. He spoke. They replied, and he came back with an unlit cigarette between his teeth and sat down again. 'It's a Rothmans,' he said. 'Australian.'

'You're still smoking?'

'Now and then. But everything in moderation.' He took up the candle between us and lit his Rothmans and sat back and blew smoke over my head. 'Nair, I've got people on my trail.'

'These guys?'

'It could be anyone.'

'Are you in trouble? What's your situation?'

'I'll fill you in eventually.'

'Stop it! Jesus!' I was the loudest one in the room. I lowered my tone, but I leaned in to his face. 'I expected you to be dealing with the big men. Moving money around. Dispensing government contracts, you know? Contracts, not contraband. Diverted aid, siphoned oil revenue, that kind of thing. Money, Michael. Money. Not pebbles and powders.'

'Don't let your speech get so strong, mate. There's plenty of time for plenty of developments. Let's enjoy the moment.' He mashed his cigarette in the candle's dish and looked away and entered a personal silence.

You had to be careful with him. For hurt feelings, Michael would stop the whole show.

I waited him out. It never took long.

'It's been seven years since we saw each other, Nair. I'm thirty-six years old now. I'm changed, I'm different. I'm new.' He turned toward me fully and placed two clenched fists on the table as if in evidence of his newness. 'I left Afghanistan four years ago. I underwent training for two years at Fort Bragg, in North Carolina, after which I was transferred to Fort Carson, in Colorado. At Fort Carson I worked as a trainer for internationals, mostly from South America, sometimes from the Middle East. They were confined to the post,

and whenever I was part of the training team for an international group, I was also kept on the grounds. Between groups, yes, I could go into town in civilian clothes. On the post I wore a US Army uniform with a sergeant's hash marks. But I was not in the US Army.'

A waiter came with a sandwich on a plate. Michael ignored him. He set it on the table. Michael ignored it.

'They promised me permanent US residency, Nair. They lied. They told me I was on a path to US citizenship. They lied. They said I would enter the US Army as an officer and go as far as my talents could take me. They lied.'

He waited for comment. I provided none. The white men across the room were drinking like Russians. They laughed like Russians.

'Listen to me, Nair. I can build you a bomb. Just give me five minutes, I hardly have to move from this spot. Just bring me matches, Christmas lights, and sugar. I can shoot a man from one thousand meters. I've done it. I am a man of courage and discipline, and the reward for that is becoming a thug for hire. A goon, a pawn, a cog in a robot who is programmed only to tell you lies.'

'Sure. We're all getting older and wiser. That's sort of my point.'

'I've looked at every opportunity for changing my situation, and I've chosen the best one.'

'Give me a piece of the plan. Anything.'

'First of all,' he said, 'we'll go to Uganda for my wedding.'

'Oh, God. Should I feel somewhat enlightened, or further confused?'

'Right. I'm engaged.'

'Not for the first time.'

'But for the last. I told you — I'm a new man.'

'Is that what I'm here for? And nothing else?'

'It's important that we keep things need-to-know and take things one step at a time. Nair, please, you've got to trust me. Remember — once or twice, didn't we make a lot of money?'

'We made a lot of money for guys in their twenties. Now we're grown-ups. We should be getting rich. Are you asking me to settle for less?'

'I'm not asking you to settle for less.' He gathered himself, so to speak, around his bottle of Guinness, and went to his depths to collect his words. 'Here is my promise to you: we are going to get rich.'

His eyes were steady. I believed him. Or anyway I was tired, tired of the struggle to

disbelieve. 'Good enough,' I said.

'So now, let's go. Let's have some dinner with my fiancée.'

As we rose from our seats, I took in the group of possible Russians — now Michael had me doing it — all of them youngish, poised, and trim. I heard one say, 'Are ya lovin' it!'

Michael left his sandwich. I drained my glass and surrendered to the hour. After all, I was getting paid for this.

★ ★ ★

As soon as we'd ordered our drinks at the Bawarchi — we'd come early; Davidia hadn't arrived — Michael started picking at a point. 'Who contacted who?'

'I had your address at Fort Carson, so you must have contacted me first, or I wouldn't have known your whereabouts.'

'Yes, yes — but after more than a year of silence between us, I had a letter from you that was forwarded from Fort Carson at the beginning of August.'

'Forwarded to what location?'

'And then I answered you, and I said, "Come to beautiful Sierra Leone!" '

'Maybe this time around, I contacted you first. Is any of this important?'

'Everything's important.'

Judging by the throng of Europeans, we could expect good food here. It was a spacious Indian place on the outskirts of town, on the beach — open-air, excepting a thatched roof — with a cooling sea breeze and the surf washing softly within earshot. The beach was fine white damp sand, like table salt. In fifteen minutes it would be too dark to make it out.

Michael's suspicions touched everyone. Now he pointed out a middle-aged Euro at the bar. 'CIA. I know him.'

'I can only see his back.'

'He was the head of the skeleton staff at the embassy in Monrovia. I knew him then.'

'You? When?'

'When Charles Taylor held the East.'

'You would have been — thirteen? Twelve?'

His face came under a cloud. 'You don't know about my life.'

In an instant the day ended, night came down, and the many voices around us, for the space of ten seconds, went quiet. A few hundred meters away the buildings began, but not a single light shone from the powerless city, and the outcry coming from the void wasn't so much from horns and engines, but rather more from humans and their despairing animals. Meanwhile, waiters

went from table to table lighting tapers in tall glass chimneys.

And as soon as they'd made everything right, Davidia St. Claire entered the scene, slender, elegant, wearing an African dress. She had the usual effect of one of Michael's women. He wouldn't have had one who didn't. Even in the Third World he managed to find them, at fashion shows and photo shoots, at diplomatic cocktail parties — at church. The gazes followed behind her as if she swept them along with her hands.

Standing up for her, I knocked my chair over backward. Michael, sitting, extended his foot and caught it with his toe, and I was able to set it right before it clattered to the slate floor.

She laughed. 'That's quite an act.'

'In honor of your dress,' Michael said. I held her chair for her, and he added, 'Nair will hold your chair.'

'I just bought it at the shop at the Papa Leone. It's from the Tisio Valley.' She modeled for us, turning this way and that. The dress was mostly white, with a floral pattern, perhaps red — it was hard to say by candlelight — ankle-length, sleeveless and low cut and soft and clinging. I was aware, everybody was aware, of her arms and hands, and the insteps of her sandaled feet, and her

48

toes. She dropped her shopping bag and sat down and smiled.

'It's almost as wonderful as you.' Michael took both her hands in his own, leaning close. 'Such eyes. How did they fit such enormous eyes into your beautiful face? They had to boil your skull to make it flexible to expand the sockets for those beautiful eyes.'

He was trying to embarrass her, I guessed. She didn't blink. 'Thank you, such a compliment.'

Davidia wore her hair short and almost natural, but not all the way, not tightly kinked, rather relaxed into close curls. She was of medium height, more graceful than voluptuous. She had a face I'd call the West African type, a wide face, sexy, cute, with a broad nose, full lips, soft chin, a child's big eyes, and she looked out from deep behind them with something other than a child's openness.

Michael took over and ordered for us all, a little of everything, more than anybody could have eaten. Two youthful waiters both wanted the honor of serving us — serving Davidia — competing for it with a kind of stifled viciousness. Davidia seemed to accept this as her right.

As striking as she was, she had an unformed, girlish quality, and I was surprised

to learn she'd interrupted her pursuit of a PhD to put in time at the Institute for Policy Studies, and more surprised to learn she'd interrupted all of that for Michael Adriko. I counted back, and this was the fourth fiancée he'd introduced me to. He didn't ask them to marry him. He asked them to get engaged.

Michael and I both talked a lot during dinner — competing to show off, I suppose, like our waiters. Michael volunteered non-facts from his store of misinformation. 'Nair has family in South Carolina.'

'Georgia,' I said. 'Atlanta, Georgia.'

'Family?'

'Everybody but me and my father.'

'His father is Swiss.'

'Danish,' I said. 'I'm half Danish.'

Michael was about to speak, but Davidia said, 'Quiet, Michael,' and then, 'I don't think I've ever met anybody from Denmark.'

'Denmark is misunderstood. I'm not sure I understand it myself.'

'I don't know what that means,' she said. 'How did you and Michael meet — may I ask?'

'We met at Fort Carson.'

'Were you in the military?'

'No.'

'Good.'

Michael said, 'When I met Nair here in 2001, he was with NATO.'

'NATO? Here? This isn't exactly the North Atlantic.'

'NATO had people here two weeks after nine-eleven,' I said.

'Are you still with them? What do you do now?'

I handed her a business card from my wallet. 'Budget and fiscal.'

'Who's 'Technology Partnerships'?'

'We crunch numbers for corporate entities interested in partnering on large projects with the public sector. In the EU, that is. We're not quite global. It's dull stuff. But I get around quite a bit.'

Michael said, 'When we met, Nair was with NIIA.'

She waited until I said, 'NATO Intelligence Interoperability Architecture.'

'A spook!'

'Nobody says spook anymore.'

'I just did.'

'In any case, I wasn't one. I sent cables in plain English. Just comparing the project to the schedule, so they could revise the schedule to fit the project and go home winners every weekend.'

'And what was the project?'

'Boring stuff.'

'Nair had something to do with laying fiber-optic cable for the CIA.'

'NATO doesn't deal with the CIA,' I said.

'It was American stuff you were putting in the ground, don't try to fool me.'

'All I did was wander around Sierra Leone like an idiot.'

'And after that,' Michael said, 'Afghanistan.'

'I was an idiot there as well.'

'I can vouch for that,' he told Davidia. 'That's where I found him after a year's separation, in Jalalabad, driving a stolen UN car.'

'You people!' she said.

'What a baby I was. I thought I was Colonel Stoddart or somebody.'

'Stoddart?'

Michael said, 'He got beheaded in Afghanistan.'

'In the nineteenth century,' I said, to dispel her shock.

'Oh, Stoddart — yes — '

'Thirty-five years old. Almost like me!' Michael said.

'To be clear,' I said, 'Michael was driving the stolen car.'

'All the UN did was cower in their compound in Kabul, and get drunk, and watch people steal their equipment.'

'Were you doing fiber-optic cable there too?'

'No.'

'Nobody realizes this,' Michael said, 'but the US military has its own internet. They have their own self-contained system of cables all over the world. And communications bunkers everywhere.'

'Bunkers? Like bomb shelters?'

'Technology Safe Houses,' I said. 'The ones in West Africa are probably rotting in the earth. Nobody cares about this place.'

Davidia was drinking wine, which I wouldn't have recommended, but she'd chosen something Italian, and she seemed to like it. Every time she took a sip, Michael and I stopped talking and watched.

'Michael,' she said, 'you've never explained what you were doing in Afghanistan.'

'Michael was my bodyguard.'

He took offense. 'I had many duties there. I transported a lot of prisoners.'

'What about now, today,' I said, 'our duties now? Somebody please tell me. Are we here for a wedding?'

Davidia said, 'Yes.'

'So, Michael, this trip has nothing to do with business.'

'Well, while we're traveling — we've always got our noses open for the smell of business.'

Davidia laughed, and I said, 'That came out wrong. But I get the message.'

Michael said, 'Davidia will be married wearing shoes of pure gold. And she'll keep them the rest of her life.'

'All this meets with your approval?'

Davidia only said, 'Yes.'

'Are we really going to Uganda?'

Michael said, 'We'll fly to Entebbe next week, is that all right? Can you come? Because in Uganda, they really know how to put on a wedding. I wish it could be a double wedding.'

'You want two wives?'

'Be serious! Two brides and two grooms. I told Davidia you're engaged.'

'On the brink of engagement,' I said.

'Aren't we all!' Davidia said. 'What does she do?'

'She's an attorney, but she works for NATO in Amsterdam — for your lot, actually. For the Americans.'

'Nair met her in Kabul,' Michael said.

'He's actually correct about that. But Tina and I weren't involved over there — just acquainted. She was a prosecutor for the UN, and Michael and I both knew her a bit.'

'A bit? She wasn't one of Michael's, was she?'

'You think everybody's my girlfriend. Do

you think I have unlimited time for sex?'

'That's exactly what I think.'

'Before the UN,' I said, 'she served as a prosecutor in Detroit. Once she took part in a drugs raid and carried a machine gun.'

'So she's dangerous. Is she beautiful?'

'Yes, but she's a little too smart for that. She keeps herself a bit plain. I prefer it.'

Davidia said to Michael, 'You'd parade me around nude, if you could.'

'Nude except for sexy platform shoes. You've got it, so flaunt it.'

'Sometimes,' she said, 'you have a thirsty face like a little boy.' She laughed. She was tipsy by now. I hoped she'd do something stupid, something to break the beautiful image. She caught me looking. 'You don't sound the least bit like Georgia. How much time have you spent there?'

'Very little. My father raised me in Europe, mostly Switzerland. I don't think he had legal custody — I think I was kidnapped.'

'Is he still alive?'

'Both mother and father are living.'

'When do you see your American family?'

Just the kind of question I like to deflect. But I found I wanted her to know. 'I've had no contact with my mother or her family since I was eight years old.'

'But you, you — ' She was flustered. 'You

see your dad, right?'

'We get together every so often. He lives in Amsterdam too.'

Michael was staring at me. 'These are things I never heard about.'

Davidia told him, 'Maybe that's because you talk more than you listen.' She said it with affection. I thought I was done, but she kept at me — 'What line is your father in?'

'He's a physician at a teaching hospital. More teacher than physician, in other words. I'm afraid he's a little crazy.'

'And your mother?'

'As I've said — no contact. I choose to believe she's happy.'

'Then I'll believe it too,' she said.

Now a beggar dressed in rags came out of the dark and wrote swiftly on the floor with white chalk: MR. PHILO KRON / DR. OF ACROBATICS. He started doing cartwheels in place while holding a platter of raw rice, never spilling a grain. He repeated the trick, now holding a glass of water, also without spilling.

The staff, the patrons, everybody ignored him, but Davidia said, 'Michael, give him something.'

Michael only offered him a scowl and said, 'Don't encourage these people.'

Davidia smiled and met the acrobat's eyes,

or one of his eyes — the other's socket was scarred and pinched shut — and this inspired him to talk, or to signal his thoughts by a series of squeaks, as he seemed to be missing, also, one of his vocal cords. 'Sometimes it's feeling like the Prophet was just here,' he told Davidia, kneeling before her, touching her hand, trembling with the intensity of his message, 'the Prophet himself, on this spot, and he went around that corner of the building there, and see, there, the dust still stirred up by the motion of his garments.' Satisfied with that, Dr. Kron took himself and his piece of chalk back into the night, and one of our waiters came quickly with a rag and wiped away his title and his name.

★   ★   ★

Later, as we hailed a car in front of the place, Davidia took my arm and said, 'What does a prosecutor prosecute in Afghanistan?'

'You mean Tina? Everything. It was right after the invasion. For a little bit there, the UN was the only law. She specialized mainly in crimes against women.'

'Was she one of Michael's?'

'Are you jealous?'

'Are you?'

'Listen, whoever his other women were

57

— you're not like them.'

'Thank you,' she said, and kissed me briefly on the mouth.

Michael said, 'Are we taking this fellow to bed with us?'

'I bet he wouldn't mind.'

'Look what you did, Nair — you got her ready for me.'

I saw them into a car and said good night and strolled home down the beach, drunk, under such a multitude of stars they gave me light to see. The small action of the waves made a rushing, muttering kind of rhythm. The moon hadn't risen yet. Occasionally a school of phosphorescent flying fish swarmed upward out of the darkness offshore.

The Papa lay about a kilometer along from the Bawarchi. I arrived still drunk and looking forward to several hours of dreamless rest, but no such luck.

The power was off, the lobby dim. The night man napped in a plush chair by the door. I got him going and he handed over my key and a handwritten message, folded in two:

I missed you on Tuesday. — H

This meant I had a date for tomorrow afternoon, Thursday, to negotiate the sale of

58

the contents of my Cruzer. I would meet my contact, Hamid, at the Bawarchi — only by coincidence, as we'd arranged these details weeks ago, in Amsterdam.

I took the stairs upward three at a stride, quite suddenly and miserably sober. I rigged my portable hammock on the balcony and lay out in the sea breeze, and came inside in the wee hours when it rained. I lit the candle and opened my laptop. No internet. Off-line I wrote to Tina —

I'm having a bad night. I miss you and even at moments your old cat and her monstrous ugly sister the dog. I don't quite yet pine for your Mrs. Landlady — what's her name? Mrs. Rimple? — but I'll probably even reach that point too before it's over.

Just tried a bite of a sandwich, and it was stale. It's only been out of the bag for two minutes. Goddamn this climate, nothing gets dry but the bread, the miserable bloody

— and heard the whining in the tone and stabbed DELETE.

* * *

As soon as day came I checked out of the Papa Leone and moved over to the Scanlon, third floor, almost where I could stomp my shoes and rock Michael's ceiling in room 230 below. Not that I'd have roused him, even if he were home. I'd had the maximum of Michael Adriko lately. And I'd only been on the continent thirty-six hours.

I stood in my room wondering how much I should unpack, not knowing the length of our stay, and deciding I'd give it all an airing —

I jumped as my door was flung open. I hadn't turned the key in the lock.

The manager stood there. Short, stocky, Arab. He looked as shocked as I must have. 'I'm searching for the cleaner,' he said.

All I could think of to say was, 'You mean the housekeeper?'

'Yes. That's right.'

'She's not here.'

He shut the door and left.

I changed my mind about unpacking everything, and got out fresh socks and underwear and kept the rest in my bag.

One of my heads said to the other, He meant to search your things, and the other head said, Don't get jumpy, people make mistakes, and the first one said, Either way, my friend, they've got you talking to yourself.

$\star$ $\star$ $\star$

'Life is short,' Michael always says, and there's fear in his face when he says it, because he understands it, he means it, this life ends soon.

Michael is a warrior, a knight. Higher-ups command him, and he pretends to obey. The rest of us live as squires and peasants.

— So my report might have said, my second, and final, report from Freetown. It might have said also:

For him the world consists of soft spots and hard spots and holes, it's all terrain, and he works it, pausing only to eat, drink, shit, piss, fuck, or treat his wounds.

Michael identifies himself as one of the Kakwa, the clan of Idi Amin Dada, and his story runs thus: After Amin's exile, when the reprisals began against the Kakwa, the boy Michael was taken to Kampala and educated by kind Christian missionaries ... But missionaries don't take a child from the village and put him in a city school. More likely he was kidnapped by a criminal gang and survived on the streets as a harlot boy.

He claims that having finished his secondary schooling, which I believe he never started, he joined the Ugandan army, entered the school for officers, and before receiving

his commission was assigned to a unique training camp along the Orange River in South Africa, where Israeli agents — from the Duvdevan Unit, he sometimes says, other times he says the Mossad — instructed him in terrorist tactics.

True or false, what does it matter? Michael's truth lives only in the myth. In the facts and the details, it dies.

And while you, my superiors, may think I've come to join him in Africa because you dispatched me here, you're mistaken. I've come back because I love the mess. Anarchy. Madness. Things falling apart. Michael only makes my excuse for returning.

And if he thinks I'd like an army and a harem, Michael mistakes me too. I don't want to live like a king — I just want to live. I can't make it happen by myself. I've got all the ingredients, but I need a wizard to stir the cauldron. I need Michael.

— So my report might have read.

As for the actual report, I banged it out quickly in the basement of Elvis Documents. The crisscross shadows of the lights' wire cages, the choking musk of the concrete walls, also the thought of Mohammed Kallon tiptoeing back and forth overhead, none of these things encouraged settling in for a lengthy chat. I wrote:

I've established contact. Changing stations quite soon. Details to follow in 48–72 hours.

'No lunch today,' I told Mohammed when I came up from his basement, only five minutes after I'd gone down.

He was already rising from his alleged chair, saying, 'I've had my lunch. What about dinner this evening? I've got some news for you.'

'Dinner? No. Just tell me.'

'Very good then,' he said with clear disappointment, 'I'm to explain something to you. Michael Adriko was attached to the US Special Forces in eastern Congo. There's a unit there, you know, chasing the Lord's Resistance Army.'

'I've heard about it.'

'Now he's absent without leave — that's what I mean when I call him a deserter.'

'All right,' I said.

And so I could have reported as well that by his secrecy, his coyness, Michael Adriko had thrown up a screen against most of my questions, in particular the first one I'd asked: If our aim was Congo, or Uganda, what on earth were we doing in Sierra Leone?

Here was the answer, from Mohammed

Kallon. Michael had landed here on the run, probably settling for any destination that would admit him with a Ghanaian passport. Not a bad choice, Freetown. Anything can happen here. Traitors and deserters can evaporate before your eyes.

Mohammed said, 'Let's meet at the Papa for dinner.'

'Halfway through you'd be saying, 'Why take me to an expensive meal? Just give me the cash.''

'Well, certainly — I could use a little cash.'

I gave him a wad of leones half an inch thick but nearly worthless, and walked out into the noontime's unbelievable heat.

One half block from Elvis Documents a man with a generator and a satellite rented time on his computer, and I sat in a collapsible chair, under an umbrella, beside his scrapwood kiosk, and found a Reuters report online. Its closing paragraph:

The LRA mission will belong to about 100 special operators, Pentagon sources said. They declined to say which unit will be assigned to the mission, but a media report in the Colorado Springs *Gazette* suggested that the 10th Special Forces Group, out of Fort Carson, Colorado, will be the one. This unit typically

handles special operations in Europe and Africa.

Despite the heat I walked to the Scanlon. I was angry. Not with Michael, as I might have been, but with Mohammed, because it was simpler.

Along my way I stopped at the Ivory Castle Hotel to talk to the baffling, inscrutable West African men who pretended to manage the air service piloted by the drunken Russians. We had to resort to the Russians because no genuine airline would take us aboard without Ugandan visas, although Uganda would issue them to arrivals at Entebbe without any problem — so Michael had assured us. I asked about the fares and schedule. The managers seemed not to understand why I would even want to know. I presented them with the white European's suffering weary smile, the only alternative to murder. Ultimately they revealed to me the prices and the times. Michael, Davidia, and I would get out of here in less than forty-eight hours.

★ ★ ★

At three in the afternoon I once again entered the Bawarchi. The patronage was light, the place was quiet. At first I thought my contact

hadn't come, and when I located him, seated at one of the smaller tables, nothing before him but a pair of sunglasses, I thought he must be someone else, because I'd only seen him in business suits. But he was Hamid, the one I'd talked to several times in Amsterdam.

He waved me over and I sat down with him. He gave the impression of being middle-aged and fond of comfort, in a loose white linen outfit with a tunic, more Arab than Euro, except for his eyes, which weren't brown, but a washed-out gray. He had his sleeve pulled back as he checked his Rolex Commander wristwatch. He wore six jeweled rings, three on either hand.

'Exactly on time.'

He handed me his phony business card, and I handed him mine.

'Do you want something to eat?' he said. 'A snack of some kind?'

'Nothing, thanks. Have you ordered?'

'Won't you join me for some tea?'

'If you haven't ordered — '

'Not yet.'

'Good. Why don't we walk on the beach?'

'Nobody hears us. We can talk.'

'I'm nervous indoors,' I said.

'Come on, don't be silly. Just tell me what you've got.'

'You know what I've got.'

66

'I want to know what I'm buying.'

'Let's walk. I don't like it in here.' I wanted us out of the public eye, because I couldn't be sure of his reaction to a bit of news I had for him. 'Do you mind?'

He sighed, and then he picked up his sunglasses.

I donned my own as well, and we passed from under the roof and into a hot, steady breeze while the sunshine crashed onto our heads. Through the soles of my sandals I felt the beach burning. In our sinister shades, the only figures in view, I suppose we looked like nothing so much as a couple of crooks plotting mischief.

When we got near the water's edge, he stopped. 'Now, before we get a stroke or dehydration or something — what have you got?'

'Exactly what I told you I'd have. Maps of the US military fiber-optics cables through-out seven West African countries. Mali is one of them. Also I have a list of the GPS coordinates for twelve NIIA Technology Safe Houses.' Including, I might have added, the safe house in the basement beneath Elvis Documents.

'You're definite about Mali.'

'Mali. Yes. That's definite.'

Mali was the current hot spot. With Mali I

had him hooked. Talk about a thirsty face.

'Let me establish something with you,' he said, 'and please forgive me: Do you know what can happen to a party who sells false product?'

'I would expect to be assassinated.'

'Your expectation is precise.'

'I'm not worried. It's very good product.'

'What about the transfer?'

'A push of the button. I have things stored away.'

'We can do it all digitally?'

'Correct. You never have to touch the goods.'

'Do you still stipulate cash payment?'

'Correct. Cash only.'

'And the price is twenty thousand US.'

'No,' I said, 'not twenty thousand. That's no longer correct.'

This was the bit I didn't like.

He started a retort, but stifled it. He must have been counting ten. 'I don't understand what you're saying.'

'The price is no longer twenty thousand. For you, out of your own pockets, the cost will be nothing — because we go in as partners.'

'Partners for what?'

'We'll be equal partners in the sale you're making. I'm providing the product, and

you're providing the client.'

He bunched his mouth in an ugly way and made a sharp noise with his tongue. 'It's completely unacceptable.' He raised his sunglasses. 'What are you thinking? You know nothing about my business.'

'I think I do. The Chinese are all over this continent, and they're paying ridiculous sums. If they're not the people you're selling to, you're an idiot.'

He replaced his dark glasses over his eyes. 'I don't like this conversation. You're too forceful. You use a personal tone.'

'I'm being emphatic, but only for the purposes of business. It's nothing personal. I'm just saying the Chinese will pay plenty for something good. And this is good.'

'It was agreed. Twenty thousand US. It was agreed.'

'We're beyond that point now. We're talking about a partnership. This is excellent product with long-term potential. Very long-term. The loss of this material will never be detected.'

He clicked his tongue again and turned his back and walked toward the restaurant, leaving me by the shore.

A dozen meters along he called out over his shoulder, 'You're a liar!' After that he didn't look back.

My head roared. Switching the price had

felt like a bold move in a sport without rules, but what was bold, and what was stupid?

I took a look at his card. CREATIVE PRODUCTIONS / Film Plus Internet / Hamid Faisel / Managing Director.

In Amsterdam he'd had a different last name but had still been Hamid. He'd been chatty, sociable, kind of fun. We'd gone to a film together, *Zero Dark Thirty*, in English, the Hollywood action movie about the killing of Osama Bin Laden. Afterward Hamid made jokes about the great martyr. 'It wouldn't be so funny to my relatives in Lebanon,' he said. 'But why should I care? Because I'm not really Lebanese. My mother is French, my stepfather also. I was raised in Marseilles. I am French. France is a happy country. Lebanon has turned into shit.' — As I say, chatty. Today, in Freetown, neither of us had any jokes to make.

I gave him time enough to get lost, if that's what he wanted, and then I went through the restaurant toward the cars out front. Hamid was sitting at a table near the entrance with a cup and a saucer before him. I headed for the front without looking at him.

'One moment, one moment. Come on.' He waved me in and I sat down with him once again. He had a pen in his hand. 'How can I believe anything you say, when you're a liar?'

'You'll have a small sample to work with, enough to understand that this represents an ongoing intelligence mother lode to anyone who taps into the cables.'

'What have they got to detect such tapping?'

'Nothing remarkable, unless there's been an upgrade in the last ten years. And there hasn't been.'

'Give me back my business card, please.'

'If you say so.'

'You might decide to get in touch.' He licked the point of his pen and took the card for a minute and handed it back with an e-address written on its blank side. The domain was dot-UK. 'Only if you want to honor the original agreement,' he said.

'Sure.'

'Don't use the twenty-five.'

He meant the AES-25 encryption standard, known as the American Standard. 'Of course not,' I said.

'And rotate your proxy every fifteen words.'

'Sure. I hope English is all right.'

'English, French, Dutch. I don't care. But choose your words — no red flags.'

I tore a page from my notepad and borrowed his pen. 'Here's mine. Maybe we can exchange ideas and reach an understanding.'

He stared down at my e-address, but he

wasn't reading. I waited. 'All right,' he said. 'Where's the harm? Think about your price and let me know later.'

And then I felt smug and thought: Of course, he can't pass this up. Not when it includes Mali.

'Send me your sample,' he said. 'Maybe I'll consider, that's all I promise. But you can trust my promise, because let me tell you,' he said, 'I'm not a liar.'

Ending it on such a note, I didn't offer to shake his hand. I went out to the beach again. The heat matched my blood, both were beating, simmering. I walked the shoreline toward other restaurants visible up ahead, where cars for hire congregated.

I took off my sandals and wet my feet in the shallows, and I watched the ocean swell and shrink and listened to it sigh.

Here the sea is warm, like a bath. It's dark, not so blue, more like black, a lustrous black.

You wade out into it until you can't. You swim out farther until you can't. Then it takes you.

★ ★ ★

At a table outside the Quonset hut from which the drunken Russian pilots administered their charter airline — with its fleet of

72

one, a commuter jet — we dealt with a young Leonean man who spoke faultless English, and as he held Michael's passport, I tried to sneak a look at it. Davidia was peeking too — at mine as well as Michael's. 'It's US,' I told her. 'I have a Danish one too, but I never use it.' Davidia's was American.

Davidia wore her safari garb, while Michael was dressed in a wrinkled suit and gray snakeskin boots. His outfit looked at first pink, but closer it was white linen with thin red stripes.

When Michael got his passport back, he let me have a look at it — a wilted Ghanaian document. 'I told you I saved the Ghanaian president.'

'A couple of times. At a minimum.' I gave it back to him. 'It's got less than two months left on it, Michael.'

'Never fear. I've got family in Uganda, and just as many in Congo. One of those places will claim me. I'll make the necessary inquiries.'

We weren't at the Freetown airport, but at an airstrip well east of the city and next to the ocean. Our aircraft waited in a field of tall grass. I said to our young man, 'That's a Bombardier Challenger, isn't it? The Royal Danish Air Force uses them for cargo.'

'Not this kind,' he said. 'This is the 600,

discontinued from 1982.'

Davidia shaded her eyes with a hand and squinted. 'Are you saying that plane is thirty years old?'

'The one you're looking at is a couple of years older,' he said. 'But it's a very good aircraft, so long as you don't overload it.'

Michael said, 'Nair — remember the Russian airline? The Freetown-Monrovia run during the war? Something Airlines? — something Russian?'

'It wasn't an airline. It was a renegade charter, just like this one.'

'They were the only ones bold enough to fly to Monrovia.'

'You mean crazy enough. Eventually they crashed, didn't they?'

'That's right, but not on the Monrovia run. That time the plane was coming from a secret rendezvous, loaded with processed uranium.'

The clerk disagreed. 'That's unsubstantiated, and in fact quite false.'

'Were you there at the crash site?' Michael said. 'If you were there, you were five years old.'

'Processed uranium?' Davidia said. 'You mean enriched?'

'Exactly right. The plane was overloaded with HEU stolen from Tenex.'

'HEU?' Davidia said. 'What's HEU? Who's

Tenex?' — and as she seemed to be talking to me, I shook my head, and she said, 'Where did it go down?'

'That's the beautiful part,' Michael said.

'It's never been found,' the clerk said. 'But factually, it only had some inconsequential cargo aboard.'

'U-235? Do you call that inconsequential?' But Michael couldn't expect to be heeded. He looked like a species of gangster in his pinstripe suit.

I tried a guess: 'Highly Enriched Uranium.'

'Nothing like that aboard,' the clerk said. By his expression, he seemed to have taken a special dislike to Michael.

The runway was visible once you walked on it, packed red dirt hidden under tufts of beach grass.

The aircraft would be booked to capacity — otherwise the Russians would postpone, and that's why the weekly charter never flew weekly. With a couple of dozen other passengers, African, Indian, Arab, a few white Euros, we waited beside the terminal, a rusty ship's cargo container open at one end, nothing in it but a row of four theater seats. Nobody would have sat inside — the heat it gave off was startling. Clouds blanketed the sky, but it was bright, and the sea reflected it so viciously you couldn't look at the water.

A white Honda Prelude arrived at the Quonset hut and stopped, and nobody got out. I recognized the backseat passenger. I said to Michael, 'Look there. It's Bruno Horst.'

'Bruno, at our point of departure. Well — nothing funny about that!'

'I can't make out the man riding shotgun, but I don't doubt it's Mohammed Kallon.'

I waved. Only the driver waved back. I recognized him too. It was Emil, who'd carried me to the Papa Leone my first day in Freetown.

Everything I'd touched, they were touching.

The clerk called our flight. As the others gathered their things I wandered over to the shore with my phone in my hand and, when the water stopped me, I opened the device and pried loose the SIM card and flicked it into the waves. If NATO Intel had a trace on it, let them trace.

On second thought, I didn't want the device, either. I made a wish and tossed it as far as I could out into the sea. I wished for magic armor, and the power to disappear.

I rejoined our group. As we boarded, a young fellow in an olive uniform ran a wand around each passenger's outline, fondling us in the places where it squeaked — that is, the

men. He didn't touch the women. We climbed onto the craft up metal treads salvaged from old passenger busses and welded into a crooked stairway. Ahead of us a frail person, an African so ill as to seem genderless and colorless and weightless, was being carried up the steps like a bolt of cloth on the shoulders of two young men. 'Going home to die,' Michael said.

I sat against the window overlooking a wing and one of the two jet engines. Michael and Davidia took the seats one row behind and across the aisle. After the engines started, one of the crew — I assumed there were two — a blond man wearing denims, white T-shirt, and flip-flops, came out of the cockpit and wandered down the aisle, saying, 'Is English okay? Okay, let's try it. I want to warn you of the safety features of this aircraft. Has everybody got the seat belt buckled? It's your choice, I'm not your mother. Okay,' he said, 'it's a trip of sixteen and one-half hours, stopping once at Kotoka International in Accra and once more at Yaoundé, and the final stop will be Entebbe. You'd better have a visa for Ghana or else for Cameroon if you think that's where you're going. If you need to get a visa for Uganda, it's all right, they can fix it at the airport without a big problem. Wherever is your destination, I think you can

expect the customs to be serious. They're always serious with our passengers. They're too serious.' He waved goodbye and reentered the cockpit and closed and locked the door, leaving behind him an atmosphere of vodka.

I'd spent five days in Freetown and learned nothing — except that I could have landed in Uganda to begin with.

The craft took off over the sea, made a tight, nauseating turn, and came in so low it bent the grasses in the field beneath. We had a close-up view of the highway heading north, and one last snapshot of Freetown: an accident on the road — a farmer talking with both hands, a twitching bloody goat at his feet, a car with all four doors open, a sign stuck inside its rear window — SPLENDID DRIVING SCHOOL.

TWO

We got our Ugandan visas at the Entebbe airport without any trouble. Hungover from the long, rocking flight, with the two stops in between, at both of which they kept us suffocating in our seats for upward of two hours while the cabin's temperature rose to match that of the surrounding tropical darkness, I, for one, wasn't sure I was still alive, felt I might have entered some intermediary realm on the way to oblivion, and the smoothness of our passage among the Entebbe officials and through the terminal and out to the hired cars only mixed me up all the more. I thought we should go back inside and double-check these visa stamps. Michael said, 'My people don't like senseless trouble. It's not West Africa. Relax.' He got us into a car, where Davidia fell asleep instantly, her head on his shoulder, and we sailed toward our beds. Cool air reached our faces through the driver's open window — cool. From Lake Victoria, I gathered.

Thanks to Michael's budgetary strictures we stayed at the Executive Suites, a place with resale-shop paintings hung crookedly,

but in all sincerity, on some of its walls, a 'bed-and-breakfast,' as Michael called it, a good two kilometers from the lake and from the real hotels. On a tour of its single story, looking for a bed that wasn't broken, I counted fourteen rooms. We arrived a bit too late for the breakfast.

I spent much of the day wandering muddy lanes in search of a phone and soon got one, another Nokia. I took a late lunch at a table in front of a quick-shop calling itself Belief Enterprises and loaded the device with minutes and sent Michael a text: 'Note new phone. Have lunch without me. I'm at a table eating chicken, while chickens wander around at my feet.'

Later Michael woke me from a deep nap by slapping at my door crying, 'Nair, dinner is mandatory.'

For three seconds I was awake, felt ready for adventure, very nearly got my feet on the floor — woke again still later with no idea where I was.

I checked my new phone. Another hour gone. Hymns filled the air outside my window, some nearby congregation worshipping in song, and then the unintelligible reverberations of a sermon through loudspeakers. By the time the preaching was finished I'd taken a cold shower and located

myself in Entebbe, and it was Sunday.

I found Michael and Davidia at a round white table in the patio restaurant embracing and cooing among the remains of their dinner, spaghetti, probably from a can. I wasn't hungry. The happy couple drank Nile beer from the bottle and I had an orange soda and Michael told us we'd traveled southeast from Freetown about five thousand kilometers and had landed five kilometers north of the equator and twenty kilometers south of Uganda's capital, Kampala, and three hundred kilometers east of the Mountains of the Moon and the headwaters of the Nile River; that the elevation was some twelve hundred meters, that we couldn't expect temperatures to get above 30 Celsius, and that we'd better set our watches ahead to 8:42 p.m., because we'd lost an hour heading east; and then in a clear, sweet tenor voice he sang most of 'Ain't No Mountain High Enough' to his fiancee, accompanying Marvin Gaye and Tammi Terrell, whose voices issued from the bartender's boom box.

I went over and got the barman to switch it off and taught him to make a vodka martini and drank one or two of them pretty rapidly.

When I rejoined my comrades with another drink in my hand Michael said, 'I was just

explaining to Davidia — we'll head north tomorrow for Newada Mountain. Or in that direction. North. Stanley explored there, looking for the source of the Nile.'

'More will be revealed,' I said. I was aware that lately I was drinking more than ever in my life. I couldn't relax or feel like myself in this region without banging myself on the head with something.

'My village is there,' he told us, 'in sight of Newada Mountain.' Next he said, 'I'm being communicated with by a spirit. Something or someone is contacting me. No, I'm serious. The spirits of my ancestors, the spirits of my village.'

'What village? I thought you were some sort of — what the hell are you, originally, Michael? Some sort of displaced Congolese.'

'I am exactly that. A displaced Congolese. And now,' he said, 'I'm going to replace myself.' He took hold of Davidia's arm as if to hand her to me in evidence. 'She's along because I'm going to marry her. I want her to meet my parents.'

'I thought your parents were dead.'

'Not my real parents. My other parents. The whole village is one family. Everyone is my mother and father and brother and sister. If the feeling is right, we'll be married right then and there.'

Davidia said, 'Wait — if the feeling is right?'

'If you're welcome. And I'm sure you'll be welcomed. The bride is always welcome, unless she comes from a clan devoted to stealing.'

'And I'll be your best man,' I said.

'The equivalent.'

'Nobody's going to cook me and eat me, I hope.'

'People don't quite understand,' Michael said, and he may have been serious, 'to be eaten pays a compliment to your power.'

A couple of whores came in and sat at another table.

The boom box was back in operation. I talked Michael and Davidia into trying the barman's martinis. They had a couple each, and danced with one another. Between numbers we listened to the song of a frog who sounded like a duck, an insistent duck.

'I knew it from the start,' I said. 'Congo. I knew it.'

'Not Congo, no, not necessarily.'

Davidia said, 'Isn't it time you told us where we're going? Where are your people located?'

'During the reprisals they were dispersed. We were uprooted and scattered. But they've reconvened. Relocated.'

'Where, exactly?'

'Where? Quite near to Arua, in the northwest corner of this country.'

'Uganda.'

'This country where we're having our supper. Uganda.'

'Not Congo,' I said.

'Not Congo.'

'And how do we get there?'

'We're taking the bus from Kampala.'

'Come on! We'll take a plane,' I said.

'It has to be the bus. You can easily see why.'

'Why?' Davidia said.

He meant Horst, and Mohammed Kallon. If for some reason Interpol was on us, they could check the flight manifests out of Entebbe. I saw the logic. I disliked the conclusion.

'You'll get to view the countryside,' he said to Davidia.

'Good! The bus!' she said.

'Arua is the birthplace,' Michael informed us, 'of Idi Amin Dada. In the month of March they celebrate his birthday.'

'What? You mean the whole town?'

'Just a handful of people. But nobody stops them.'

The bus . . . Out of pity for us all, I didn't laugh. 'So we simply climb aboard,' I said, 'and go away.'

'Yes. Day after tomorrow. Can you just come with me?'

'Sure. I'm drunk enough.'

'Good. Stay drunk.'

'What about you,' I asked Davidia — 'are you drunk enough?'

'I'm in love enough.'

She had a somber glow about her, a smoldering vitality that warmed the air. She made me hungry. I wanted to smell her breath.

And the nightclub girls, one of them wearing a curly blonde wig, like a chocolate-covered Marilyn Monroe . . . The bartender didn't talk to them and they ordered nothing, they only watched me, and waited.

Michael's tongue was tangled in martinis — 'I don't want to be a thumb,' he said, 'in the turd in the punchbowl of life.'

'What?'

Michael was drunk. That meant he was in pain. He gripped a pen, he was writing something on a napkin. He tapped me on the shoulder and handed it to me. In the pleasant darkness, I couldn't make out the letters.

I told him, 'I wouldn't have expected you to marry black.'

Michael shook his head as if to clear it. Davidia stared at me. 'What did you say?'

Right. What had I said? 'The drinks are

clobbering me. It's the altitude.'

'You should have put food in your stomach,' Michael said.

Davidia said, 'Explain your remark.'

'You mean defend it.'

'Fine. Defend it.'

'I'll explain it,' I said.

'We're waiting.'

'He's always had a weakness for the Middle Eastern type, that's all. The Persian princess sort of female. I apologize for talking out of turn. I do apologize.'

She laughed. She was angry. 'Don't twist yourself in knots.'

It was only for Michael's sake I was trying to smooth things, but Michael wasn't even listening. 'Back to another subject,' he said. 'I never answered your question about the Tenex corporation.'

'Tenex?'

'Do you remember? At the Freetown airfield. We were talking about uranium. Tenex handles U-235 material from dismantled Soviet warheads. Dilutes it to ten percent pure and barters it to the United States.'

'Jesus, Michael — again, the U-235?'

I've always thought it a laugh, Michael's obviousness when he means to be sneaky. No stage villain ever looked more the conspirator,

leaning forward into his face's shadow, his head cocked toward the game, the trick, his right eyebrow going up, his lip curling in a sneer.

A quick, horrid intuition assaulted me.

Davidia placed her hand on my forearm and asked if I was okay. I said, 'I'm fine, except I need to be smarter.'

'Smarter isn't always better though, is it?'

'Good night.'

I went over and made an arrangement with the whore in the blonde wig. She stood up, and hand in hand we journeyed to my bed.

She was drunk, also in some way drugged, and she passed out when we were done — perhaps before we were done, and I simply didn't notice.

★ ★ ★

Later I woke as the woman was leaving, and I locked the door behind her and lay in bed watching the Chinese cable station, a piece about fourteen baby pandas in the Shanghai zoo. A sudden rainstorm hit the roof like an avalanche and killed the city's power and sent all of existence back where it came from. I thought of the woman wandering around out there in the roaring dark.

On my nightstand I found the napkin

Michael had written on. By the light of my cell phone I made out the words, but not their meaning:

He's my panda
from Uganda
he's my teddy bear
they say things about him
but I don't care
Idi Amin
I'm your fan!

— I read it several times. The rhyme scheme interested me.

★　★　★

Not long after six in the morning I heard, through the papery walls, the buzz of Michael's clippers and the shower running next door, and soon I heard someone going out. A few minutes later came a light tapping. I was heating water for instant coffee — the Suites provided a drip brewer but nothing to brew in it, only a jar of Nescafé. The tapping came again, and I realized it must be Davidia.

I got close to the wall and said, 'I'm awake.'

Her voice came quite clearly. 'Come and see me.'

'Should we meet in the restaurant?'

'Let's talk in here,' she said. 'Come over. Or around.'

'I could easily come right through.' Talking through the wall like this, I felt how close our faces were.

The lights in the hallway flickered on and off. The door stood open. In the random illumination she waited in a yellow silk robe, barefoot. She stepped aside and I entered bearing my cup and my jar of Nescafé.

'Where's Michael?'

'Taking his morning run.'

The air tasted damp from the shower. Her underwear was lying around. I smelled her perfume. But she said, 'It stinks in here. Sorry. Sometimes he sits down and smokes half a dozen cigarettes one after another. Doesn't say a word. Lost in his head.'

She picked up a cigarette from the nightstand and put the end in her mouth. Looked around. Perhaps for a lighter.

'Do you smoke?'

She threw it in the pile of butts in the ashtray and said, 'I'm so stupid.'

'Let's have some coffee. Do you have bottled water?' She gave me a liter jug and I set about heating water in the brewer.

She sat on the bed. 'We had a fight.'

'I'm surprised to hear that. I mean to say

— you were pretty quiet about it. I had no idea.'

'He wanted to be quiet. So he could hear you through the wall.'

'Hear me?'

'You and the girl,' she said.

'We were quiet too,' I said.

'We're a stealthy bunch of idiots,' she said. 'And I mean idiots.' She got up but didn't know where to go. 'I've been wanting to see you alone.'

'Why?'

She paused. 'I don't have a ready answer.'

'Did you have something you wanted to say?' Seeing I wasn't helping, I added, 'I'm only trying to help you figure it out.'

'I wanted to see what we were like together.'

'Oh.' I devoted myself to the cups and spoons and Nescafé. 'What were you fighting about?'

'I thought Kampala was the destination. Now we're going on to Arua.'

'But last night at dinner you were ready to swing with it.'

'"Swing with it"? Who are you, Jack Kerouac? You reach way back into the last century for your Americanisms.'

'Nevertheless.'

'Sure, last night I was a real swinger.

Alcohol affects me too. I didn't realize he wasn't telling us anything.'

'Michael doesn't draw up plans. He weaves tales. Just let him be mysterious. If there was any way of hurrying him along, believe me, I would have found it by now.'

'This is why I had to talk to you — to compare notes. Can I trust you? No — I can't, can I? — I mean, trust you to be straight with me. What are we doing? I mean, specifically, you two — what are you up to? There's something going on, and he won't tell me what.'

'There's nothing going on in the sense of — going on. We're traveling together.'

'Why do you tag along?'

'I'm one half of the entourage.'

'He assumes you're devoted to him. I'm not so sure.'

'He assumes I'm devoted to getting rich. You know — exploiting the riches of this continent.'

'And is that really you? A cheap adventurer?'

'Why do you call it cheap? Adventure is glorious. I don't understand why people put it down.'

'I can't believe you just went off with that poor woman, in her silly-looking wig. Did you think to use protection?'

'This is a little crazy. Don't you think it's none of your business?'

'No. But don't you think I have reason to be crazy?'

'Drink this coffee,' I said.

'Something's wrong with him, Nair. In the middle of the night he gets these sort of, I don't know what, nightmares, sleepwalking, talking in his sleep — really, I don't know what.'

'Actual sleepwalking? Walking around in his sleep?'

'No, but — talking, thrashing — talking to me, but talking crazy, looking right at me, but he looks blind when I shine a light on him.'

'Night terrors. Right? Violent memories.'

'It's driving me nuts. It's scary.'

'Tell me something: When did you arrive in Africa?'

'Tomorrow will make it two weeks.'

'Just short of two weeks. Right on schedule for a meltdown. Nothing serious. A tiny low-grade implosion, let's say, of your American personality.'

'I've traveled before. Don't condescend to me. I'm crazy about a man who's driving me crazy because I'm crazy about him. He won't tell me anything. He took my cell phone.'

'Really? Jesus.'

'He won't let me call home.'

'Your people must be frantic.'

'There's only my dad, and we don't correspond much anyway. He's bitter at me since I started doing work at the Institute. Still, I mean, if I could call him — I would. If Michael would let me. Why won't he let me? Is he always like this? Because it seems like something new.'

'It's nothing new.'

'You've seen it before. Paranoid suspicions. Taking away people's cell phones.'

'I've been analyzing Michael Adriko for a dozen years. First of all — you realize he's a war orphan. He was born into chaos, and he's pathologically insecure. He keeps a stranglehold on the flow of information because then it feels like his life can't get away from him. But whatever you absolutely need to know, he tells you. Even though sometimes I'd like to torture him with electricity.'

'Don't joke. He's been tortured before.' It was true.

Davidia stood there holding her cup with two hands looking alone, and pitiable, and stupidly I said, 'Are you really going to marry him?'

'That's what I'm here for.'

'Do you really love him?'

She said, 'Do you know who my father is?'

An unexpected query. 'I guess not.'

'Michael didn't tell you? My dad's his CO — the garrison commander at Fort Carson. Colonel Marcus St. Claire.'

'Oh my lord,' I said, 'oh my lord.' I jumped up to say something else and only said, 'Oh my lord.'

'Until I met Michael, I'd only known two loves: love for my father, and love for my country. Now I love Michael too.'

'But you said your dad and you were on the outs.'

'It's complicated. It's family. I'd say we're estranged. All the same, he loves Michael as much as I do. Everybody loves Michael. Don't you love him, Nair?'

'I can't resist him. Let's put it that way.' And I added, 'Oh my lord.'

★ ★ ★

I went to the lobby, more on the order of a vestibule, and ordered some coffee. Soon Michael came through the doors in a powder-blue sweat suit and put his hands on his knees and bowed like that, breathing heavily, showing the top of his big muscular shaved head. Then he stood and whipped off his sweatband and wrung it out over the floor.

I waved to him. 'Come here, will you?'

He came over.

96

'Sit down.'

He sat down beside me on the divan, his leg against mine.

'Michael. You're pissing me off.'

'Never!'

'Tell me once and for all, in full detail. What's this all about?'

'Do you like Davidia?'

'I don't want her here.'

'What-what!'

'Not if you're up to what I think you're up to. And if it's what I think, then you're fucking up, man. You're fucking up.'

He stared down at the palms of his hands for a bit and then showed me his face: a soul without friends. 'Let's walk around. I'm still cooling off.' But first he went to the counter and called for the clerk and begged a cigarette and stuck it behind his ear.

I followed him out the doors and into the wash of red mud that passed for a street. The brief stretch of morning had already baked it hard. At this elevation the air was cool enough, but the equatorial sunshine burned on my back. It was crazy to walk.

Michael strolled beside me gripping my arm with one monster hand and with the other massaging my neck, my collarbones. His face shone with joy and sweat. 'It's good to speak honestly to you, Nair! Now it's time,

97

now I can do that. Now I'm happy. I was desolate, but now I'm happy. Ask me anything.'

'Jesus, Michael, where do we start? How about your military status?'

'I belong to nobody's military. I was an attaché merely.'

'There's a US Special Forces unit hunting around eastern Congo. Looking for the Lord's Resistance. Were you attached to them?'

'That's correct.'

'Did you run off?'

'That's an ugly rumor.'

'Did you run off?'

'I didn't run off. I moved away in support of my plan. My beautiful plan — and yes, yes, yes, we're going to get rich, how many times do I have to tell you? Be patient. Soon you're going to see something. With one stone, I'm killing a whole flock of birds.'

'Cutting through the muck — your status is AWOL.'

'Detached. Detached is more precise.'

'Next question. Are we messing around with fissionable materials?'

'Hang on, my brother.'

Over the last few days his speech had lost its American flavor, and his stride, I noticed, had an African man's swivel now, and his

shoulders rolled as he walked, like an African's. The lane climbed steeply here. He stopped to get a light from a vendor and then he was many paces ahead, on a rise, jogging toward the crest while puffing on his cigarette. I caught up with him and he said, 'My brother, do you think our wedding ceremony involves U-235?' — with a false and sickly grin. What an amateur. When it came to fountains of falsehood — a bold artist. But a simple denial, one word, a flat lie? No talent for that.

'Hold on,' I said, 'let me catch my breath.'

A shirtless beggar in khaki shorts approached, smiling and dragging one leg and crying, 'Sahibs!' The leg was enormous from elephantiasis, as if another whole man clung to him.

Michael yoked the man's throat with one hand, in the web of his thumb and finger, and lifted him so his horny yellow toes dangled a few inches off the ground and said, 'Nothing today. Ha ha!' and set him back down. We walked on. To me he said, 'I jog at six every morning. Do you want to get in shape with me?'

'No. I want you to tell me about U-235.'

'Not yet. What else? Ask me anything, Nair.'

A bit more, not a lot, had been revealed.

No sense driving further against this foam-rubber wall. 'How about this one: You're marrying the camp commander's daughter?'

'The garrison commander. Yes.'

'This is too wonderful. Where's the unit from the Tenth?'

'Close by Darba, Congo.'

'If we go up there — won't he want her back?'

'Whether we go or not, he'll want her back.'

'He won't get a bunch of vigilante Green Berets on our tails, will he?'

Michael was silent in a way I didn't like.

'Will he? I'm not up for risking any bloodshed. 'Any' means not one drop.'

'No, no bloodshed. They won't suspect we're anywhere near them.'

'Let's just not go.'

'Not go?' He turned in a complete circle, seeking a witness to my folly. 'He says 'Not go'! Do I have to make it clear? Then I'll make it clear. Let me make it clear about my clan. It's as if I left a man for dead and ran away to save myself. Then the next day he walks into my camp covered with blood, ready to go on living. Can you imagine the shame you would feel looking in his eyes? That's the shame that makes me go back to my village. Can I make you understand? I'm

going to marry Davidia. She'll be my life's mate. We've got to launch our lives together properly, with the blessing of my people. How can I make you *understand*? This is essential, it's not a gesture, it's not a nice idea — it's the essence of the thing. Without it, I'm nothing, and she's nothing, and we're nothing.'

As he expressed these ideas he followed them with his eyes, watching them gallop away to the place where they made sense.

'And we're going somewhere called Newada Mountain?'

'Near there. I haven't yet learned the exact location.'

'And yet you're sure your people have reconvened.'

'I just know they had to come back together. It's the natural thing to do.'

'It's essential.'

'Yes. Essential. You say it like an empty word, but the word is full. It's the truth. It's about the essence of things. Nair, I can guess where you got your information about me. From Horst, or Mohammed Kallon. Fuck them. Officially I've deserted, but in truth I'm returning to the loyalty I ran away from. What is desertion? Desertion is a coin. You turn it over, and it's loyalty.'

I agreed. 'My, my. You've been thinking.'

'A soldier must never think. In fact, when you're forbidden to think, it comes as a relief. Why did my mind start thinking?' His face was swollen with misery. 'Nair, you're the most important friend I've ever had.'

* * *

At five the next morning Michael had us traveling in a hired car through the darkness toward Kampala. As we approached the capital the traffic got thicker, and the air itself, with the smoke of breakfast fires and diesel fumes, and we raced under the attempted streetlights, many of them burning, turning the smoke yellow. Somewhere around here we'd get on a bus that would take us to the country's northeast corner. We hunted up and down unnamed streets until the driver gave up and put us out, and then the three of us stumbled over gutters and potholes among the hordes of street denizens waking up to the long slow overclouded African dawn, begging for assistance — we begging; not them. Michael got us to the booking office of the Gaagaa line, as it was called, a five-by-five-meter space completely covered with people asleep, who didn't mind being stepped on by others making for the clerk's cage. The clerk showed us a seating

chart, and I wrote my name where I wanted to sit, up front near the driver, and Michael put himself and Davidia across the aisle.

As we boarded the craft I looked up and realized it must have been dawn for half an hour, but the sky was so cloudy no real sunshine made it through. It was good having a cushion to sit on, even a gashed and moldy one, but I couldn't understand Michael's cheery attitude, his eagerness amid this fleet of debauched luxury liners exported from Malaysia or Singapore in freighter-size lots of wreckage, throttled and punched into taking a few more gasps, filing onto the roads with their busted television sets and torn-off seat belts, full of Michaels. We stowed our gear in racks overhead and Michael made sure Davidia and I each had a bottle of water and a box of Good Life butter biscuits. From some sort of church in the building behind us, on the second floor, above the public toilets, came a chorus of singing. Davidia arranged her long African skirt and pillowed her head on a folded scarf against the window and fell asleep. The passengers settled in all around, pulling their cell phones to their heads and talking. They smelled of liquor and urine and armpit. Michael now placed himself among them, resuming the mantle of African poverty — the way a civilized African

does, relaxing the shoulders and calming the hands and letting down the veil over his heart.

The bus's woman conductor stood in the aisle and addressed us, giving us her name and town and then bowing her head to pray out loud for one full minute in the hope this journey wouldn't kill us all. She invited everyone to turn to the next passenger and wish him or her the same thing, and we did, fare ye well, may this journey not be your last, although one of these journeys, surely, will send us — or whatever parts of us can be collected afterward — to the grave.

Our captain was a small man in a crisp white shirt and gray trousers, with a beard and turban. He sat down and started the engine and rattled the gearbox, and in just a few minutes the speedometer, I had a clear view of it, topped 100 kilometers per hour.

Somewhere behind us in Kampala, somewhere in Entebbe, I could have found Wi-Fi, I could have sent an encrypted summary-of-activities to NIIA . . . Goddamn, such an SOA might have begun, you perfect assholes. You sent me into this mess but told me nothing relevant. Fully half of what I've learned, you already knew. You didn't mention any U-235, did you, though I'm willing to bet you'd heard rumors, and that's

why I'm on this thing in the first place. And I'm not the only one on it, as I'm sure you're also aware. You said nothing about Interpol's interest, and as for Michael Adriko's desertion, I had to hear about that from Mohammed Kallon, a cheap Leonean grasser. Are you after information? I might inform you that Michael Adriko travels incommunicado with his bewildered fiancée, who happens to be the daughter of the camp commander for the US Tenth Special Forces Group, and that yesterday I saw her brassiere lying around and it was white, imprinted with tiny pink flowers, but you probably know all about that too. In any case, if there's something I know and you don't, anything at all — you can wait for it at the bottom of Hell . . .

Three hours along the route, the highway changed from two lanes down to one. The rate of speed stayed at 100. Smaller vehicles drove off the road as ours sailed toward them. The big lorries, the twelve-wheelers coming at us with their manifestos painted on their faces — AK-47 MONSTER — FIRE BASE ONE — GOD IS ABLE — LIVE FOR NOW — gave us half the road's width, and on our left side our own wheels traveled into the muck. None of these maneuvers required any reduction of speed on the part of anyone.

We slowed down only for the accidents, getting on the margin to steer around a small wreck, later another, and then we met a big one that stopped traffic both ways. I'd been nodding off and opened my eyes on a smashed lorry, a smashed pickup truck, a car upended and torn down the middle and sprouting limbs and dripping with blood. Pedestrians peered into the shattered windows without too much discussion or excitement. It must have just happened — ours was the first vehicle to come along, nothing to block the view. A baboon crouched on the bank of the roadway watching. A second observed from fifty meters on. Neither acknowledged the other. I noticed a bicycle bent in two tossed down on the grass. Michael clicked his tongue. 'They just won't slow down.'

While we waited for some force of civilization to take charge of the catastrophe, people descended from our bus to stretch their legs, eat their snacks, laugh, talk, relieve themselves. The three of us joined them at the roadside. Davidia shaded her eyes with a hand and studied the baboons studying us.

Michael said to Davidia, 'He's talking to you,' pointing to an old man who approached us. 'He is a magician.' He looked less than magic, instead looked tiny and silly, sucking

on a long purple sugarcane. 'He says we are all captives of this world. We were stolen while we were asleep and we were carried here, and now we're held captive in this world of dreams, where we believe we're awake.' While Michael translated, the magician laughed and hacked at his stalk of cane with his two or three teeth, snorting. He smiled brightly at someone he recognized across the road and turned away from us as we vanished from his mind. Michael said, 'Someone just has to drag that pickup truck to the side, and we'll pass through.' He went back into the bus. In twenty minutes the driver sounded his horn. People began climbing aboard. Michael told me, 'It's not as bad as West Africa. But it's still a hard land.'

All were aboard but one. In the field beside us Davidia, herself, was peeing — she gave everyone a big smile as she rose from her squat and dropped her hem and hitched her waistband with a very African, very female shimmy of her hips. I felt I was seeing her for the first time.

* * *

In Arua we took rooms at the White Nile Palace Hotel. Here was the palace, but we'd crossed the Nile twenty kilometers ago. We

arrived at night and formed no impression of the surrounding neighborhood except by its sounds — goats and cattle, arguments and celebrations. Surveying the parking area and later the tables in the café, I judged we'd come among missionaries and relief workers — Médecins Sans Frontières sorts of people with good, big SUVs and clean hiking shoes. The grounds were well-kept and our quarters were comfortable. I hadn't quite expected that.

At dinner Michael was nowhere in evidence. Davidia and I shared a table with an elderly, exhausted French woman of Arab descent who told us she studied torture. 'And once upon a time before this, I spent years on a study of the Atlantic slave trade. Angola. Now it's an analysis of the practices of torture under Idi Amin. Slavery. Torture. Don't call me morbid. Is it morbid to study a disease? That's how we find the cure for it. What is the cause of man's inhumanity to man? Desensitization. The numbness of the perpetrator. Whether an activity produces pleasure, pain, discomfort, guilt, joy, triumph — before too long the soul grows tired and stops feeling. It doesn't take long. Not too long at all, and then man becomes the devil, he laughs at his former scruples, he enslaves and tortures without compunction.' The woman's taut,

quivering neck, her mouth opening and closing . . . Halfway through her dessert of ice cream with chocolate sauce, without a word, she got up and left the table.

'Is she coming back?'

'No. She's paying her bill,' I said.

'She seemed possessed.'

'You attract a certain type, don't you? Orphans and magicians and circus people. You draw them to you. I don't know how.'

'I'm interested, and they feel it.'

'Where's Michael? I haven't seen him since we checked in.'

'As soon as we dropped our bags on the floor, he went out.'

'Where?'

'I don't know. 'Seeking word.' That's all he said.'

'More will be revealed.'

★   ★   ★

But not revealed immediately. Whatever Michael was working on, it kept him away a lot the next two days. When it wasn't raining Davidia read airport novels by the pool, in a tropical two-piece with a wraparound skirt, while I sat in the thatched shade with my laptop open on the bar, looking busy. The pool was kidney-shaped. Why? Why shaped

like a human organ? Frequent downpours kept it brimming over. People rarely swam in it. An arm's length above its surface, pairs of mating dragonflies whipped to and fro. Once in a while Davidia unwrapped herself down to her bikini and dipped herself in the water.

For restaurant and poolside music, American country tunes with a dash of rockabilly, the same forty-five-minute tape played all day long.

I wrote to Tina:

Well, no internet this AM at the White Nile Palace (Palace for Whites) Hotel. Writing off-line at the moment. No Wi-Fi here. We have to queue up for internet at the manager's office.

A light rain began. Davidia left the area with a wave. She had very high, very round breasts. She wore sandals whose red color against her brown feet looked somehow violent. I reached beside me for my coffee and knocked it from the bar, and it shattered all over the tiles. I'd put myself on a seventy-two-hour moratorium — no spirits, no wine, no beer. A somber young waiter with a push mop came to look after the mess.

In its relationship with Emmanuel, the

manager, the office computer is sort of a cartoon villain, coming up with some new way to thwart him every time he approaches it — this time it was a warning beep that wouldn't stop — and his procedure is to start whacking whatever parts look whackable and twisting wires like they've been bad little wires and taking hold of the monitor with both hands and shaking the shit out of it, and today he gave the wall plug a good hard kick — not so stupid, really, because you do often get new results around here by wiggling the wall plug. Or snapping it with your finger. The people who work under him all know how to handle the computer just fine, and if the network's up, they can make it happen, but Emmanuel, he just starts right in on the contraption like he's carrying out an old vendetta, and I've learned not to ask him to try, except for entertainment.

I tried and deleted several ways of getting onto the next topic, and finally wrote —

Have you heard anything from Grant or that Major Kenworth guy, or any of those other boys in Sec 4?

— Section 4, Internal Inquiries, counterintelligence, the spy catchers. They hunt the traitor.

Let me know if anybody comes over from there just to say hi. I'll tell you what it's all about later on, when we're together again.

— and deleted the final sentence and wrote instead, 'I've put in for an opening over there, to tell the truth,' and deleted *to tell the truth*, 'and if I have a shot at it, if they're interested in me, they'll probably do a little snooping.'

★ ★ ★

I woke and dressed fast without showering, ridden by a desire, an absolute lust, to get it all done this very moment, plus a feeling I wouldn't get it done at all. I skipped breakfast and flagged one of the motorbikes waiting outside the hotel, and we traveled as fast as the engine could propel us toward the Catholic radio installation. Gripping my laptop with one hand and my life with the other, I made up my mind not to ride one of these things again. The night's rain had slicked the road going into town, and quick maneuvers around potholes or out of the way

112

of death sent us gliding in zigzags over the red mud. Bursts of adrenaline drained me and calmed me. The forward charge slowed down as we mounted a long steep hill toward three large towers in a compound of low buildings, the Catholic communications center.

At the gate a uniformed guard searched me, and a laminated security pass went around my neck. The guard walked me over to the nearest of several adobe buildings, and there a kind woman in a nun's habit led me to a large room and sat me down before one of three computers at a long counter against the wall. She took a chair by the door. For the moment, it was just the two of us. I logged on with a password and immediately logged off.

While I waited, I heard the roar of a soccer game drifting up from the school at the bottom of the hill.

Pretty soon a blue-uniformed Ugandan soldier entered the room. I sensed him coming but stared at the screen until he touched my shoulder and said, 'Please come,' and led me to the Secure Communications Environment, the 'SC lounge,' or the 'SC café.' It looked like the room we'd just left. Only one computer console here.

This place had nothing to do with NATO, except in the way of 'courteous exchange,' as

it's called in the business. The safe communications here were an operation of the British, MI4 or 5 or 6 . . . May I reveal a fact? I don't know how many MIs there are. In any case, it was nothing to do with NIIA. As far as I'd been allowed to know, NATO maintained no safe sites anywhere in Uganda for communications. The Americans like to say 'commo' — I think it's silly. Using my own laptop, I checked my list of e-mails. One from NIIA. I didn't open it.

Another one, from Tina: a photo taken in a mirror, her face hidden behind the camera and her breasts exposed. Not a word of text.

I sent her what I'd composed off-line, and added:

Nothing has happened since I wrote the above. I've spent my time listening to the BBC on a little radio or watching the images of Al Jazeera on the satellite TV, when the TV works. Emmanuel has permanently bested the hotel's computer and it just sits there half dead. Nobody can use it now. It's not a communication device anymore, it's capable of making a few high-pitched noises understood only by itself. Therefore I just took a half hour's trip across town to the Catholic radio station compound, where they have

a media center with three computers & Wi-Fi.

Don't forget to let me know if you hear from Sec 4.

— and felt I was hitting the thing too hard and deleted the last line and wrote:

I thank you from the bottom of my scrotum for the glimpse of your beauties. I hope I can assume they're yours.

Nothing from Hamid. I'd expected nothing. It was my turn to talk.

I switched to my own keyboard. As he'd suggested, I didn't use the American Standard. For a lark I used PGP, and in accordance with Hamid's wishes I rotated my proxy after every fifteen words:

230K dollars US.
50–50 split.
Currently in transit.
Will return to site of previous meeting when we have a deal.
Suggest date exactly 30 days following previous meeting.
Sample product: Basement Elvis Documents Freetown.
NIIA safe site. Check and see.

Don't answer until the answer's yes.

Having suggested a date, I heard the clock start ticking. Today was October eleventh — I'd have nineteen days to wrap things up with Michael and find my way back to Freetown. An easy schedule. But Africa wipes its mess with schedules.

I opened the communique from my boss:

Let's not overlook opportunities for filing. Check in daily. I don't add 'when possible.' Check in daily.

No amount of detail is too great. Err on the side of inclusiveness. Give us an abundance to sift through and ponder each day. Every day. Daily.

From this point forward, consider that a mission imperative.

I replied:

Nothing to report.

— and closed the window.

★ ★ ★

The rain came hard. The dining room's fine vaulted ceiling apparently leaked profusely,

and when Michael and Davidia and I entered that evening looking for dinner, the maitre d' came at us with a push mop, driving a minor flood before him out the doors. On a hoarding on the step, a list of the cocktails on special — 'Safe Sex in the Forest,' mostly vodka, and one called 'The Pussycat,' whose main ingredient was identified as Baboon Whiskey. Time to lift the drinks moratorium? My thirty-dollar Timex watch said not even close.

The musical fare had changed — today, fifties pop, specifically 'Smile' as rendered by Nat 'King' Cole. Nothing else. Just 'Smile.' Over and over. 'Smile' . . . 'Smile' . . . 'Smile' . . .

Michael had turned up two hours before, dangling a set of car keys. 'Toyota Land Cruiser. Four-wheel drive. Full of petrol.'

At dinner Davidia wanted to know when we'd go riding. 'Soon. It's all ours.'

I wasn't so sure. 'Where did you get it?'

'From Pyramid Environments.'

'Pyramid? Who's that?'

'Pyramid Environments. Security. I know all those guys. The manager's office is in Arua. I know him from Fort Bragg.'

'Bragg? I thought you were at Fort Carson.'

'And Bragg — I told you that. At Bragg I trained Colombian commandos. The US

assists them in going after the drugs racket down there. Everything was done through translators. Let me tell you something you already know ... working in simultaneous translation is exhausting. It's like walking everywhere on your hands, and never your feet.'

'So you've told me many times,' Davidia said.

'I don't like the situation over there,' Michael said, meaning the situation at another table. 'These guys don't look right. They're up to something.'

'Doctors Without Borders.'

'Then why don't they go someplace and play doctor? First we see them at lunch, and now at dinner.'

'Good lord. Is it possible we're following them?'

'Perhaps we should be.'

Davidia glanced at me as if to say Help.

'Nobody's spying on you,' I told Michael.

'Wait a minute. That one is Spaulding. Remember Spaulding?'

'I remember. That's not Spaulding.'

Michael got up and went over to them.

'I hope he's not about to be rude,' Davidia said.

'He's just being Michael.'

'He's getting pretty crazy, Nair.'

'You know what? I think he's right. It's Spaulding.'

'Who's Spaulding?'

Spaulding possessed a great mop of platinum hair. I wouldn't have guessed such a thing, and I hadn't recognized him. As it happened, I'd never before seen the top of his head.

Michael brought him over. Spaulding didn't sit down. Pretty soon Michael would tell us he'd been the one to give Spaulding his very first sight of death. He'd told me this story many times.

'Here's Spaulding.' To Davidia: 'Spaulding is MI6.'

Spaulding didn't mind. 'He introduces everybody as some kind of spy.'

'Have you chucked your turban?' I asked Spaulding.

'A turban's all right in Afghanistan, in the winter.'

'So you were never actually some kind of Sikh?'

'Just keeping my head warm,' Spaulding said.

'What's your religion, then?' Michael said.

'Lapsed Catholic.'

'I myself,' Michael said, 'am a lapsed animist. This is Davidia, my wife-to-be.'

'Congratulations, then, the two of you.'

'Davidia — Spaulding is with MI6.'

'I don't hang out with MI6,' Spaulding said, smiling. 'They're all homosexuals.'

Michael said, 'I showed Spaulding his first dead body. In Mogadishu.'

Spaulding said, 'It was more like two hundred dead bodies. All laid out neatly side by side in the street. Fresh-cooked.'

'Remember the dust devils? Two kilometers high. That's where the legends of genies come from.'

'You couldn't have been more than thirteen or fourteen. Your voice hadn't changed.'

Michael produced a soprano: 'Ayeeeeee! — My voice will never change,' he went on in his man's baritone.

'I didn't meet Spaulding till Afghanistan,' I said.

Spaulding studied me. 'Really. Have we actually met?'

'Here comes our food,' Michael announced. 'None for Spaulding.'

'Have a lovely evening,' Spaulding said, mainly to Davidia, and rejoined his table.

Davidia said, 'Jesus Christ. You people!'

I looked at Michael — looking back at me. 'And there you have it,' he said. 'It's already time to leave town.'

★ ★ ★

The White Nile Palace Hotel had proved in one respect far too proper for my taste, but that afternoon, as I sat at a table near the bar trying to make sense of the hamburger I'd just been served, a little brown slut with a wig of short red hair came in and stood within reach of my arms and started wrapping and unwrapping the skirt that covered her bathing suit as she queried the bartender, ignoring me and inflaming me, and I thought, Thank goodness, at last, a reasonable woman. I got her to sit down with me and asked her name. It was Lucy. She was friendly enough. I felt us on the brink of striking an arrangement.

The PA played 'Jingle Bell Rock.' Two American-sounding women swam up and down the pool with gentle strokes, side by side, conversing about the Bible and God and spiritual challenges.

Michael Adriko turned up at the pool's far end. He wore black bathing trunks. I supposed he could swim, but I'd never seen him at it.

He was talking to a Euro, a white man. It was rare to see Michael looking serious, rare to see him listening intently. I wished I could read the man's lips. He was of middling height and middling all around, mid-thirties, with thinning, colorless hair. Rimless spectacles, a short-sleeved dress shirt tucked into

dark corduroys that had come untucked at the back — a civil servant sort, he seemed to me, except that he wore the shirt half unbuttoned to display a thick gold necklace.

I moved to the bar and tried to catch Michael's eye, wondering if I should be introduced. I didn't catch his eye. I wasn't introduced.

I took up my cell phone and asked Lucy to excuse me, I had to make some calls. She said, 'Maybe you need to call your boyfriend,' and went to the bar to pout and say nasty things about me.

The two men each sat on the edge of a recliner, heads bent toward one another. I took a stroll around the pool pretty much in the manner of someone who had no idea what he was doing, passing behind them in order to — what? Smell what might be brewing — hostility? Conspiracy? Conspiracy, I thought.

I walked past them and out the back gate onto the grounds, and I took note again of the man's heavy necklace, which had tainted his neck's flesh with a greenish collar. I walked around a bit, then came back past the pool and through the bar, heading for the restaurant.

'Just give me a minute,' I said to Lucy as I passed her. 'I won't be two minutes.'

I took a table in the restaurant and kept an eye on Michael and the other. Again the PA was playing 'Smile' and had been playing it, I realized, for quite some time.

After one more full turn through the song, the man got up and came toward me through the patio door, staring at me hard. He looked no more dangerous than a mathematics instructor, but my face flushed, I felt it — he passed me by and went out the front way. I watched out the window as he left the grounds by the gate, waving to the guard.

Michael was coming into the place.

'Join me for one second,' I said.

He glanced around strangely, apologetically, and I realized that in his swimming shorts, he felt undressed.

I said, 'Michael. What-what?' He sat down across from me and I said, 'Who was that guy?'

'Well, he's a businessman.'

'Are we in business with him?'

'Exactly.'

'Do you want to tell me what it is?'

'Right. Things are in motion. It's time for full disclosure.'

'Tell me.'

'Come to my room in ten minutes.'

I nearly exploded in his face. 'If now is the time, why ten fucking minutes?'

'What's your hurry?'

'There's a girl I want to talk to.'

'This is slightly more important.'

'Why ten minutes?'

'Davidia's napping. I'll kick her out.'

After he'd gone, I went back to the pool after Lucy — she was lying in the big rope hammock cuddling with a fat African fucker.

★ ★ ★

At the Palace the rooms occupied circular bungalows modeled after the local huts, but a great deal larger and roofed with rubber shakes, not straw; four rooms to a bungalow, each room a quarter circle, each with a verandah, a door, a bathroom, two windows side by side. This one had a bed, a desk, a TV, and a standing electric fan, just like mine. A couple of shelves and hangers on a rod — no closet.

I looked around for evidence of Davidia. The room had been cleaned, and everything was stowed, or hanging. It didn't look as if anybody could have been napping here.

'Full disclosure.'

Michael unfurled a black shopping bag and dumped the contents on the bed: bright yellow electrician's tape wrapping a package the size of an American softball.

'Pick it up.'

It was heavy for its size. 'Feels like a couple of kilos.'

He went hacking at the tape with a penknife and soon laid out before me a shiny lump of metal no larger than my thumb, on a rag of odd-looking material.

It looked like gold. I assumed it was gold. I prayed it was gold.

'What's this stuff it's wrapped in?'

'That's a bit cut from the smock you wear when you get an X-ray. It's lead-lined.'

'Oh, shit,' I said.

'That's right.'

'Uranium.'

'Very correct.'

'U-235?'

'No. It's polished, but it's just ore. As long as it fools a Geiger counter . . . Superficial authenticity, that's all we're looking for. It comes from southern Congo. The Shinkolobwe mine.'

'Not from a crashed Russian cargo plane.'

'No.'

'You don't actually have a planeload of enriched uranium.'

'I told you — full disclosure. There's nothing else. Have you heard of the Manhattan Project?'

'Sure.'

'The uranium for that came from the same mine, there in Shinkolobwe.'

'Looks as if a dog just squeezed it out its ass.'

'A little lump can make a very big bang.'

'If I touch it, will I get cancer?'

He laughed. I held it in my hand.

'I'm in the process of parlaying that bit of dog business into one million dollars US.'

As if he'd opened a gash in me, all the tension ran out. I dragged the chair away from his desk and sat down. 'So it's a scam.'

'Of course it is. Do you think I'm running around with enriched uranium? If there was any U-235 on the market, New York City would be nothing but a crater already.'

'And who's our friend, with the fake gold necklace?'

'Fake?'

'Didn't you see his neck? He's probably poisoning himself with gold spray-paint. I didn't like the way he came at me in the restaurant.'

'He's calling himself Kruger, probably because he's South African. He saw you cruising around us. And Nair, it's genius. The minute he saw you, I improvised something: you're the bad scientist.'

'I'm the mad scientist?'

'The bad, the bad, the bad. You're the

renegade engineer who recently examined the crash site for the Tenex corporation. You reported to Tenex there was nothing there. No uranium material. But you lied. It's there. You kept the truth to yourself, and you're selling the crash site's coordinates. Just a few numbers on a piece of paper. For one million cash US. It's too brilliant, Nair.'

He paused for my reaction.

I couldn't see where to begin. A bit of rain started on the roof above and the leaves outside, and we listened to that for a while.

'You're the verification,' he said. 'We meet with Kruger and his partner, who's bringing a Geiger counter. We give them this shiny radioactive object as proof of possession, and you verify what I say about the crash site. Then on to the big swap. One million.'

'But, Michael, have you thought this through? Or thought even a little? How would this scam work? Take me through it, step by step. What are the steps that lead to the moment when the money's out on the table?'

'By the time the money's on the table, we'll have a lot of guys to help us. After our meeting with Kruger and his partner, we'll have twenty-five K US as our payment for proof of possession. With some of that money,

we'll get a squad together. Congo is full of brigands. M23, Lord's Resistance — plenty of warriors, and nothing to do all day.'

'And then what? Cowboys and Indians? The money's on the table, and a bunch of guns come out?'

'I'll handle that part. You'll just handle the oily parts, because you're good at that. But the answer is yes. Armed robbery.'

'You skipped over my real question. How do you get the money on the table?'

'When we meet with Kruger and his partner, we'll tell them that as soon as they have the big payment prepared, we'll be prepared to turn over another X kilos, say five kilos, and that's all we could carry from the crash site. We promise them the coordinates to the rest.'

'And for telling them this fairy tale they'll give you twenty-five K?'

I heard him say, 'Twenty-five,' and then the rain outside came harder and washed out his words. I said, 'What? What?'

'Twenty-five K immediately, Nair. In our pockets. Then we go from Arua to Congo and we find my villagers, my family. A beautiful wedding takes place. Then we make arrangements for the final contact and the rest of the payment. It's going to be a big payment, Nair, very big. Big.'

'Right. One million. You already said.'

'I haven't said it to them yet. Maybe I'll say two.'

'Who's going to let you string them along all that way with just this little piece of dogshit?'

'The question to ask is — who could pass it up? Who could say no? If the claim is at all credible, they have to give it the full treatment.'

'Credible? It sounds completely and obviously false, Michael — can't you see that? What words can I use? Nonsensical. Impossible. Out of keeping with reality.'

'Reality is not a fact.'

'Around here it certainly isn't. God.'

'Reality is an impression, a belief. Any magician knows this.' Like a cartoon villain, he rubbed his hands together. 'Oh my goodness, Nair, you just tickle them in their terrorism bone, and they ejaculate all kinds of money. If you mention the name of one of the Muslim Most Wanted — boom, they put on a circus for you.'

'You've skipped another question, haven't you?'

'What. What's the question?'

'Who is this 'they'? Are they a fantasy too?'

'Of course not. Kruger works for them.'

'Who? Who are we dealing with besides this

Kruger? Do you even know?'

'We're dealing with the Israelis.'

If I'd had to stand up from my chair at that moment, I'd have failed. I was that shocked, and that much afraid. 'Then you're dealing with the Mossad.'

'Their involvement is likely.' And he seemed proud of it. He smiled with all his teeth.

'You're scamming Mossad.'

'They know me. If I say I have it, they've got to take me seriously and get together the cash.'

The rain roared, or it was my head, but in any case the sense of things rushed away on a flood. 'Michael . . . Michael . . . '

'Nair. Nair.' He got his face close to mine as if he thought I couldn't hear. 'I know those people. You *know* I know them. I was trained by them.'

'Michael, be quiet.'

'Let me tell you about it.'

'No. I'm feeling bewildered. Please shut up.'

He complied. I didn't say a word. In the silence, which was nevertheless quite loud, his folly bore down on us like a tremendous iceberg. Its inertia was irresistible. In this room, in Africa, reasonable arguments were just mumbo jumbo.

'Is that enough quiet? Can I talk now? Because I want to explain one thing: I've got contacts, I know Mossad — ever since my training in South Africa. I can call them anytime that we want to cancel, and the whole thing's canceled. Never happened.'

'Well, Jesus Christ, man — call them now, and call it off. Cancel everything. Mossad? You're insane.'

'All right. I'll cancel if you say so.'

'I just said so.'

'But let's wait until we take it one tiny step further along. Let's meet with these guys and their Geiger counter, and walk away with twenty-five K. Then no more. Nothing further than that.'

'No brigands versus Mossad. No showdowns at the table.'

'Exactly. And if they don't like our lump of shit tomorrow — no loss. At least we tried.'

'Tomorrow?'

'Yes — tomorrow. I told you, full disclosure.'

'Fuck it, Michael. I'm done.'

I got up, making a loud noise with my chair, and headed out the door toward a place to be determined later.

'How done?' Michael called after me.

* * *

In two minutes I arrived at the bar pretty nicely drenched. I took a table where I could watch the storm.

At the bar sat Spaulding, his cranium wrapped in a big white turban. He pointed at it. 'What do you think?'

What I think — I thought to myself — is you're spying on me.

I checked my watch. Time to lift the drinks moratorium. An hour past.

As I looked around for the barman, Spaulding came over to me. 'Shit, Nair, I sort of didn't recognize you yesterday. You know — without the uniform.' He set a full drink before me, saying, 'Cheers, mate. It's made with Baboon Whiskey.'

Like that, I drank half of it down. 'Have a seat.'

'I really can't. Car's waiting. I'm checking out.'

I nearly said, Good. 'Where are you off to?'

'Oh, God knows. The itinerary's a bit complicated. Entebbe to start. What about you?'

'Just here. Then home again.'

'Home again to — '

'Amsterdam.'

'Amsterdam! I love the hash. Do you go to the coffee shops?'

'Every day. Wrap up in my turban and get

out my hookah and set fire to all manner of shit.'

He laughed and said, 'Happy trip, Nair,' and headed off briskly, with a sort of half salute that knocked at his stupid head-wrap.

A bit sweet, but the drink had a kick. I signaled the barman. 'Let's try a vodka martini.'

Rain swept across the pool's face, and then it stopped. The sky was half-and-half — one storm had passed, another was coming. My first drinks in three days were going to my head, expanding my consciousness. I didn't like it. I gulped the vodka without tasting it and made my way to my bungalow and changed into shorts and a long-sleeved shirt and lay down. The TV lit up when I tried it. I watched Ugandan news, a report about a pair of twins conjoined at the shoulder — in other words, a two-headed baby — who had died, and then one about a child whose face had been eaten by a pig. Its fingers as well.

This information drove me out to a chair on the verandah. The sky was stuffed with thunderheads nearly black. I shut my eyes yet felt aware of the garden at my elbow, the blooms opening as if in a time-lapse, the stalks lengthening. Blossoms like dangling red bells, blossoms like tiny white fountains, fuzzy

yellow caterpillars on brown twigs, a squad of snails lugging their small shelters up the spears of a plant.

The moment was dark as evening, but all was bathed in a great vividness. The rain shot out of the sky, hard as hail. A wondrous assurance lifted me, a force positively religious invited me to stand and shed my shirt, to drop my shorts and kick them from my feet. No need of clothes when clothed in African magic, and I walked naked across the grounds through the booming and the lightning with the sweet rain pouring all around, and soon I stood looking down into the swimming pool. Everybody else was indoors, and through this whole experience no other person was visible anywhere in the world except the bartender, all alone behind the bar under his awning a few yards from the pool-side, watching as I jumped into the water and drowned.

From this dream I woke to another: I lay on my back beside the pool while Michael Adriko kissed me, breathed fire into my mouth and down my throat. I rolled over retching and coughing, my lungs tearing.

I came awake again on a lower rung of reality, still lying on my back, but now in my hotel room, wrapped in a shroud, shivering. Michael sat beside me on the bed.

I said, or tried to say, 'You spat in my mouth.'

'What happened to you, Nair?'

'Somebody drugged me.'

'You didn't drug yourself?'

'I had one whiskey and one martini. Maybe the olive was bad.'

'Bad? You mean evil?'

'What? Stop talking to me.'

'Davidia is here,' he said.

'Where?'

'Where? Here!'

'I'm not there,' her voice said, 'I'm here, on the verandah. Can you hear the crickets? Are those crickets?'

All around the music, like little bells. 'Some sort of insect, yes,' Michael said.

'Spaulding did this to me. Was it Spaulding, do you think?'

'It could be anything. A virus, a bite from a spider, or even a spell, a curse — people have such powers. I've seen too much to laugh at it.'

'That fucking towel-head dosed my martini.'

Michael laughed with such vigor that Davidia came in and looked at his face and said, 'Are you all right?'

'You should have seen Fred's expression!' He meant the bartender. 'Like the aliens were

135

landing in his pool! Seriously,' he said, 'he must have dragged you from the pool himself. He was wet to the waist. His shoes are ruined.'

'I'll give him some money,' I said.

The rain had stopped, and Davidia was correct — the creatures had resumed, the bugs that chimed like porcelain, frogs that belched like drunkards, and now more frogs, snorting like pigs. A suffocating sleep fell over my face. I came under its shadow convinced that Spaulding had poisoned me.

★　★　★

The next morning I asked for Spaulding, and Emmanuel, the manager, said he'd settled his account and left in a taxi for Arua's small airfield. Flying where? No commercial planes this morning, according to Emmanuel. Only the UN plane to Yei, in South Sudan.

I continued on to the restaurant for my appointment with Michael Adriko. I'd promised to meet him there and tell him my decision.

There he was, near the blaring television, doing nothing, not even watching it. 'Well?'

'I haven't decided.'

'Take your time. Up to ten more minutes. Don't sit down. Walk with me,' he said,

already moving, 'I've got to see about the gas.'

'Is it a long drive?'

'Just into town, over by the market, but you know the rule — half a tank is empty. You remember the rule.'

I remembered.

When we came to the parking lot, he paused. 'As of right now, the process is halted. You see how easy it is?'

'I get uncomfortable when you stop in the middle of walking to make a point.'

'At any moment in the procedure, we can say 'enough.''

'I understood the point.'

'Then understand this one: Do you really want to go back to that boring existence?'

'Never.'

This much was true, the only true thing between us.

By now we'd reached his borrowed Land Cruiser. We both got in. The engine caught quickly, first try.

The guard held the gate wide open for us.

It was a years-old model, much like the blue-and-white Land Cruisers we'd often borrowed from the UN in Jalalabad, sometimes Kabul. Too much like. It even smelled the same inside, like spilt gas and dirty clothes.

'Are you ready?'

'No. For this? No.'

★　★　★

We stopped at a filling station where a woman topped off our tank, and we waited.

'Near the market, you said?'

'That's all I know. They'll call me with the meeting place. What time is it? — eleven-thirty-three,' he informed himself. 'They'll call me in the next half hour.' We sat side by side on the vehicle's rear bumper, Michael studiously smoking, blowing white puffs upward through the brown fumes and the red dust, under the yellow Shell insignia. After the call, he pocketed his phone and threw down his cigarette and stomped it like an insect. 'We're off.'

We left the SUV in front of a place called Gracious Good Hotel, under care of the taxi drivers loitering there. Michael, a bright red zippered daypack slung over his arm, guided me across the street toward the market by way of a narrow alley with light at the far end, its crevices roiling with crippled beggars — many were blind, and as for the others, they seemed to look through your own eyes and down your throat. Ahead of me Michael was a bent silhouette, handing over a crumpled

bill. 'My name is Michael,' I heard him say, 'pray for me.' An old woman caught the money between her leprous paws and turned her sightless eyes up toward him and her lips moved below the noseless hole in her face, praying, 'Michael, Michael,' not for him, but rather to him, to the deity Michael . . . And crash, back into the daylight — it never happened . . .

I caught up with Michael at a clothier's stall. He was looking at a coat of fake black leather too hot for this region. He set his mirrors on his scalp, gripped the sleeve, touched the fabric with one finger. I didn't know if he was trying to buy something or just delaying, looking out for a tail.

The latter. When we left the market square he led the way into a dry goods store across the street. Inside we made our way directly down the center aisle to the back of the store, where a woman napped in a collapsible chair, and we asked her for another entrance. She pointed through a curtain, we passed through it and out into a side lane, then up to the left — and I recognized the street, and saw our Land Cruiser parked just a block away.

He handed me his daypack. 'Take charge of the little morsel.'

'Of course.' Lethargy and nausea overtook me. It felt like it weighed fifty pounds.

Michael said, 'I go first. Wait until you see me come out again, then you'll come and join me. It may take a few minutes.'

'What's going to happen in there?'

'Before I bring you on the stage, I'll say I want to see the cash. They'll say no, but this way I get to review the environment.'

'And then what?'

'It's two South African guys — Kruger is one, you saw him. You'll verify everything I tell them, right? Then I'll go with them. You can stay there — it's that café there, you see it? I'll go with them, we'll sit in their car or something with the sample and their equipment, and we'll make the exchange. And I'll come back in and collect you, and then back to Nile Palace.'

'Where's their equipment, do you know?'

'Ah — you're thinking smart now. If it's not in their car or somewhere we can walk, I'll make them go get it. I'm not driving off with them.'

On this sunny street, where earth-moving machines worked over piles of red dirt, improving the surface, and generators clattered in front of the shops and schoolchildren in green-and-white uniforms walked home for lunch, all this sounded reasonable.

'Stop breathing so fast,' Michael said.

'I'm fucking nervous.'

'Good. It helps you look the part. Just don't faint.' He left me standing there and in order to keep my mind off itself I studied the nearby billboard exhorting the use of condoms and followed the progress of a small car over the ruts and small boulders from one end of the block to the other, its horn playing the first six notes of the 'Happy Birthday' song. Looking around for something else, I spied Michael already back outside, standing in his own spotlight in his aviator sun shades as if in support of the warning stenciled beside him: DO NOT URINE ON THIS WALL 30,000 FINE. And he wore the fake black leather duster from the market. I was nervous to the point that I hadn't even seen him make the purchase.

Michael must have sensed it. He took my arm and kept me going as we went inside. I was living one of my persistent nightmares: I step onto the stage, it's time to speak, I don't know my lines. In this particular bad dream the stage was a four-by-four-meter dirt space enclosed in ironwork and roofed with tin, with a sign on the left saying SIMBA DISCO / PHONE CHARGE ACCUMULATOR AVAILABLE and on the right a Bell Lager clock with one hand, counting only the minutes, and wooden tables and benches. We sat down across from the South Africans.

They were a half-and-half team, like Michael and me. The black one, I assumed, was Zulu, and could have been one of Kruger's math pupils, but he looked in his thirties too. He wore his sunglasses on the back of his shaved skull. In most other respects he seemed to be trying to resemble an American rapper: a hooded sweater, baggy hip-hop shorts I hadn't seen anyone wearing in Uganda. A word about this Zulu's shoes. They were purple joggers, elaborately designed and, by the look of them, enclosing enormous feet. There's no explaining why I should have been so penetratingly aware, at this moment, of anybody's fashion choices. Kruger suggested a drink, and I certainly concurred, and now came the moment when I discovered the East African quick-shot — a square plastic envelope that would fit in your palm and holding one hundred milliliters of, in this case, Rider Vodka — Sign of Success. You chew off a corner and slurp. I bought several, several. The floor was tiled with discarded packets.

Michael produced a cigarette and called for a light, and the barman brought over several for sale. Michael had to try three or four of them before he got one that worked.

Kruger said, 'Everything here is fake.'

Michael said, 'Only my heart is real,' and put away his cigarette.

I wasn't taking in much, only the Rider Vodka. Remarks were delivered, there was talk of a Geiger counter, the location of their car, mention was made, in fact, of roentgens, but of all this I registered one exchange only: Michael said, 'Nice necklace, brother,' and Kruger said, 'I like yours too,' and when Michael thanked him, Kruger added, 'It looked good on my friend before you stole it,' and Michael said, 'Who? What friend?' at which point, as if time had skipped forward, the three of them were standing up and fighting. The Zulu had Michael from behind in a bear hug, or was trying to pin his elbows, while Michael twisted side to side and the Kruger fellow thrust with a knife at Michael's chest and belly, then at Michael's throat.

Another skip — the Zulu lay on his back, wide-eyed, struggling to take a breath. Michael had hurt him somehow. I had an impulse to act, an image flitted through me, I saw myself taking two steps, jumping onto the man's chest, standing on him, keeping him down. No part of me acted. I experienced it as a question only — shouldn't I, shall I. I didn't. Now the seconds passed more fluidly, as if a stuck film had caught in its sprockets,

and I watched the movie, which wasn't like the movies after all, not even like a boxing match on TV. I heard the initial thumps, then my hearing turned cottony, and I remember Michael's eyes — they watched, they looked, they moved here, there, they gauged — when he had his target, he locked on Kruger's face, not on his hands, though one hand gripped the knife in preparation for downward thrusts —

Michael danced backward, knocked a bench over between them, plucked at the table — a salt shaker in his hand; he threw it hard, it struck the man's chest, and Michael followed its arc, picking up the bench as he closed on his opponent, ramming the flat seat against him. Kruger fell backward as Michael's feet left the floor, one hand at Kruger's throat, the other still holding the bench in place, and his weight stuck the man to the table. His fingers closed on the carotid arteries, and Kruger lost conscious swiftly — a matter of a few seconds — managing to slash at Michael only once with the knife, which sailed to the floor, along with the bench, as Michael stood and snapped Kruger's arm over his knee. The breaking of the bone was quite pronounced. Deaf with adrenaline, I nevertheless heard that sound crisply. I heard it echo back into the room

from the surrounding hills.

Michael wasted no time continuing the contest. He signaled me, I stood still, he came close, gripped my wrist, and before I formed even my first thought about what was happening, we were both in the Toyota and moving along as Michael steered with both hands, saying, 'Wrap my arm, wrap my arm.' His right forearm bled in spurts. He extended it across his chest toward me, steering with his left hand, and I understood at last, and found my bandanna and wrapped it around a long gash that showed the yellowish bone. I tied it with a square knot. 'That's going to need stitches,' was his first remark since the action had begun. 'So much for South Africa,' was his second.

★　★　★

Michael pointed out the White Nile Palace as we passed it. 'I want you to drive back here after you drop me at the hospital.'

'Where's the hospital?'

'I've seen the signpost up here a couple of kilometers. We go to the right. After that I don't know.'

We rumbled across a wooden bridge. Ahead of us a pedestrian, an old man, jumped up on the railing to save himself.

'Well,' I said, 'I wasn't much use to you, was I?'

'But, Nair — what's there, between your feet?'

'For goodness' sake.' His red daypack.

'You grabbed my bag. You saved the most important thing. The valuables.'

A couple of minutes off the main road we found the hospital, a campus of one-story structures of concrete and brick, the Church of Uganda Kuluva Hospital, according to the sign at the guard post. The guard waved us down and peered through the window and waved us through when he saw the blood. 'Nurse is coming,' he said. 'Proceed to Minor Theatre.'

The door to the building called Minor Theatre was locked. Michael squatted on his haunches with his spine against the wall, smoking, while the blood seeped from his bandage and pooled between his feet. His eyes were bright and he gave off a certain energy.

He looked, I have to say, in better shape than I felt. I stood upright, but only to prove I was able. 'I wish I'd made one tiny fucking move to help.'

'I didn't need help. Did you hear his bone breaking?'

'God. I didn't even drive the car. I've

always known I've got zero courage, but I don't like to be reminded.'

'There's no such thing as courage. It's a question of training. You know, I'm not merely trained in unarmed combat — I'm the instructor.'

'Maybe you should instruct me.'

'I instruct you to stay by my side. You'll win more fights that way.'

At the entrance to the grounds a car came to a sharp halt, and the man calling himself Kruger more or less fell out of the passenger door into the arms of his driver and the guard. The guard dragged the chair from his shack and sat Kruger down in it, and he and the driver — who was not the Zulu — carried Kruger in it toward another building with his shirt off and his arm bound up in it all bloody.

Michael waved with his own wounded arm. 'No hard feelings, mate — next time I'll kill you.'

Kruger sailed past in his chair with his eyes closed, chalk-faced and uncomprehending. His partner was nowhere around.

'I don't know what kind of mess we're in,' I said.

'I think we're better off in Congo now.'

'How did all this come about, Michael? Who were those characters?'

'I'm sure of this much: they weren't Mossad. Just a couple of jokers Mossad has on a string.'

'In other words, Mossad has you marked for death.'

'If Mossad wanted me dead, I'd be dead. Mossad works very tight. They use teams of six or seven or even more and they train and plan very carefully, and they get it done every time. They don't use idiots who attack you in a café. These guys were just associates, like me. But I believe them this far — I believe Mossad gave them money. That's why that fool pulled a knife. They wanted to keep my payment for themselves.'

'This scam is over,' I said, 'finished, okay?'

'Agreed.'

'Because it pisses me off when I go along with stupid ideas.'

'You're pissed off now. I see that. Okay.'

'I wish I had transcripts of the conversations that led to this,' I said, 'the conversations you had with those guys. I bet I could show you a dozen places where they were obviously — obviously — playing you.'

'In the end, you have to go by instinct.'

'You trust too Goddamn much.'

'Is that really a fault?'

'What? Yes. A fatal one. The life you lead, the people you deal with — do you think it's

just teddy bears hugging marshmallows?'

He laughed at me.

I wished Kruger would stab him again. 'You trust the wrong people,' I said. 'Believe me.'

★ ★ ★

This hospital had been established in 1848, according to the sign at the entrance, and originally as a place for lepers, according to Michael's nurse, who prepared the sutures and such on a tray. No doctor arrived. She stitched the wound herself. 'We will close the laceration in two layers,' she told Michael. 'It's deep.'

'How long do you think this will take?' I asked.

She was jabbing a swab down into the damaged area. 'The sutures must go close together.' I took this to indicate a lengthy procedure.

'If I had some water, maybe I'd clean up the car a bit.'

'There's a stream there' — she pointed with her chin — 'running behind the morgue.'

'Where's the doctor?'

'The doctor is sick.'

The guard abandoned his post and found me a bucket and led me to the creek behind

the small brick mortuary, the stink of which came over the transom and into the afternoon, but nobody seemed to notice. I went back and forth with the bucket until I'd flooded the car's floorboards and turned the bright red mess into a faint pink mess, and then I went about peeping in windows. In a dirty concrete room behind a door labeled MATERNITY WARD, I saw Michael's assailant, the fool who'd pulled a knife, true name unknown, stretched naked on a bare mattress on a metal bed. He was alone in the room, the only occupant of a dozen such beds. The maternity ward's only patient. He had a round, simple face, and he breathed through his mouth. His arm lay out beside him, still bandaged with his shirt.

Michael's nurse, when I returned to them, was being assisted by a young girl dressed in the green skirt and white blouse of the local schools. Work on the wound seemed to have ceased while Michael chatted with a police officer in a close-fitting uniform, all of it — even boots, belt, and helmet — crisply white. His large sun lenses gave him the face of an inquisitive insect.

'Officer Cadribo is making a report.'

'Ah,' I said. 'Good.'

'My friend Roland,' he told us all, 'will bring my fiancée. Did you see the route? It's

just through the gate to the road, then turn left, then right at the main road.'

'Hannington Road,' said Officer Cadribo.

Michael told him, 'We're staying at the White Nile Palace. We'll meet you there around suppertime, all right? The incident is hardly worth mentioning, but you have to make a report, we understand that. Let's make it an occasion. We'll buy you dinner.' He wrapped my shoulder in his good hand and drew me close. 'Go to the hotel, collect our things, and get Davidia. Check out and come back here.'

Just to be talking, I said, 'How's the wound?'

'We're waiting for just a few more cc's of Xylocaine,' the nurse said.

Michael said, 'We tried finishing without it, but God — it hurts! I can't hold my arm still.'

Michael and the cop began talking Krio or the local one, Lugbara, faster and faster, laughing, their remarks ascending to the tenor register.

As I left them, Michael said, 'Remember — you're driving on the left!'

★ ★ ★

Packing was nothing, three changes of clothes — and now one less, as my bloody jeans and

T-shirt went in the trash. I called the desk and asked how to call a room and they said they'd patch me through.

Here, as in West Africa, land-line phones were answered by saying, 'Hello?' and then taking the receiver away from the ear and staring at its silence before replacing it to the ear to listen a little more to the silence.

'I said it's Nair.'

'Nair. I hear you. Where are you?'

'I'm in my room.'

'Go ahead.'

'Can you handle it if things get a bit more up-tempo?'

'What are you saying?'

'Well — just that we're breaking camp. Would you mind getting all your gear packed in the next few minutes? I'll help you carry everything to the jeep.'

'What's going on? What's happened?'

'Michael's moved up the schedule a bit, that's all.'

'Moved it *up*. *What* schedule?'

'We really should leave in the next few minutes.'

'God. God. God. Is Michael there? Let me talk to him.'

'He's tidying up some loose ends. I'll come round as soon as I'm packed.'

'Nair, this is ridiculous. I'm not going anywhere.'

'Then at least pack Michael's things for him, will you, please? I'm coming to your room. I'll see you in a few minutes.'

When I knocked on the door, she said, 'It's open,' and I found her sitting sideways on the bed. She was dressed, except for shoes.

I saw no evidence of packing. 'Do you mind if I shut the door?' She gave a little wave, and I shut us in and said, 'The journey resumes.'

'I don't think so.'

'If we're going at all, we really should be pretty brisk about it.'

'I'm not kidding. I've had it.'

'All right. But I've got the Land Cruiser, and if we're going, now's the time.'

'Where's Michael?'

'I left him in conference with some of his cronies. We'll stop and pick him up.' She didn't move. 'I'm your chauffeur.' Not even her hands. 'Sorry if the news is sort of sudden.'

'So here's a piece of news,' she said. 'The lyrics for 'Smile' were written by two guys I've never heard of named Turner and Parsons.'

It seemed to me they had two soft suitcases and two knapsacks. 'What if we just shovel

your worldly goods into your luggage?' I took some shirts off the rod. 'Do you want the hangers? Let's leave the hangers.'

'But the melody was written by Charlie Chaplin for his 1936 film *Modern Times*.'

I stopped messing around. 'How did you find this out?'

'I went online in the manager's office. It was driving me crazy. I thought maybe Irving Berlin — I was rooting for Irving Berlin, I don't know why. I guess I've always liked the name.'

'I see. Did you get a chance to catch up on your e-mail, then?'

'No. Michael doesn't want me to. You know that.'

'Have you been in communication with anyone?'

'No! I just said no!'

'Right. I just wondered.'

'Is it any of your business?'

'That's just the thing, Davidia. Our business is getting all mixed up together now. Yours and mine. I hope you realize that. If you realize it, this is going to be a whole lot easier.'

'What is? What's going to be easier?'

'Can I take a chair?'

'You're taking my things. Why shouldn't you take a chair?'

I sat down. 'There's a lot you haven't been aware of. Nothing sudden is happening here. More is just suddenly being revealed.' I took a moment to frame my thoughts. I don't know why. I'd imagined telling her this many times. 'We talk about how the world has changed since the Twin Towers went down. I think you could easily say the part that's changed the most is the world of intelligence, security, and defense. The world powers are dumping their coffers into an expanded version of the old Great Game. The money's simply without limit, and plenty of it goes for snitching and spying. In that field, there's no recession.'

'*That* field? *Your* field. It's obvious you don't work in some bank. It was obvious all along. You're CIA.'

'Goddamn it. Ma'am, I am not in the Goddamn CIA. Don't lump me in with that lot.'

She seemed about to speak, then didn't. I got up and sat beside her on the bed.

'You're sitting too close.'

I moved closer. 'But the truth of it is you're partly right. I don't work in a bank. I'm still with NATO intelligence. I'm here on assignment, actually, and the assignment is Michael Adriko.'

'What? *Why?*'

'Michael's in trouble.'

155

'Oh, Jesus. What's he done?'

'He may get out of it. You know Michael. But I think we'd better get out of it first. You and I.'

'You and I?'

'I'm leaving on my own, and I think you'd better come with me.'

'What for?'

'For whatever it's worth.'

'For how long?'

'As long as it lasts.'

'As long as what lasts?'

'Let me get you out of this.'

'To where?'

'Back to Freetown. For a start.'

'Why?'

'I've got business there. I can set us up.'

'Nair, there's nothing between us.'

'Come here. Let me hold you.'

'Are you crazy? Stop touching me.'

I had to stop, or I couldn't talk. The feel of her skin took my breath away. 'I've known Michael for almost twelve years, and all this time I've thought I was infatuated with him, and I was wrong. All the time I've known him I've been infatuated with you. Waiting in infatuation for you to materialize. For him to produce you, conjure you, bring you, fetch you.'

'Oh God,' she said, 'you're complicating

this impossibly. You're making it impossible. Why do you have to be crazy too?' She stood up and started piling things on the bed. 'What's Michael's plan? If any.'

'He's going to Congo.'

'And you're not.'

'That depends on you.'

'I think I'd better go.'

'I think we'd better not. There's no law over there. The government has no writ. The cops, the army, psychotic warlords — they all take turns robbing anyone who's not armed.'

'Then why don't you leave us now?'

'Because I can't. I couldn't bear it. Not without you.'

'This is awful. Shut up.'

'Once you've had a look at the place, you'll want to come with me.'

'I'm going with Michael. Take me to Michael.'

'I'll take you wherever you want.'

'I've got to. I can't just disappear. I have to hang on till Michael's situation is . . . stabilized or something. Or at least clarified.'

She put a bag on the bed and started filling it like a pit.

'Hold up for a bit. Will you? Okay?' She didn't. She kept packing. 'Davidia. I didn't mean to scare you.'

'Well, you did scare me. I'm scared — of you.'

'I got crazy. I don't want to make you crazy too.'

'Too late.'

'Have I forced you into this decision? Because I didn't mean to put you in a corner. Wait a minute.' She didn't pause. 'Stop packing for a second.'

'I'm going with Michael now, and I think you'd better take me to him.'

'Are you sure? Are you sure?'

'Yes!'

'All right, fine. Just a minute. Look at me.' She settled down. 'I shouldn't have said what I said.'

'I agree.'

'I'm crazy.'

'I said it first.'

'So we agree on that too. So will you keep all this quiet?'

'Quiet?'

'Don't tell Michael.'

'I've promised Michael I won't talk to anybody, now I promise you I won't talk to Michael — is that what you're saying?'

'Let me be the one to come clean with him, that's all.'

'When?'

'Not right away.'

'How long do I have to betray him, then?'

'Not long.'

'How long exactly?'

'Two days exactly.'

'Forty-eight hours.'

'Correct.'

'Promises to him, promises to you, and everything is secret from everybody else. This is what we call a situation.' She seemed to see some humor in the thing.

★　★　★

To make ourselves more visible I lit the headlamps. Nobody else did such a thing, none of the bikes or vehicles set themselves apart.

Davidia said, 'This is blood, isn't it? How badly is he hurt?'

'He needed quite a few stitches.'

'Where's the hospital?'

'Actually it's back that way.'

'Then why go this way?'

'Couple of errands.'

For these conditions I drove too fast. It was nearly 4:00 p.m. I had no idea how late the Catholic communications center might be open. Nevertheless I stopped at a vendor's shack and bought all his hundred-milliliter packets of spirits. Then I stopped at another vendor, and I did the same thing. Still I had less than a couple of liters. Before I left the

hotel I should have gotten the biggest bottle of rum, or tequila, whichever had the bigger proof. Baboon Whiskey, if that's all they had. But I'd forgotten.

On the way up the long hill in the middle of Arua I nearly stopped again for another such transaction, but the sight of the towers at the top lured me on. 'I'm stopping up here at a place with internet,' I told Davidia. She said nothing.

Across the road from the gates, I turned off the engine and said it again. 'If you have someone you want to communicate with, here's the place to do it.'

'Just hurry up. I'm worried about Michael.'

'You can wait with the guard.'

'I'm fine right here.'

When I got out, I went around to her window. She didn't roll it down. 'Will you be all right?'

'Will I?'

'If you get uncomfortable, lock the doors.'

I heard them locking even as I turned away.

★ ★ ★

I had two e-mails, the first from Hamid:

Firm and final offer is cash funds 100K US for you.

If your answer is yes, we meet same place same hour.
Cash takes time.
Your share 100K US. Final offer.

I liked his figure. I didn't like his next one:

Will meet 4 weeks following date last meeting.
Not 30 days. 4 weeks exactly. No fallback. One chance.

On the one hand, the money was set, and it was good money. But with his other hand he'd ripped two days from the calendar. I closed my eyes and set about composing a comeback, a counteroffer, and then scotched it. I had nothing to offer.

I opened the second e-mail: several hundred angry words from my boss at NIIA. Before I'd read half, I deleted it.

I banged at the keys: 'Hello, you idiotic shits. Are you waiting for my report? You can wait till Hell serves holy water.'

I pressed DELETE.

Again I banged on the keys, this time at some length:

Goddamn you. You smiled sweetly while slipping a rocket up my ass and lighting

the fuse. Now you want to dress me down?

Would you cunts please explain what British MI is doing at my hotel?

Would you cunts care to describe Mossad's involvement in — what shall we call it — this affair? Investigation? Cluster-fuck?

All of you, go fuck yourselves. Fuck each other.

I hold the rank of captain in the Army of Denmark. What has any of this got to do with Denmark? What has any of this got to do with me?

Why have you put me in a position to be murdered?

For three seconds, four seconds, five, my finger hovered over the DELETE key, and then I pressed SEND.

★ ★ ★

I logged out, plugged in my own keyboard, and went to PGP. I wrote back to Hamid:

Sold.

THREE

[OCT 15 11PM]

All right, Tina. The chief captor, the witch doctor, the general, the jailor or kidnapper or whatever he is, has just showed me my favorite thing in East Africa, a plastic baggie that would fit exactly in a shirt pocket, and shows me the label, '40% Volume Cane Spirits 100ml,' before biting off the corner and sucking it dry, explaining, 'It's for the cold,' and tossing it aside, and I notice, right now, that the dirt floor of this big low hut we're in is littered with similar packets sucked empty and tossed aside — paved with them — 'Rider Vodka' and 'ZAP Vodka' and the Cane Spirits. I'm familiar with these packets, in fact many of these empties were mine-all-mine as recently as one hour ago, when they stole them, yet I don't perceive any gratitude in the black lacquer faces of these drunken soldiers all around us. What I do perceive is that this place smells powerfully of unwashed humans.

I just saw a single firefly flash upward. Or a capillary exploded in my brain. The truth is

I'm a little drunk too. And this won't be one of those pitiful attempts to explain 'how I got into this mess,' because there's no sense calling it a mess until we see how it all turns out. Sometimes you just get stuck. That's Africa. Then you're on your way again without any idea what happened, and that's Africa too. And while you're stuck, if they give you a pen and paper? — you might as well.

As to why I have no computer, it isn't because they took mine away from me, but because as Michael and Davidia and I headed toward the Congo border in a Land Cruiser borrowed, now stolen, from Pyramid Environments, with our guide or abettor, a Congolese whose name I didn't catch, Michael stopped the car on a bridge over some tributary of the White Nile River and said, Here we'll toss our communications, and threw his phone out the window. Davidia chucked hers as well, and I was glad to get rid of everything (although my laptop and second keyboard were guaranteed GPS-untraceable, and my phone was already a replacement. I didn't want the weight of them anymore, that's all). It was sunset. Below us people washed their vehicles in muddy water up to the axles, the drivers splashing the red dirt off their rumpled pocked and sagging

Subarus and such. Davidia said only one thing: 'How long do you have the car for?' — 'What?' — 'When do you have to return this vehicle?' — 'Oh — it's flexible,' Michael said with a wide smile, as if describing his mouth, 'it's quite flexible.'

My friend and your friend Michael Adriko, that is, and his fiancée, Davidia St. Claire. You knew I went to Freetown on a hunt for Michael. I found him all right, with Davidia on his arm, and I'll catch you up on all the rest as time allows. To put it in shorthand, Michael's enthusiasms, let us say, had us leaving Uganda in a rush for DR Congo on Oct 13, just a couple of days ago. We'd jumped from Freetown to northwestern Uganda, a town called Arua, where I last heard from you by e-mail and where I last saw your breasts, and I wish I'd downloaded them ... Earlier, at Kuluva Hospital in Arua, while getting his flesh stitched together after a fight it's pointless to explain, Michael had enlisted a guide to show us a hole in the border, because none of us had Congo papers. When Davidia and I got to the hospital, Michael introduced this man, a skinny little guy in bright blue trousers and a T-shirt that said, I Did WHAT Last Night? and told me to give him one hundred dollars. — When he's got us through to

Congo, I said. — Fair enough, Michael said.

Daylight was almost gone as we got near the border, a good circumstance for people smuggling themselves, and we passed among groves of tall eucalyptus, Michael driving like an African, far too fast for the crumbling red-dirt surface, I mean fast, 90 or 95 KPH mostly, scaring the bikes to the side by means of constant beeping, using the horn much more than the brakes, oblivious to the children, goats, ducks, trucks coming at us, the overloaded busses appearing around road bends, leaning on two wheels, and women walking down the road balancing burdens on their heads, mostly basins full of 'white ants' — centimeter-long termites they sell in the market as snacks. I've never tried them, but it's a comfort to realize that every couple hundred meters or so across this land, a chest-high berm teems with nutrient morsels. One of these women crossed our path, her right hand raised to steady the pan on her head, blocking half her sight, she couldn't have seen us, she kept walking into the road, Michael tried to veer, and we *hit* her, we struck her *down*, I heard her say 'uh!' in a way I've never heard it said, never, and the jeep swerved, bounced, straightened, and kept on . . . I looked back, she was flung down on the clay pavement in the dusk, she

looked lifeless. Davidia said, 'Michael! Michael! She's hurt!' — 'She wasn't watching!' he said angrily, going faster now. His shoulders hunched as he pushed the accelerator hard, and we were racing away from — what? A murder, perhaps. We'd never know. 'Michael, Michael,' Davidia said, but Michael said nothing, and she said, 'Go back, go back, go back, go back,' but we wouldn't go back, we couldn't — not in Africa, this hard, hard land where nobody could help that poor woman flopped probably dead in the road and where running away from this was not a mistake. The mistake was looking back at her in the first place.

No words among us now, just Davidia's sobbing, and then her silence. Michael drove a bit more soberly as we skirted the border, heading north. If we didn't find our hole soon we'd come to South Sudan. The surface got terrible. I'm not sure it was still a road. We came into a village, and the guide muttered in Michael's ear, and we went quite slowly now. Michael switched off the headlamps — he was only using the parking lights anyway — 'Let's enjoy the moon!' It was just past half-full, with that lopsided swollen face, that smile at the corner of its mouth. People strolled around under its strange orange glow.

Kids played tag as if it were daytime. We went slower than the pedestrians through this crowded twilight, this thickly human evening. Sudden laughter from a hut, like a soprano chorus. What have they got to laugh about? Bikes without headlights floating out of the dimness. A man leans against a shack, cupping the tiny light of a cell phone to his ear.

The guide said, 'Stop.' He got out, shut the door, walked around to Michael's window and spoke low.

Michael told me, 'Give him fifty.'

'Not till we're in Congo.'

'We're here. This is Congo.'

'I thought you said one hundred.'

'He's quitting early. Just fifty.'

I handed Michael a bill. The man folded it up small, then turned away and walked toward a hut, crying softly, 'Hallooo.'

'Who's coming up front — Nair?' Michael asked.

'I guess I am,' I said more or less to Davidia. Her face was invisible. For the last two hours she'd said not a word. We left the village behind and lurched along a half kilometer farther and stopped.

Michael said, 'The main road's over that way, but we'll never find it till we have some daylight.' He fiddled with his watch. 'Set your

time backward one hour. We've crossed into another zone.'

We sat in the car saying nothing, thinking and feeling nothing, or trying not to, while the weather changed and the stars disappeared. The moon burned right through the overcast with a curious effect, seeming to hang just a few meters above us while the clouds lay behind it, much higher in the sky. Michael switched off the engine. We heard a multitude of insects ringing all around us like finger cymbals. The ringing stopped. Raindrops exploded on the roof and streaked down the dirty windshield.

Stupid, stupid Michael said, 'Congo! Here, we're not in any trouble.'

[OCT 16 2AM]

How much time do I have to catch you up? They won't move us tonight, surely. The party's over and everybody's snoring, sleeping on top of their rifles. The only one awake with me is a radio somewhere — a DJ talking French full-speed and spinning American country music. And two or three mosquitoes making their rounds. Very few mosquitoes at these East African altitudes, though when Michael and Davidia and I came aground in

171

the dark just inside the Congo border, he, Michael — to pick up the journey again — said, 'Many voices on the air tonight,' and rolled up the windows against the insects, because as a child he suffered malaria and a mosquito is the only thing on earth, I believe, that scares him.

The car was stifling. I slept, or only suffocated — I saw the woman in the road in more detail, the wrap that covered all but her arms and shoulders in a pattern red or purple, in the dusk it could have been either, and her basin of ants rolling on its edge away from her like a toy, and she lay there as limp as her towel — the white cloth, that is, she'd rolled into a bun to cushion her head — stretched out straight beside her.

Sometime in the night came Michael's voice: 'I'm moving.'

We were both awake I'm sure, Davidia and I.

'It's very subtle. But there is definitely movement.'

Davidia said, 'Michael, quiet.'

'I'm sliding down. I'm sliding off.'

'Sshh.'

'I don't know what I'm going to turn into once I'm on the floor.'

She: 'To hell with this. To hell with you.'

'I itch all over.'

'Don't start your scratching. Don't scratch.'

He squirmed and clawed at his ribs, elbows knocking the steering wheel. 'I'm in a cocoon. What will I be when I come out?'

Davidia said, 'He's going mad. We'll be holding him down while he screams bloody murder before it's over.'

'I'm coming out of my skin!' he screamed. Writhing. He bumped the horn and it honked and we all jumped, and then he got hold of himself and we got quiet again.

When daylight came we found ourselves parked behind a church in the middle of a field, a big crumbling adobe building, salmon-pink, its tin roof corroded red. Beyond it lay a proper dirt road and a collection of low buildings, dark inside, the wind blowing through. But pots steamed and fry pans sizzled on cookfires all around. Without talking about it the three of us got out of the car and made our way toward the possibility of breakfast. I watched Davidia walk. Her long African skirt swayed and the hem danced around her feet as she floated ahead of me. People wandered around, others were just waking up, crawling from under a couple of lorries, dragging their straw mats behind them. Nobody remarked on us. Michael found us some corn cakes and hot tea served in plastic water bottles. He said,

'Last night I became a lizard. Now I know what we have to do.'

He went exploring, running his electric clippers over his scalp and his cheeks and his jaw as he walked around talking to folks.

Davidia and I sat on a bench outside a shack called The Best Lucky Saloon and she said, 'Boomelay boomelay bommelay boom and all that.' — 'What?' — 'Vachel Lindsay. Or Edna St. Vincent Millay or somebody.' — 'Oh.' — 'It's a poem about the Congo.' — 'Oh.' We watched a woman sitting on a stool, working on the hairdo of a little girl sitting on the ground between her knees, while behind her, standing, another woman worked on *her* hair . . . The buildings and shacks were gray and brown, everything streaked with red mud. I recall three green power poles, one broken and leaning and held up apparently by the wires alone.

Michael came back with several bread rolls for each of us and said, 'Some lizards can fly, so you pick up information if you become one,' and went away again.

Davidia said to me, 'You haven't seen this before?'

'What — seen him go through magical transformations, you mean, in the jungle night?'

'Well,' she said, 'when you put it that way'

— she was kicking at a rock — 'then it sounds as troubling as it really is.'

'Maybe it's a chemical problem. Are you taking something for malaria?'

'Once a day. It's called Lariam.'

'Lariam causes nightmares. I take doxycycline.'

'You said 'transformations in the jungle night' — but where's the jungle?'

'The people cut it all down. They burned it to cook breakfast, mostly. And to make way for planting.'

A hundred years ago it would have taken an hour to hack through ten meters of undergrowth. Now huts and footpaths and small gardens cover the hills. By 9:00 a.m. we were passing among them, back on the road, driving on the right side now instead of the left. Within 20 minutes we had a flat tire.

Very briskly Michael raised the car on a jack and attacked the nuts with a tool and got on the spare — a different-colored wheel and a wrong-sized tire lacking any tread at all.

We saw very few motorized vehicles. An occasional motorcycle, an occasional SUV, always, it seemed, stenciled with a corporate or NGO acronym. Passenger busses coming like racecars, nearly capsizing as they careened around the curves toward us, slinging dust bombs from under the wheels. A

few lorries bearing cargo, laboring slowly; other lorries with smashed faces dragged among the trees and abandoned. Many, many pedestrians strolling on the margin or crossing side to side, looking up from their daydreams only at the sound of a horn. It was the holiday of sacrifice, Eid al-Adha, and Muslims walked on both sides of the road, some of the women lugging prayer mats as big as house rugs.

The point is, our Land Cruiser stood out, and we couldn't possibly face any officials. Before we reached any sizeable town, Michael drove off the road to detour, along little more than footpaths, down into gulleys, through patches of agriculture, knocking over stalks of corn and bushes of marijuana to get around the checkpoints and then back onto the real road, along which he sped as if he hadn't only yesterday slammed this jeep into tragedy, again proceeding African style, all honking, no braking. A little boy ran right in front of the car, running at top speed as if hurrying to get killed. Michael swerved in time, mashing the horn and crying out the window in English to the boy's family, 'Beat that child, beat that child!' I watched to the side, keeping my eyes off the future. The fields were a light green, the color of springtime in the temperate zones, soft and even-looking,

with here and there the slow white smoke of trash fires strung over them like mist. Late that day Michael pointed at the hazy distance and claimed he saw the hills of his childhood, the Happy Mountains, called by the missionary James Hannington, in frustration and disgust, the Laughing Monsters, and Michael told us of a forest in those mountains 'where you'll find pine trees about a dozen meters in their height, Nair. Bunches of ten evergreens, fifteen, twenty or more together. What do you call a bunch of trees — a copse? Copses of pines about a dozen meters in height, Nair. And these aren't common evergreens, but their needles are actually made of precious gold. And you can gather all the needles you want, but if you get pricked by one, and it draws blood — you will lose your soul. A devil comes instantly at the smell of your blood, and snatches your soul right — out — of your heart. Remember,' he said, 'when I told you never to have anything to do with the voodoo? Now you're going to find out why.'

'Michael,' I said, 'was it your people who martyred Hannington?' and he only said, 'Hannington was stabbed in the side with a spear like Jesus Christ.'

The wedding would be blended into the Burning of the Blood, a weeklong ceremony,

he said, 'when we put away the bad blood of the war, and drink the new blood of peace. I tell you it is an orgy! Many babies are made. A boy conceived in that week will be a man of peace among his people. But only within wedlock. No bastard can be a man of peace.'

At one point, as the dusk fell on us, he said, 'Any moment now we'll reach Newada Mountain. Tear out my eyes, and I could find it by my heart.'

We turned onto a road that got muddier and muddier each kilometer until we were just mushing along through patches of gumbo separated by horrifyingly slick hard flats, but at least it wasn't raining. 'Fifteen kilometers more to Newada Mountain,' Michael announced, and after a couple dozen kilometers, three dozen, many more than fifteen, certainly, we took a shortcut, a footpath that delivered us into a wasteland, a stinking bog of red gumbo, the sort of mud you can't stop in, even with four-wheel drive, or you'll sink and never get going again. By full nightfall we'd determined that the stink came not from the bog, but from our vehicle. 'I smell petrol,' Michael said, and the engine began to miss. 'I'm not sure about the fuel pump,' Michael said, and the engine died. He cut the headlamps, and in the blackness quite vividly I perceived how an

English missionary like James Hannington might have stood up to his buttocks in this sludge and wept, and heard the mountains laughing.

The dead engine gave out small noises as it cooled. With the headlamps switched off we could measure the darkness, which was deep and thick, without moon or stars. Every now and then the frogs started up all around, and then stopped. From far off came a wild, syncopating percussion.

Davidia said, 'Are those jungle drums?'

'Probably someone's idea of a disco,' Michael said.

'Well — let's go,' she said, but we all three felt the impossibility of moving off on foot into the dark and the muck. Michael closed the windows and we slept the same suffocated sleep as the night before.

And woke at dawn in the foundered jeep, with no better plan than to get out of it and pee.

Michael and I stood on the driver's side, Davidia squatted on the other. We'd arrived, we now realized, nearly at the limit of the red muddy lowland, at the feet of the mountains we'd seen by day, within sight of a place of twisted trees and lopsided shacks.

'Take your packs,' Michael said. 'Walk soft.'

He meant us to understand that by a light

tread on the superficial hard spots we might not break through into the gunk, although in many spots we broke through anyway. By tacking in search of better footing we spent half an hour making a few hundred meters.

The village lay between a field of corn and a banana grove. Michael had called it exactly right — the main shack, among squat huts and other shanties, was the Biggest Club Disco, with a generator on the ground outside, not running. Michael took a tour while Davidia and I sat on a bench and watched the village wake up, men and women fussing over cookfires beside the huts, children, chickens, goats, all going softly and talking low in the chilly dawn. Michael turned up with three Cokes and quite a few biscuits wrapped in a page of the *Monitor*, a Ugandan newspaper, and said, 'Watch these people. We don't know their hearts.'

'Why don't you just say they're not your tribe?'

'It's more complicated than that.'

'No it isn't,' I said. 'Is this your clan, or not?'

'All right, the simple answer is yes — they're speaking my dialect, but it's not my close family. It's not the right time to reveal myself.'

'Who do you think you are? Long-lost

Ulysses?' Then I felt embarrassed for him. I could see by his look that he thought exactly that. 'Michael, is this Newada Mountain?'

'By my reckoning, it's very near.'

Davidia wasn't suffering any of this. 'Get us some real food,' she told him.

'Sit there,' he said, as if we weren't already slumped side by side on the bench.

When he'd gone I moved close to her, hip touching hip. I said, 'He's using you for something. Something mystical, superstitious.'

'Like?'

'I don't know. Kidnapping one of the gods and coercing the others to . . . rearrange the fate of us all.'

She made a sort of barking noise, with tears in her eyes. 'You're crazy.'

'As crazy as he is?'

'No. Once in a while.'

'It's time I got you out of here.'

'You don't have to say it twice.'

'Then let's go.'

'Go how?'

'We'll walk.'

'Where?'

'Uganda's that way — east.'

'How far?'

'I don't know. But it isn't getting any closer while we sit here.'

'What will he do?'

'Nothing. He can't hold us at gunpoint.'

'Why not?'

'Because he hasn't got a gun.'

Something was happening, suddenly, to every person in the village — as if they choked on poisonous fumes — and their voices got loud, and we heard a vehicle in the distance. Davidia asked me what was wrong, who was coming, what kind of car. 'I don't know,' I said, 'but I don't give a shit — we'll hitch a ride out of here or kill them and take the fucking thing.' Then we heard other engines, several vehicles, none of them visible yet. Somebody had a gun: one shot, two, three . . . then the rest of a clip. At that point our own jeep, three hundred meters away and to the right of us, burst into silent brightness — the boom of the explosion came a second later.

Davidia and I stood up simultaneously from the bench. We watched a white pickup truck scurrying across the landscape at a tangent to us, driving hysterical villagers before it, sparks of rifle fire bursting from the passenger window and soldiers standing up in the back and firing too, when they could manage it, as they bounced and swayed and hung on.

I turned toward the nearest copse of larger

trees, and discovered that it was besieged by other vehicles. I felt relief when Michael came toward us in a hurry calling, 'Let's go, let's go, let's go.'

The banana grove seemed a possibility. Anywhere, really. We proceeded in a sort of innocent, unprovoked manner, nothing wrong here, just walking.

We entered the grove. Behind us came a hush, then a man's rapid voice, many gunshots, and the uninterrupted keening of a woman somewhere, and soon the whole village, it seemed, was crying out, some of them screeching like birds, some bawling, some moaning low. Every child sounded like every other child.

As soon as we'd put a little distance between us and the din of souls in the clearing, I sat on the edge of a pile of adobe bricks and wrapped my arms around my middle. 'My stomach's a sack of vomit.'

'I'll give you ten seconds. Then double-time.'

'Where's Davidia?'

'I'm right here.' She was behind me.

A woman burst onto the path ahead of us with eyes like headlights, running with her hands high in the air. Bullets tugged at the banana leaves around her.

I lost my head. I see that now. We'd moved

a hundred meters along this path, breathing hard, our steps pounding, before I formed any clear intention of getting up and running. Of my panicked state I remember only others panicking, the faces of tiny children swollen into cartoon caricature, the long wet lashes and pouting lips and baby cheeks and the teardrops exploding like molten gobs in the air around their heads. I remember shoes left behind on the ground — flip-flops, slippers, whatever's hard to run in.

Michael collided with my back, gripped each of my elbows from behind, and propelled me along. Davidia kept pace, clawed at our clothing, at the banana fronds too, and got in front of us, then away from us, and Michael steered me off the path and hugged me, stopped me.

'You can't outrun bullets.'

'Yes I can!' I meant it.

He pointed amid the grove and said, 'Go ten meters and get down.' He watched while I obeyed, then was gone.

Multiple guns now, and many fewer voices.

I lay on my belly. A few steps from my face the grove ceased, and to the right the gumbo bog took over, and for an unquantifiable period I watched a heap of something burning out there before I understood it was our vehicle. Part of the driveshaft remained, a

wheel with its tire, and around these two things only the shell, still giving out small flames, and surrounding that, the red earth steaming and smoking.

Michael came along leading Davidia by the hand.

I stood and followed them along the edge of the grove and toward a cornfield. We stopped to watch the white pickup truck charging at us, plowing down the stalks until it slid to a stop almost in our faces, a spiffy little truck with fresh gold lettering across its front windshield: ALL EYEZ ON ME. Soldiers leapt from the back of it, and the three of us walked before their guns.

We waited in front of the disco while they wrapped up the looting. Most of the villagers had escaped — no more screams, only the soldiers' whoops, their panting and shouting, and much laughter. The young recruit responsible for us drifted some distance away, dazzled by the excitement, but rather than running, Michael and I sat Davidia on the bench and stood in front of her as camouflage because we didn't want anybody noticing us, noticing Davidia, raping Davidia — and they raped a couple of women behind the disco, a young one and her mother, who in their terror seemed almost apathetic, almost asleep, and who afterward walked away

brushing the dirt from their bare arms and the fronts of their torn shifts. It took the commander a full hour to bring his troops to order. He mustered them in front of the disco, thirty or so young men in green cammy uniforms, and went from face to face lecturing bitterly, pointing often at the shreds of our Land Cruiser out in the wasteland. Apparently rape and looting were lesser crimes than blowing up a good machine.

Michael said, 'Did you see the fireball? Petrol vapors. I told you the fuel pump was ruptured.'

[OCT 16 6AM]

I know Michael's sleeping. He'll sleep through a barrage. I don't know where he's being kept, or Davidia. I hope they're together. I'm in the main hut with the commander, along with ten or twelve other men, the number changes, they come and go. It's a spacious hut, an open-air corral, really, with low adobe walls under a thatched roof, a cafeteria table, a tattered couch, three broken chairs.

They've got my pack, my extra clothes, passport, cash — 4K in US twenties, fifties, and hundreds. They left me my Timex watch, out of contempt for the brand or perhaps for

186

the concept of time itself. They stole my penlight too, but they've lent it back so I can write by its tiny glow.

Why take everything but the watch and the light and my ballpoint pen, and then give me this lined paper torn from a schoolroom notebook, 42 sheets of it? I've sat up all night scrawling on them because I'm too terrified to sleep. The liquor's worn off and I'm going mad. When I've filled these pages they'll be included, I suspect, with some sort of ransom demand.

The roosters are calling. Nobody's stirring yet but one person out by the latrines — a young woman in a dirty linen shift, barefoot, hardly more than a girl, hacking a trough in the earth with a vicious-looking short-handled hoe, a trough in the earth shaped, I'm afraid, quite like a grave.

[OCT 16 8AM]

The commander claims to be regular Army but could easily be lying, or just confused. His cammy uniform bears no insignia. Beneath his open tunic he wears a T-shirt with the faded emblem of a bottle on it, soda or beer. He calls himself a general, won't say his name. Drives his own little cream-colored

Nissan truck, the one that says EYEZ ON ME.

He takes me for the leader, because I'm the white one.

Last night, after discovering that my bad French and his own bad English render idle conversation impossible, he nodded toward the small cassette player on his table and punched a button, and it played a song called, I believe, 'Coat of Many Colors,' by Dolly Parton, over and over. Just that one song, repeating. This wasn't psychological warfare, but a sincere attempt at hospitality.

This morning he shared with me his general's breakfast: strips of tripe in a broth smelling pretty much like kerosene. It took me a while to get it all down and set the bowl aside. The meal came with dessert, a sugary pudding sprinkled with the legs, if not more, of some sort of insect.

[OCT 16 12 NOON]

After breakfast, when I thought everybody was still sleeping off last night's liquor, they all jumped up on the general's shouted orders and mustered in the clearing among the huts for the very quick court martial of the recruit who blew up our Land Cruiser.

When they'd made a circle and wrestled

themselves to attention, all thirty or more of them, the general's aide-de-camp, his main henchman, dragged the youngster out of a hut barefoot and stripped down to ragged gray shorts and stood him up before the fresh-dug grave. His hands were tied behind him with a winding of black rubber. Perhaps from a tire's inner tube.

I made up part of this audience of dazed, half-dressed soldiers. Davidia and Michael stood across from me. They were many feet apart. Davidia looked unhurt, unmolested. The magic of her US passport must be working.

Michael, with his Ghanaian document, enjoys no immunity. He caught my eye and turned sideways — his arms were bound behind him, but I couldn't see his hands for the press of the crowd. He smiled and shrugged.

Our general faced us taking a similar posture, hands behind his back and feet apart, and addressed the whole group briefly — in a localized French, I think — before tearing off his sunglasses and turning on the malefactor and lecturing him in the face for five or more minutes, screaming into the kid's open mouth, right down his throat. During this harangue the general's henchman strutted back and forth in his mirrored sunglasses

and helmet, slapping his pistol against his palm, until it was time to push the kid to his knees and put the gun to his head. The youth wept and bawled while the general shouted him down to silence. When all was quiet, he counted down from trois! — deux! — un! and the henchman's hammer snapped on a empty chamber.

The general laughed. Then the troops all laughed too.

The general pushed his henchman aside and drew his own pistol and raised it high and pulled the slide back as if demonstrating how to cock this particular weapon and pushed the barrel hard against the kid's neck and forced him down onto his face, and bent over him like that while he sobbed into the dirt. Some of the troops exclaimed — the general would get it done! . . . He stared hard one by one at each face, saying nothing, until he'd forced them all into a state of pensive sobriety. He worked his shoulders. Shifted his stance. Planted his feet. Still playing, I felt sure of it. But the pistol was cocked, and one small mistake makes a murder, and in Africa, so the old hands assure me, the first one pops some kind of cork, and they don't quit after that.

Ten seconds passed. Once more the boy spoke out — a pitiable, wrenching sound, his

face like a newborn's — trying to direct his words backward to the man about to dispatch him.

The general fired one loud shot into the sky. Again the exclamations — fooled us two times! He turned his back on the youngster and leveled the weapon at the crowd, aiming in particular at Michael Adriko's face.

Michael bared his teeth and wagged his head and played the clown. Nobody laughed. On either of his shoulders lay a black hand, but his guards seemed not to know who the general referred to when he cried in English: 'That one!'

Or maybe they didn't know the words. He said that one, that one, that one until the two men unslung their rifles and prodded Michael forward to the edge of the ditch. The general held out his hand and wiggled his fingers for one of the weapons, an AK, the kind with a folding stock and a pistol grip, and he swung it around and jabbed the barrel at Michael's chest.

Michael stepped backward into the ditch and stood with the young recruit in a ball at his feet while the general put the barrel's mouth against one of Michael's eyeballs, and then the other, and then the first again. Michael dodged his head and clamped his mouth around the barrel and sucked and

French-kissed it with his tongue, the whole time looking up into the general's face as if wooing a woman. Oh, Michael. If one voice laughs . . . Perhaps the general would laugh. But the general had been carried beyond his instincts and had to wait for Michael to decide what happened next. Michael drew his head back and averted his gaze, and the general seized on that as a sign of surrender and returned the rifle to its owner and stooped, hooked a hand into Michael's armpit, and helped him out of the ditch. He spoke softly to Michael, and Michael answered softly. I don't know what they said.

Another minute, and the party was over, everyone dismissed, they were taking Michael back toward the smaller huts. Apparently they kept him separate from Davidia.

As he passed, he said to me, to Davidia, to the sky's blank face — 'We'll be fine. I'm talking to these people. A few of them are Kakwa, like me.'

Somehow he'd not only cheated fate, but also coaxed it to lend him a cigarette, which one of his guards was lighting for him as they dragged him back to his prison. Puffing, squinting, he hopped along as if often in the habit of smoking with his hands tied behind his back.

I got close to Davidia. Before they

separated us again, I said to her, 'Are you all right?'

She said, 'Yes. Yes. Are you?'

[OCT 16 1:30PM]

I'm back in the general's quarters. 'Coat of Many Colors' — 'Coat of Many Colors' — 'Coat of Many Colors' —

My pen's got a fresh cartridge, but the ball keeps skipping. This encourages more deliberate penmanship.

Tina, —

Tina. I doubt you'll see me again in the flesh. I may as well embrace candor. With every stroke of this pen I've wanted to say it: I've lost my heart to this woman. I'm in love with Davidia St. Claire. The sight of her blinds me. This morning, the nearness of her outshone everything going on among these violent men.

Right now I feel two ways. I'm grateful Davidia's all right. I'm sorry that Michael isn't dead.

FOUR

Online again — bathed and shaved and revived after eleven hours' sleep, plus three cups of coffee brewed American style — I wrote to Tina:

You'll be hearing from the boys in Sec 4, and I suspect you've been briefed to some extent already by your own bunch.

I regret your involvement, nothing else. But your involvement — deeply.

I don't mean to be curt, just brief. I don't know how long I have the machine.

They'll intercept this communication, I suppose, and blackline half of it — but friends, please, let me tell her this much unredacted:

Listen, Tina, when the boys from Sec 4 come around, remember you work for the US, not NATO, not really. I'd urge you not to speak to them. In fact there's no reason why you shouldn't just go back right now to DC. Or even home to Michigan.

Thanks, chums. Thanks for letting me

transmit that bit of advice.

I just want to be careful not to overstep with my hosts. Who are they? Well fuck, as we Yanks like to say, if I know. Friends of Intelligence. Meaning allies of stupidity.

That was snotty. They've been cordial. I should delete it.

— But I saw them coming for me and pressed SEND.

★ ★ ★

On the afternoon of the second day, my backpack, my own toiletries, and freshly laundered underwear — also my own — appeared on my bed. But not my watch.

And not my clothes. We still paraded around in red pajamas of cotton-polyester, the same material as the white sheets on our beds — not cots, but barracks beds. And we still possessed the olive socks, shorts, and undershirts they'd issued us. We'd been allowed to keep the shoes we'd arrived in.

'We' being myself and one tentmate, a Frenchman, Patrick Roux, not Patrice, a tiny man with a sparrow's face and giant horn-rim spectacles, and a five-day beard and bitten fingernails and a personal odor like that of

linseed oil ... or was my sensitive nose merely sniffing out a fake, a plant, a snitch?

The Congolese Army couldn't reach us here. I could sleep knowing I wouldn't be prodded awake with a gun barrel and then shot; though I rather expected to be greeted one morning with some delicious coffee and informed of my arrest on a charge of espionage.

★   ★   ★

After supper on the second night, I wrote to Tina online:

> I won't outrage you with pleas for forgiveness. I hope you hate me, actually, as much as I hate myself. And no explanation — nothing you'd understand — only this: the other day Michael asked me if I really want to go back to that boring existence. I said No.
>
> They've reviewed and returned some dozens of pages I filled by hand. None of it, apparently, impinges on their plans for world domination. If I somehow crawl free of this mess, I'll transcribe and transmit those pages to you, and I may even take time one day to set down an account of things, everything, beginning

— 17 days ago? Really, only 17 days?

They've made a few things clear. I'll get one hour's online access per day, sending to NIIA recipient(s) only (including you), and I'd better be careful not to compromise in any serious way what they're up to down here — or else what? They'll take away my red pajamas?

Right now I can tell you I'm still in Africa. Behind loop-de-loops of razor concertina wire, shiny and new. Behind barricades four sandbags thick and nearly four meters high.

I suppose they'll redact this too, but for what it's worth: I'm here thanks, I'm sure, to Davidia St. Claire, thanks to her relation with the US Tenth Special Forces Group, in whose hands I now find myself. I believe yesterday I caught a glimpse of their fearless leader, Col. George Thiebes himself, out there on the grounds. Commander of the whole 10th. I'm pretty sure I was meant to.

This isn't a prison. My tentmate and I are the only ones in red pajamas. The setup for the fifty or so African detainees (they wear white) seems makeshift and temporary — they're rounded up and soon released.

Our pajamas say 'Nair' and 'Roux' —

handwritten with textile markers — but none of the personnel wear name tags on their utilities or have names stenciled on their T-shirts.

Even during meals, Roux removes his glasses frequently and spends a lot of time breathing on the lenses and polishing them with his shirttail. He speaks to me only in French but rolls his *r*'s like a Spaniard. I gather he returned from business in Marseilles to find that his wife, a Congolese, had gone missing, and while running around looking for her he did something, he can't guess what, to bring himself in conflict with the American dream.

Nobody stops me from having a walk around, but whenever I do, one or more large enlisted men go walking around the same places.

Davidia must still be here. I have no reason to believe they've taken her elsewhere.

Michael Adriko is elsewhere. He never got here. He's gone. He got away.

* * *

After two days' grilling, I got a break.

Off-line, I finished transcribing the hand-written letter to Tina. The notebook pages

ended with this quick entry:

I've slept two hours with my face on the table and just woke up to find everything changed. The general returned my pack and clothes and even several hundred of my 4K dollars — all the twenties.

Michael's sitting in the back of the general's pickup — hands unbound. I saw Davidia getting in the front. The day has turned. Whether it turns upside down I

Much activity — time to go —

. . . All right, Tina, there you have it. My rise from terrified prisoner to confused detainee.

Michael or Davidia must have told the Congolese Army about her connection with the 10th Special Forces. And only about Davidia's connection, surely, because when Michael disappeared, nobody cared.

Last time I saw Michael I was getting in the truck, up front, with the Congolese so-called general and Davidia. Michael leaned over the rail, nearly into my window, and handed me a pellet of chewing gum. 'Here. Keep yourself busy.'

When we made our rendezvous that night, it was like a magic trick. During a

rain, the men in the back of the general's pickup had covered themselves with a dark plastic tarp. They whipped the tarp off. Michael had vanished.

Our escort were three US infantry Nissan pickups, just like our general's, only olive rather than white.

As Davidia and I boarded, one of the youngsters who'd guarded us said to me, 'Newada Mountain.'

'Yes?'

'I am from there. I am Kakwa.'

'Yes?'

'Your friend is there.'

'Michael? My African friend?'

'Yes. He left to Newada Mountain.'

'Oh!' I said — getting it for the first time — 'New Water Mountain.'

As for lately, Tina: no activity to report. I've spent the day in idleness, in limbo, in hope. I've made a proposal, and wheels may be turning. We just might forge an arrangement. In any case, they haven't said no, and they've given me a day off. I can use one — my head still spins, and I slept very little last night, and before that I had no appetite for dinner, as my lunch was interrupted when this American, wow, a genuine asshole — attached to NIIA I suppose,

but he withheld identification — dropped out of the sky.

I was sitting at a table with Patrick Roux, my tentmate and alleged fellow detainee, when we heard what must have been this new man's chopper landing but thought nothing of it, choppers come and go. Ten minutes later he entered and bumped across the cafeteria like a blimpy cartoon animal, I mean in a state of personal awkwardness, as if balancing a stack of plates, but he carried only his hands before him, at chest level. A blue checked shirt, khaki pants, brown loafers. 'Come and talk to me.' — And I said, 'No.' He had a fringe of brown hair with a big bald spot. He had fat cheeks and soulful, angry eyes. Reasonably young, mid-thirties.

He stood by my place leaning on the table and looking down at me until a sergeant and a private came and lifted me by either arm from behind. As they quick-marched me out, he went over to the serving line, apparently for some lunch.

Online, just before I pressed SEND, I added:

The soldiers took me to a tent, and the

sergeant left, and the private stood at ease by the tent fly, and I sat on one half of the furniture, that is, on one of two folding chairs.

The sergeant returned with a chair of his own, unfolded it, and sat down and stared at me. Together we waited thirty minutes for my first interrogator.

I said nothing, and the sergeant said nothing.

He was present every minute of every session, and he always said nothing, and he never stopped staring.

My answers had to come fast. He who hesitates is lying.

'We've been getting a lot of NTRs from you.'

'We?'

'Your reports have been forwarded to us. They were all NTRs.'

'If there's nothing to report, that's what I report. Would you rather I make things up?'

'Why would you transmit two identical NTRs with a thirty-second interval between them?'

My stomach sank down to my groin. It irritated me that I couldn't control my breath.

'On October second you sent two NTRs in

a row from the Freetown facility, thirty seconds apart. Why is that?'

'It was my initial utilization of the equipment. I chose to double up.'

'But on October eleventh you sent an NTR from the Arua station. Weren't you utilizing that equipment for the first time?'

'It didn't seem necessary to be redundant. I had confidence in the equipment because the setup there seemed more robust — was obviously more robust.'

'Why don't you go Danish if you're working Danish?'

'Pardon?'

'If you're working as a Dane, why don't you travel as a Dane?'

'I thought I was working for NATO.'

'You're an army captain.'

'Yes.'

'In whose army?'

'Denmark.'

'Flashing a US passport.'

'A Danish passport is something of a risk, because I hardly speak Danish at all. It makes me look bogus.'

'Two NTRs thirty seconds apart — isn't that a pretty crude and obvious signal?'

He was right. I kept quiet.

'Who intercepted that crude and obvious signal? Who was it actually meant for?'

'This is boring. Can't we just talk?'

'I see you're in red.'

'You're noticing only now?'

'White is for the grown-ups. Red is for the noncompliant. Gitmo protocol.'

'Guantánamo Bay?'

'Yes.'

'All those nifty short forms — I hate them.'

'Give us a location on Michael Adriko.'

Here I counted to five before admitting, 'I've lost him.'

'General location. Uganda? Congo?'

'Congo.'

'East? West?'

'East.'

'Close to here?'

'I could only guess.'

'Then do so.'

'I believe he has reason to be in the area.'

'You had him, you lost him, he's reachable. We should know that. Isn't that something to report?'

'From what facility? We've been in the bush.'

'I'd call it something to report.'

I raised a middle finger. 'Report this.'

'Believe me, I will.'

'Good.'

'Now we're getting somewhere,' he said. 'Do you smoke?'

'No.'

'Smoke pot? Opium?'

'Never.'

'Which one?'

'Cut it out.'

'What about alcohol?'

'Yes.'

'Correct. You were reported drunk in the restaurant of the Papa Leone there in Freetown on . . . ' He consulted his notepad.

Fucking Horst. Old Bruno. 'The evening of the sixth,' I said.

'So you agree.'

'I agree on the date. Not on my condition. I didn't take a Breathalyzer.'

'What about when you sent the meltdown message, rockets up your ass and 'go fuck yourselves' and all that, were you drunk?'

'I'm sober now. Go fuck yourself.'

He said, 'Captain Nair, in March of 2033 they'll give me a gold watch, and I can retire. Till then I've got nothing to do but this.'

'I'm through answering questions.'

'As you wish. But you and I will stay right here.'

'When can I see an attorney?'

'As your legal status evolves, you'll be afforded that opportunity.'

'And my legal status is — what?'

'Evolving. In accordance with the progress of this interview.'

'Well, the progress has stopped. When can I leave?'

'Right now you're being detained without recourse to counsel under US antiterrorism laws.'

'Which law in particular?'

'You can expect to be informed of that as your status evolves.'

'Okay. Suppose this interview sails smoothly along. What can you offer me?'

'A good listener.'

'Then I'll be the one to make the offer,' I said. 'I'm going to tell you everything, and then I expect you to bring in somebody higher up. Somebody who can deal.'

'I'm not considering any offers.'

'Then I assume you're not authorized.'

'I don't recommend you make assumptions.'

'But surely you can send me up the chain.'

'Also an assumption.'

'Fine. Offer withdrawn. Let the silence begin.'

Our bodyguard, the sergeant, was one to emulate. On taking his seat he'd rested his hands on his knees, and he hadn't disturbed them since.

Within half a minute I had to wipe sweat

from my upper lip. Why had I begun this contest? And did it matter what I told them? They're only digging for lies, and when they turn up the truth they brush it aside and go on digging, stupid as dogs.

The interrogator had the sense not to let it go on. He looked at his wristwatch, which might have been platinum. 'Here's an idea, Captain Nair. Why don't you repeat your offer, and why don't I accept it?'

★ ★ ★

Our tent had a good rubber roof without leaks. A strip of mosquito gauze running under the eaves let in the searing light all night, the disorienting yellow-ochre sunshine without shadows. Except for the microwave and satellite towers the base resembled an expanse of sacred aboriginal rubble, sandbag bunkers, Quonset huts emerging from mounds of earth bulldozed against them, and in the midst of it all two monumental generators that never stopped. No fuel or water reservoirs in evidence — they must have been buried. An acre of trucks and fighting vehicles, a hangar like a small mountain, a helicopter bull's-eye. Mornings and evenings a live bugler, not a recording, blew reveille and taps.

Our sandbag perimeter could have accommodated three more tents, but ours stood alone. My tentmate liked to sit on the wall and stare across the way at the chain-link enclosure full of Africans, nearly fifty of them, Lord's Resistance, I should think, or collaborators, women on the north side, men on the south. No children. The men spent their time right against the divider, fingers curled on the wire, laughing and talking, while the women formed a single clump on the other side, never looking at the men. Once in a while a down-pour drove them all under blue plastic canopies strung up in the corners. Quarrels erupted often among the women. I never heard any voice that sounded like Davidia's.

Patrick thought he might spot his wife among them, so he said. Still paying out this line. I didn't buy it.

We took our meals with everyone else. Officers and enlisted men ate together in a large Quonset along with civilian guests and Special Ops helicopter crews and detainees from NATO countries, of which Patrick and I were the only ones, the only people modeling red pajamas.

The Special Activities Division sees some sort of advantage, I think, in starting the questions when your fork is halfway to your mouth. Just grab you up, goodbye hamburger

211

sandwich, and it's off to the interrogator.

This one was new. And that was good.

★　★　★

We met in a Quonset hut, in an office with a desk, two aluminum dining chairs, and some empty cardboard boxes and a cardboard barrel of MREs I could have stood in up to my neck. 'Meal Rammed in an Envelope,' he said. 'Care to suck one down?' I declined. He served me black coffee. I could have chosen tea and milk.

I said, 'Where's Sergeant Stone today?'

'Sergeant Stone?'

'I don't know if his name was Stone, but he certainly seemed to be made of it.'

'No sergeants here.'

'He never introduced himself. Neither did the civilian.'

'Under current regulations, that's not a requirement.'

'But under the circumstances, it might be courteous.'

'Sure. Agreed.'

'So — who are you?'

'Let's skip over the courtesies for now. Can I suggest we do that, without irritating the shit out of you?'

I was too irritated to answer.

212

He used a lot of motions getting a bag of tea into a cup. He seemed older than the first one, but in a way he looked younger, looked barbered and tailored, in dark trousers, a nice white shirt — I wouldn't know silk, but it might have been — and cuff links. He looked the way I try to look.

He sat down facing me with our knees nearly touching. We observed each other's manner of drinking from a cup.

'Captain Nair, I'd like your opinion.'

'I'm full of opinions.'

'Good. Well. In the fullness of your opinion — does all this you've been telling us the last couple of days sound like a desperate, unbelievable lie?'

I counted to three. 'Yes.' Counted again. 'Now can I ask you a question?' Silence. 'Where are you going?'

'I'm not going anywhere.'

'Why not?'

He sipped his tea.

'In case I'm telling the truth.'

He drained his cup. 'Or in case you stop lying. More coffee?'

'No, thanks.'

He stood and set our cups aside and pulled his chair behind his desk and sat down. 'I've reviewed all your written material,' he said, opening a drawer and

taking out a manila file folder.

'Yes.'

He laid it apart before him. Printed e-mails, and my long note to Tina. 'The Congolese Army threw you quite a party.'

'Yes.'

'Stressful.'

'Yes.'

He spent a few minutes perusing the pages of the letter, pages crusty from sweat and tears. 'Sometimes I wish I had the balls to say this stuff. I don't even have the balls to think it.'

I didn't reply.

'Another way of putting it is that we're seeing a lot of anger, and that's not characteristic of our expectations. No matter what the level of stress.'

'I don't deny it — lately I've been out of sorts.'

'Sure, that's another way to put it. If you think all this is funny.'

'Well, I was dispatched to this region on an assignment, and now two weeks later I'm being dealt with as some kind of terrorist.'

'I think you're regarded as absent from your assignment.'

'But I'm not absent, I'm present. Here I am, waiting to get back to work.'

'A Special Forces attache goes AWOL,

starts making alarming noises about enriched uranium. You're sent to make contact, deliver one report that you've done so, and you immediately go silent.' He raised a printed e-mail by two corners and faced it toward me. 'Until this maniac salvo.'

'I've been pursuing my assignment according to my best judgment.'

'And this meltdown message? 'Cunts' and such?'

'Everybody likes to quote that one.'

'I know. It's very compelling. But why did you send it?'

'Theater,' I said.

'Really.'

'I'm dealing with some rogue Mossad agents. I had to make it look good.'

'A rogue Mossad agent, you're saying, was sitting beside you while you transmitted insults to your NATO colleagues.'

'Didn't the last guy tape our interviews? Yes? Have you heard them?'

'I've read highlights of the transcript.'

'Then if you want the details, you can read the whole thing. Don't ask me to rehash.'

'And all of this, the crazy transmission, tossing your commo equipment, getting rounded up by the Congolese Army, all of this was in fulfillment of your superiors' request that you keep a close eye on this

fellow. And you say your mission's momentum has declined sharply. And you propose a strategy to reboot.'

'Yes.'

He sat back with an empty-handed shrug. Shaking his head. Smiling. 'Hard to know what to make of all this.'

'I want to ask about Davidia St. Claire.'

'On that subject I've got nothing to share with you. I mean really — I just don't know. But she's not in any trouble. I'd be more concerned about the one you sent the notes to. Tina? Is that her name?'

'You can read the name right there. I can read it, upside down.'

'This would be Tina Huntington. Works for us in Amsterdam.'

'Who's you?'

'Who — me?'

'You say us. Who's us?'

We both laughed.

'We the Americans, from the USA,' he said.

'Right. She works for you. You're NATO?'

'Nope. I'm a US naval attaché.'

'Rank?'

'I'm attached. Not in. Just attached.'

'So you don't need an ocean.'

'I have an ocean. I'm actually assigned to a ship.'

'In the Indian Ocean? African Atlantic?'

'Well, it moves around. It has propellers.'

'A carrier?'

'Naw. A command ship. Floating office complex. Just about a luxury liner. USSOCOM.'

'I don't know what that is.'

'USSOCOM? US Special Operations Command. The ship is the regional command center.'

'For this region.'

'Yes.'

'Meaning — DR Congo? East Africa?'

'For AFRICOM. Africa. The whole continent.'

I felt, suddenly, in love. I leaned closer to study his face. 'Who are you?'

'I'm the person who can deal.'

'You still don't have a name?'

'The name I have is Susan Rice.'

'You're not black enough to be Susan Rice.'

'Plus, she's a woman.'

'I was getting round to that.'

'I'm the closest thing to Susan Rice.'

She was the current national security advisor in the White House. The queen, in other words, of the secrets and the dark.

He placed his hands on the desk before him. He liked this part. 'Well, Captain Nair, you've rubbed the right lantern.'

* ★ ★

Patrick Roux and I sat on our sandbag wall observing a gang of men creating more sandbags — not all men, actually. We often saw women wearing US uniforms. And of course we saw women among the white-garbed African prisoners. Never any kind of female civilian. Never Davidia.

In the motor lot I counted twenty-two Nissan pickups with canopy shells. One dozen Humvees. Four Stryker fighting vehicles, each worth millions. The helicopter hangar probably housed a chopper big enough to devour them all.

I said to Patrick, 'This was more amusing when it was science fiction.'

He appeared not to comprehend.

The sandbag detail worked in three-person teams — the digger, the sacker, the stacker — filling bags from a heap of dirt and loading them onto a flatbed truck. I remembered reading, as a child, during the first Gulf War, that in order to supply such sacks for their emplacements the Yanks were shipping thousands of tons of American sand across the seas to the Arabian Desert.

Within our perimeter we had a chemical port-a-potty and a vestibule containing a proper shower that ran hot water up from

under the ground. Always hot. You couldn't run it out.

The mess served excellent fare. Real eggs, real potatoes, American meat. In the mornings we smelled the pastries baking.

We had two sets each of the red pajamas, underwear, bedsheets, and towels, and our laundry was collected by enlisted personnel and returned clean eight hours later. That we made our own beds began to seem unreasonable.

★ ★ ★

For nearly an hour I sat alone. When my host arrived he didn't sit down, hardly entered his own office. 'I've gone over the transcripts in detail.'

'Very good,' I said, but he'd already left the room again.

In five minutes he returned, shut the door, and occupied his desk. I waited for an offer of coffee. He plunged into a period of meditation in the manner of Sherlock Holmes, elbows on the table, fingertips on his temples.

'What makes you think we'd pay you off and let you stroll out of here?'

'You'll have to help me figure that out.'

Silence.

'I'll need a convincing story.'

Silence.

'But if I turn up with a good enough story, and if I've got a bag of money to vouch for it, then the thing is in motion again, and the direction of that motion is toward something that has to be taken extremely seriously. Don't you think?'

'We're taking it seriously. No matter how unlikely. This shit story from Michael Adriko — Adriko? Or Adriko.'

'Accent on the second syllable. Adriko.'

'A ton or more of HEU. You're really alleging that?'

'I can only personally vouch for the existence of two kilos, approximately — judging by its weight in my hand.'

'You held it in your hand.'

'I did so. Yes.' He was silent. 'I don't know anything about nuclear devices or their manufacture.' Silent. 'I'm wondering, though, if a couple of kilos wouldn't go a long way.' I wished I'd stop talking, but his silence was working on me. 'I mean in terms of explosive capability. I have no explosives training. But possible damage. Destructive potential.' Still silent. 'So even if two kilos is all he's got — '

'Would you submit to a polygraph?'

'Oh. Well. Where — here? When?'

'It wouldn't be hard to arrange. Can I arrange it?'

'Of course. If it amuses you, fine, sure, but I mean — I can tell you now, you'll get an Inconclusive. I mean to say — I've been telling so many lies and listening to so many lies until I don't know what's true and what's false. And we're in Africa, you realize' — shut up shut up, I told myself, shut *up* — 'and you realize it's all myths and legends here, and lies, and rumors. You realize that.' I bit down on my tongue, and that worked.

He waited, but I was done.

'All right. Excuse me for just a minute. Help yourself to coffee. Ten minutes max.' He left the door halfway open behind him.

The coffee urn waited within my reach. I drew myself a cup — yesterday's, room temperature. I couldn't form a useful thought. I kept tasting the coffee, expecting it to turn hot and fresh. Without a watch I could only guess, but it seemed rather closer to thirty minutes than ten.

When he came back in, he drew himself a cup too and sat behind his desk, sipped once, said, 'Jesus,' and then went silent.

He interrupted his thoughts only once to say, 'No polygraph.'

He got up and went to the door and called out, 'Clyde?' and sat down behind his desk

again. 'Take these cups, will you?' he said to the private who arrived. 'And bring us a fresh service. Not the whole bucket. Just a carafe or something, okay? Leave the door open.'

The silence resumed. I had the impression nothing in the world could happen until we had coffee.

'I'm authorized to tell you Davidia St. Claire is on her way home.'

'Oh . . .'

'You can assume she's been debriefed. Queried. Meticulously.'

'You mean she's already left?'

'Let's concentrate on the people in this room.'

'Just tell me — is she gone?'

'If she's not, she will be soon.' The private took a step into the room and paused. 'Thank you, Clyde. Is it Clyde?'

'Yes, sir.'

'Thanks. Pull the door shut as you leave.' To me he said, 'I want to hear you say it.' He let the carafe languish on his desk. Poured no coffee. 'I want to hear exactly what you're proposing.'

'Well, just what you said a few minutes ago, what you suggested.'

'Which is?'

'That you pay me off and let me stroll out of here. And I get back to what I was doing,

222

and see if the deal is still in motion, or if the deal can be started up again, and, see if we can bring the parties together as arranged.'

'The parties to this proposed, this alleged, this fucking unprecedented criminal conspiracy.'

'Yes. Those parties.'

'You, and these Israelis, and the people Sergeant Adriko represents. If such exist.'

'That would be the objective.'

'A sting operation.'

'That sounds,' I agreed, 'like the applicable terminology.'

'I think we've already deployed the applicable terms, fairy tale, for instance, and bullshit, what else, God,' he said, 'there's not a shred of doubt in my mind. You are fucking with us.'

'And yet — here we are.'

'I can't deny it. Since nine-eleven, chasing myths and fairy tales has turned into a serious business. An industry. A lucrative one.'

'Are we talking price now?'

'What a silly, silly man.'

'But if we were.'

'Then I suppose this would be the moment when you say a number.'

'They want two million.'

'Cash? Or account?'

'Gold.'

'They expect gold?'

'Would that be possible?'

'Gold. What's the price of gold these days?'

'Around forty-five a kilo, US.'

'Forty-five thousand. So, forty-some kilos. Forty-four plus.'

'Call it forty-five.'

'Forty-five kilos of gold.'

'Could you do it?'

The look in his eyes made me sorry for him. 'Do you want to hear the truth?'

'Yes.'

'We can do anything.'

★ ★ ★

Early afternoon. I lay on my bed. I heard the sound of a helicopter coming down.

The walls of the tent rippled. Then they convulsed. I determined to stay inside and avoid the dust, but I was visited with an intuition. I knew. I went outside.

I stood by the sandbag hedge and watched the man I still believe to have been Colonel Thiebes, now in officer's dress, heading for the chopper as it swayed in its descent, a duffel grip in his left hand, his right hand cupping the elbow of Davidia St. Claire.

Davidia and her protector stopped and let

the red cloud overwhelm them while the machine completed its landing. It was a utility helicopter, but not a Black Hawk, something smaller, I don't know what kind. Davidia leaned toward its skis as they felt for the ground. She concentrated on that vision. No backward glance. The chopper had hardly touched down before they were in motion toward it.

I ran to overtake her. I called her name. She couldn't hear me for the roar of the blades. I called again — 'Davidia!' I screamed it many times over.

I gave up running and turned my back against the dust. In a few seconds the wind fell off and the noise got smaller. The craft must have been traveling low, because when I looked around again I could hear it, but I couldn't find it in the sky.

I went back into the tent and closed and zipped the flap and sat on my bed, blinking my eyes and beating the dirt from my hair hand over hand.

★ ★ ★

I felt a touch on my shoulder, and I woke up frightened. It was dark, quiet — very late.

Patrick Roux said, 'These are your clothes.'

He sat there in our only chair. I could see

he held something in his lap. 'It's time to get dressed.'

He was speaking Danish.

'What?'

'It's time to go. Right now the way is open.'

'Wait. Wait . . . *what?*'

'It's time to go. Just take some items for grooming. What you can fit in your pockets. Here's your wristwatch back.'

Great joy powered me out of bed. 'You fucker,' I said. 'I knew it.'

'You prefer English?' he said in English.

'Or German,' I said. 'I went to Swiss schools. The truth is I hardly speak Danish at all. Is this my shirt? I went to English-speaking schools.'

'We have six more minutes.'

'They've shrunk my shirt.'

'Let's be prompt.'

★ ★ ★

When I'd kicked my pajamas aside and dressed and was all ready to go, we delayed, I on my bed, Patrick in the chair, with nothing to do, it seemed, but listen to the rumble of the generators and the giant buzzing of the floodlights outside. He peered at his wristwatch. My own watch, the cheap dependable Timex, read 1:15 a.m.

226

After two minutes he said, 'Now we'll go.'

We stepped into the orange glare and a soft, glittering rain. Patrick zipped the tent's fly behind us and we walked across the grounds and right through the open gateway, passing without a challenge between two gunnery emplacements, five soldiers on each, in their helmets and night goggles and armor. The gate rolled shut behind us and we entered the dark.

The rain let up, but still we had no moon. For thirty minutes we walked along the road without flashlights, going north, feeling with our feet for the ruts and the boggy soft spots. We didn't talk. The din of the reptiles and insects, our steps and our breaths, that's all we heard.

Headlights came up on the road far behind us. Shortly afterward, we heard the engine.

We stepped to the side, and the headlights stopped fifty feet short of us, and Patrick went to the vehicle, a Humvee, I thought, but I couldn't really see, and in a minute his silhouette came toward me and then disappeared as the car turned around and accelerated back the way it had come.

Now Roux directed our steps with a small flashlight. I could make out a sizeable package dangling from his arm. He slung it over his shoulder. As we walked it gave out a

kind of clicking and muttering.

For quite a while the vehicle's aura remained visible behind us. I would have expected them to run blackout headlights, but they didn't seem to care.

When they were well away, Roux said, 'We'll get off the road here, and take a rest.'

'Let's not drown in a mudhole.'

'No, it's good ground.'

He found a spot he liked, laid out a handkerchief, and sat with his back to a tree. Between his knees he set down the package, a canvas haversack. He unbelted the flap, and I knelt beside him while he unpacked the contents by the beam of his penlight — it showed eerily on his eyeglass lenses, like two sparks in his face.

On top, a large manila envelope, inside it a map of the Democratic Republic of Congo. And cash. US twenties. 'This is my money.'

'Your funds when you arrived. It's all there.'

No wallet, no cards of any kind. 'Where's my passport?'

'You don't need it.'

Also, a manila folder — the one I'd seen on the desk of the man from USSOCOM — holding, as far as I could tell in the dark, printed copies of my e-mails, as well as my handwritten pages, and not copies, but the

originals themselves. 'They're dusting their hands of me completely, aren't they? I bet they're burning my pajamas too.'

Roux made no answer while I looked at some items wrapped in a hand towel. A metal fork and a spoon. A folding knife with a single blade. A penlight. 'But what about a cell phone? How will I stay in contact?'

'They'll be able to locate you.'

'Of course they will.'

At the bottom of the sack rested two one-liter bottles of water, and at the very bottom, a cloth bag. Roux set the bag on the ground and opened it and trained his light on a lot of metallic lozenges, each wrapped in tissue paper.

I held my light in my teeth and unwrapped one. Considering its heft, it was small. Three fingers would have covered it.

A kilo of gold.

I said, 'Goddamn! Goddamn!' and the light dropped from my mouth.

'Captain Nair, listen to me. In the first place, these are only twenty kilos.'

'That's still a million dollars' worth. Goddamn!'

'Stop saying Goddamn.' Roux set down his penlight and paused to polish his glasses on his shirttail. Squatting over my pile of riches. 'In the second place, these are not genuine.'

'Well, then, fuck. Fuck and Goddamn. Not genuine?'

He unwrapped another, shone his light on it, turning it in his dirty fingers. 'The plating is copper and nickel, with some gold. Inside it's only lead.'

'Who's going to fall for crap like this?'

'Nobody. It works only with complete amateurs — you know, drunken tourists lured in by pimps, that kind of thing. It's not for serious ruses, it won't pass any kind of knowledgeable inspection. It's something you can flash, nothing more. It's just for you to flash.'

'This is outrageous.'

Roux laughed and said, 'I laugh because you're entertaining. I'm going back now.' He scooped up the contents and fastened them inside the pack and stood up. He seemed in a rush. 'Yours to carry.'

I donned the pack. The load was heavy, but it was good equipment. Thick straps. I could probably hike a long way without chafing my armpits.

Facing him I understood, only now, that he was perhaps as tall as I. But he had a tininess of personality, and a sparrow's face, also tiny. So then even his size was an illusion. His Frenchness, his bag of gold, his lost wife — all fake.

'I'm instructed to tell you to get physically close to certain parties, keeping this material with you.'

'That was my understanding.'

'They'll maintain a fix on your location at all times. Remember that.'

'Is this a drone operation?'

'I'm not aware of such a thing.'

'Sure.'

'I'm only a messenger, but I can assure you personally you won't be harmed. We don't fight like that, harming our own people.'

'Sure. Except when you do.'

He said, 'Don't worry. Never worry. And don't drop your mission.'

'I wouldn't consider it.'

'If you do,' Roux said, 'if you drop out of contact — you'll be in an unacceptable situation. A kind of hell. Always hunted. Never resting. Nobody who tries it can last very long. You know it, don't you? Nobody ever lasts.'

* ★ ★

The US Army kept their garrison well out of the way. I had the road entirely to myself. By the fragrance, I guessed it cut through a forest of eucalyptus. The sack's contents clicked rhythmically and with every step I

said yes, finally, yes, at last: I'm done with you all, done with your world, done with you all, done with your world.

Twenty kilos of nonsense on my shoulders. How many pounds? Better than forty. More like forty-five. How many stone? Something like three. Right around seven hundred ounces. Yet the pack felt weightless, until my giant excitement gave way to the question why I wasn't getting rid of it. Some item among the contents called out uninterruptedly to a global positioning satellite, a chopper full of Special Ops, a Predator drone, a fleet of drones — called out, after all, to the people who would either bring order to my affairs in a prison or murder me and solve my life.

I trudged for five hours, covering in that interval only a few miles. The dawn had begun — as always this near the equator very gradually, and even doubtfully — before I spied any huts among the trees.

I reached a slick soft spot I couldn't skirt unless I ranged far into the wood. I sidled left along its edge and came to a sucking, lethal-looking red-and-yellow mudhole sprouting dead limbs around its border. In such a pit anything might be drowned. I shrugged off the pack and opened it at my feet. I set aside my papers and cash, and the map, and

the water. I gripped one strap and spun myself to get the pack whirling and let it fly ten meters. It slapped the surface, skidded, rolled slowly under.

My Timex said it was 6:17 on the twenty-sixth of October. Five days, nine hours left in which to find my way to Freetown. Plus an hour I'd pick up changing time zones. I unstrapped the watch from my wrist and pitched it underhanded into the muck.

Five thousand kilometers. One hundred thirty hours.

I drank down a liter of water as I stood there, tossed the bottle, kept the other, which wouldn't stay with me much longer. While the pack sank with anything metal — penlight, camp knife, phony kilos, the lot — I removed my shirt and used it as a bindle for the rest. I thought about tossing away my belt with its suspicious metal buckle, considered also the buttons on my shirt and trousers, realized I might as well go naked — what certainty would it bring? There's always something more to be rid of. Something inside.

★ ★ ★

I wondered about Michael. I expected him to turn up at my side having lingered in the area

all this time, watching for some sign of me or of Davidia. As soon as I thought of him, there he was, Michael, crouched at the base of one of these tall trees just ahead — but it wasn't Michael. Only a termite berm. As the day came on it revealed many more such berms feeding on the eucalyptus, and I thought I saw blurry figures or ghosts crouched in the grove, watching me, and soon the woods were full, indeed, of people moving among the trees and poking slender sticks into the mounds, harvesting the white ants. I was joined on the way now by dozens of mud-spattered, stately women balancing baskets on their heads, taking the insects to the market. None of them spoke. They had the manner of ghosts. Possibly one of them had sprung from the corpse of the woman we'd struck down in Uganda. But their feet padded on the clay. I heard them breathing.

I followed them out of the woods and into Darba, a town without electric light, without even useless wires, just old power poles broken at the tops like huge dead stalks. The place materialized around us in a haze of cook-smoke, a city of sturdy French colonial buildings without panes in the windows or doors in the doorways, concrete husks into which people had moved their animals while they made shanties of twig and adobe for

themselves in the yards.

I stopped at a café, really a tent. I gave the barman a twenty-dollar bill and he left me sleeping on my face at his only table while his small daughter looked after the establishment.

I woke when a guy came in flying on what looked like the greatest drug ever made. He was speaking in tongues, his feet didn't touch the floor, he was just being lugged around by his smile; it turned out he was merely drunk on a few baggies' worth of 'spirits' branded, in this case, as Elephant Train.

I bought him another and another, and as many for myself. When I asked him if he spoke English, he said, 'Super English.'

'Where is Newada Mountain?'

'You need to go La Dolce.'

'How do I find La Dolce?'

'Go to Newada Mountain.'

'No. No. Ou est La Dolce?'

'La Dolce!' I heard the two Italian words, though he might have said Ladoolchee.

'Is La Dolce near Newada Mountain?'

'She is the mother of Newada Mountain.'

'A person? A woman? Une personne? Une femme?'

'Yes. The mother. Oui. La mère. Oui.'

Elephant Train. I spread out my Congo map, and together we searched for Newada

Mountain as we bit into many packets and sucked down the contents, but the map got smaller and Congo grew larger, and soon we were lost.

The barman returned and presented me with a pair of slip-on jogging shoes, blue in color, a pair of black denims called El Gaucho, and a yellow T-shirt with a woman's brown face on it. Who is the woman? I said, and he said, Très jolie! I said, Oui oui. He gave me my change in Ugandan shillings. I said, No Congo francs? and he said, Le franc? — c'est merde.

When I asked about Newada Mountain he said, It's there, pointing north, but I don't know how to get there. Go to the coffin maker. He's going to Newada. He's next to the church.

Yes, I see the church.

He's going to Newada Mountain. Follow the coffin maker.

The clock on the post stretched its hands out sideways, nine-fifteen. I'd walked for five hours, slept for one. Spent another getting drunk. Out back of the café I found a dry spot of earth to stand on among the puddles, and got myself into the new wardrobe. The jeans and T-shirt sagged quite a lot; the blue shoes fit perfectly over my grimy socks.

Behind the Église du Christ I found a man, a very small one, perhaps of the Mbuti, one of the Pygmy groups, dressed in a sports shirt and clean trousers and shiny plastic sandals. He stood with his hands on a green bicycle, rolling it backward and forward as if to check its worthiness. I said, 'Are you the coffin maker?' He didn't understand. I tried to remember the French word for coffin but I never knew it in the first place. Somebody called to him, he abandoned me for a fool, and I followed him as he walked his bike along the crumbling tarmac street.

On sawhorses out front of his lean-to rested five bright purple coffins, two of them, I'm afraid, quite short. These were the two he was concerned with. He parked his bike's rear tire on a notched block to steady it and mounted both coffins — equal in length, about a meter — sideways behind the seat and fastened them down with black rubber straps, which he tightened and yanked and tightened again.

He high-stepped over the bar of his conveyance and straddled it while he rolled it free of the block and set his feet on the pedals. For a moment he stood in the air, then descended as he produced a forward

motion. He knew I was watching. I don't think he liked it.

I followed some distance behind him, out of the town and into a small rain, then under a hot blue sky. The tarmac ended in a fog of red dust out of which the vast faces of speeding lorries exploded one after another, saying I AM LOST — TOUT AU BOUT — REGRETTE RIEN — coming within half an inch of touching us, as if some superstition required it. I lost him in the choking clouds until he left the highway for a sidetrack, and I glimpsed a bit of purple a quarter mile off to my right.

For some time I floated along like a marionette. I had no reason for believing these two small coffins were headed for Newada Mountain. We had the sun traveling toward our left, and therefore, it seemed, this track took us north, and north felt reason enough to be doing anything — that is, some particle of my memory put Newada to the north of where I'd first entered Congo with Michael and Davidia.

I had no problem keeping up, as he stopped often to get his strength. On the upward slopes he got off and walked his bike, and I pulled ahead of him. I never said hello or the like. My shoes held up, though my socks were falling to pieces. No blisters. The

bottoms of my heels felt raw, but only slightly.

About three hours along, many kilometers from the highway, the green bike's rear tire went flat — perhaps owing to some sabotage, as the puncture happened in front of an establishment consisting of a bench and a bicycle pump, open for business, which business was tire repair. The repairman pried the tire loose from its rim, pulled out the inner tube, and went about patching it with a remnant cut from another inner tube.

While this went on I had the sense to find a kiosk and buy a bag of breadrolls and some candles and matches and two liters of water and a yellow number-two pencil and a small kitchen knife wrapped, for safety's sake, in newspaper. I paid with a five-thousand-shilling bill, and the proprietor and his wife shuttered their store and went to canvass their neighbors for the balance. They hadn't returned before the coffin maker set out again.

As far as I know, during the rest of the journey, as much as fifteen kilometers, I believe, the bearer of the coffins took no water. I ate my bread and drank down my two liters and then started dying of the drunkard's thirst.

I let him blaze the trail into another spell of rain and out again. We entered open

farmland. In the mud, the tread-prints of goats and barefoot humans. The wet fields shone hard enough to burn my eyes. We passed boys as they stopped hoeing to throw themselves down in the corn rows with their arms flung wide and their chins in the dirt, praying toward Mecca, but they sounded like coyotes howling. Just afterward, the coffins disappeared over a rise, and when I'd climbed to the top I looked across a landscape of rolling hills and silhouettes — the lumps of huts, a few skeletal, solitary trees, and three cell phone towers with much the same lonely and distinguished aspect, one in the north, two others beyond it in the northwest.

The coffin maker, already free of his cargo, charged back down the way he'd come. I moved to block his way. He skidded to a stop and leaned on his handlebars, tipping his bike to the side with one short leg outstretched and a toe on the ground, and when I asked him if this was Newada Mountain, he spoke his first words to me, saying, 'Oui, c'est Newada,' and kicked off again, gaining speed down the hill, and I gathered he'd reach the wider road before full dark. A bit along in his descent he turned his head and spoke once more, calling, ' — le lieu du mal!' which I think means the bad or the wrong or the evil place.

ATTENDEZ EN ANGLAIS:
FINDER PLEASE DELIVER THIS MATE-
RIAL TO THE UNITED STATES MILITARY
GARRISON NEAR DARBA, CONGO

TO WHOM IT MAY CONCERN (US
MILITARY PERSONNEL):
PLEASE FORWARD ATTACHED MATE-
RIAL TO
DAVIDIA ST. CLAIRE
C/O GARRISON CMDR COL. MARCUS ST.
CLAIRE
US 10TH SPEC FORCES, FT. CARSON,
COLORADO, USA

WITH GRATITUDE — KAPTAJN ROLAND
NAIR (CAPT.) JYDSKE DRAGONREGI-
MENT, HRN (ROYAL DANISH ARMY)

[OCT 27 ca. 12 AM]

Davidia,
I wish I could record this silence. It's like
the bottom of the sea. In silence like this, my
head makes its own noise — I can hear the
moon, I can hear the stars. Once in a while a
sick child croaks in one of the huts.
(I started to write this a couple of hours
ago. I lit a candle, but the flame drew the

241

nocturnal insects, including a moth big as a sparrow that batted out the flame in its forays and then crashed at my feet with its paraffin-spattered wings on fire and lay there flailing and burning for several minutes — all because of its infatuation . . . And then I saw the half moon coming up, so I've waited for its light to write by, sitting in the doorway of this hut. I'm guessing as to time of day, but the moon's been waxing fatter and rising later and I remember it rose around ten pm when last I owned a watch.)

I won't bother catching you up. Someday I'll attach this to a full account. I'll wrap it all in brown paper and tie it with string and plunk it in a DHL pouch addressed to you, or to Tina Huntington. Which of you am I writing to?

To you, Davidia. Just letting you know (should only this fragment reach you) that as of the date above, I was still alive.

For the third time in ten days, I'm a captive — not held by others, but stuck, no option for movement. In my universe, time and space converge on 3 pm Nov 2nd at the Bawarchi Restaurant in Freetown — remember the Bawarchi? — 5000 kilometers and 112 hours from here and now. Not a clue how to get there.

I have some candles and matches, but as I

say — the crashing bugs. I've got paper and pencils and a knife. The clothes on my back. 720 US dollars. 60K Ugandan shillings. No credit cards or plane tickets, no passport, no documented actuality. No pills against malaria. Every day, more African.

I think when the wind shifts I may be hearing the brook at the bottom of the hill, or people down there laughing, or weeping.

Several hours ago, Davidia, at dusk, I climbed this hill and arrived at the village of New Water Mountain. I stood among a couple dozen huts. No mountain visible. Hooves and feet had beaten the hilltop's ground into a flat, muddy waste. The only splashes of color came from yellow twenty-liter water jugs — they lay all around. And two bright, child-size purple coffins. Beside the coffins, two old men scraped at the ground, one with a hoe, one with a spade, both men barefoot but wearing long sleeves and trousers.

Nearby, a man and a woman seemed to be taking apart one of the dwellings, removing its thatch, setting the materials aside. The woman stopped, laid her head back, and put her face to the sky — I expected a mournful howl, but she only trembled a bit, then settled her mind, it seemed, and returned to the work.

A giant leafless tree, an arthritic-looking horror, dominates the vicinity from the top of the rise (I can hear it creaking in the breeze right now as I write). Four people stood at the tree's base, hallooing up toward the highest branches like hounds. One of them, a white woman, met me as I approached, and she said, 'Are you wondering where the chickens went?' — I said I wasn't — 'And the goats? They're all dead. And most of the children. Dead. Are you lost?' — I said a little — 'You look disturbed.' — She meant drunk. I said I was.

She'd walked among several villages with these others, two women and a sturdy-looking man with a machete on his shoulder, all Africans. She alone was white — white and plump, probably in her thirties — and grimy from hiking, but hale and upright.

I said, 'Jesus, I know you.'

'You know Jesus?'

'I saw you at the White Nile Hotel, didn't I? You were swimming in the pool.'

'My husband Jim and I are from the North East Congo Mission of the Seventh-day Adventist Church.'

'I had the impression it was something like that.'

'It's the Lord's work,' she said, 'but every day you want to kill somebody.'

The man with the machete said, 'We must go, Mom.'

'I know. I just said so.'

She told me her husband had spent the day in Darba trying to find someone from the Ministry of Health so they could get some action up here. 'Or the Red Cross or somebody. What a laugh. But we have to try.'

'What about Doctors Without Borders?'

'He'll check with them too, but they like to stay close to Bunia for supplies. Close to the airfield. And the brothels. We call them Doctors Without Pants.'

The woman continually waved her hands and flicked her fingers as if battling with cobwebs, and I feared for her sanity as much as mine. She said, 'We've looked at three other villages in the last two days. It's the same thing for fifty kilometers around. The people are crazy, the water is poison, everybody's dying. We've convinced them to evacuate — all but this bunch. They've got a queen who rules them from the treetop. Come over here and you can look.'

We joined the others. Several meters above us, between two large boughs, a chair was hanging. We could see the bottom of the chair, and a pair of feet, in white tennis shoes, dangling below it, and in the boughs above the chair were bunches of thatch, evidently to

protect the owner of the feet.

'She won't come down till morning, but we can't wait for that. We're meeting the reverend in Kananga. It's two kilometers down that path. Or more.'

The feet up above seemed quite still. 'Is she asleep?'

'I don't know what she is. Are you gold, or hydrocarbons?'

'Pardon?'

'Are you with one of the companies? Which particular corporation?'

'None. I'm here looking for a friend of mine, but I haven't spotted him. Or much of anybody, actually.'

We stood on a patch of brown earth littered with corn husks and cassava peelings. To the west I saw a couple of distant cell towers, lone trees, many huts — all in two dimensions, flat against the sunset. In the other direction, everything was bathed in a somber metallic light, and the two child coffins, ten steps away, seemed uniquely purple, a purple without precedent. Beside them, the two old diggers had nearly disappeared into the earth. I went over and looked. The margin between the twin graves had crumbled to make a single large hole. As they smoothed its sides with their tools, the men sloshed up to their ankles in muddy

seepage, maybe the very stuff that had killed the poor tots.

She said, 'Usually when somebody dies they do a big wake with a lot of howling and drumming, but they've had too many, and now it's just a chore. The whole region is toxic, thanks to the lust for precious metals. This is the outworking of a spiritual travesty. Are you any kind of believer?'

'No.'

'We're getting out of here day after tomorrow, and I am Goddamn glad.'

'How are you traveling?'

'Walking, for now. Jim has the Trooper. We'll make one more swing through the villages, and then back to Lubumbashi. We'll take a plane from Bunia.'

'Look,' I said, 'if I find my friend, we'll need a ride out of here. I don't mind paying, and I don't mind begging.'

'It depends on how many come in the car. Where are you going?' — I said I didn't know — 'Any decent hotel, am I right?' — I said yes — she recommended Bunia. 'There's quite a bit of UN activity there. Peacekeepers and such. It's a UN town.'

'How far away is Bunia?'

'A couple hundred kilometers. It's the nearest airstrip. The UN uses it, and some charters.'

'Please, ma'am. Please. We don't need seats. Put us on the roof. Really. This is Africa.'

She thrilled me by saying, 'We'll probably come right through here day after tomorrow. We'll do our best to take you aboard. Look for a blue Isuzu Trooper with the top painted white.'

'I'll be looking for it, believe me.'

'In the meantime, you'll meet the queen. Maybe they'll elect you king.'

'Are you laughing at me?'

'After a while,' she said, 'everything's funny.' For one second — I think because of her bright anger — she seemed sexy. She turned to her friends. 'Next is Kananga. Only a couple of miles, yes?'

They walked on, four abreast. I watched them get away. Toward the bottom of the hill a flashlight came on, and its spot trembled over the ground . . . I hadn't learned the woman's name or told her mine or even asked if she'd seen anybody like Michael.

The sun had set. The West turned a densely luminous terrifying aubergine. I stood alone beside the queen's tree. I tried shouting Michael's name and got no answer. As far as I could tell, the queen slept on undisturbed.

I looked into one or two huts. The people inside them ignored me, even when I called to them.

Then the night came down, and I found this hut empty and came in and sat inside, right here on the dirt floor, and this is where I've lived for the last few hours — maybe till I die — probably of thirst. I haven't had water since noon. Soon I'll go down and drink from the toxic creek.

[OCT 27 ca. 7AM]

When a woman's screaming disturbed my dreams I thought nothing of it — there's always some woman or infant or animal screaming — and I stayed under the darkness in my head as long as possible before I woke up thirsty and frightened in this hut. I'm crouched in a corner. The female screams go on. A sound of hammering or chopping too — not rhythmic, just violent. I have to piss. I need water. A man screams also.

This thirst is murdering me. Give me sewage — I'll drink it. But I can't look for the creek now. I'm afraid to leave this hut.

★ ★ ★

Davidia. I've had a look. It's Michael out there. Adriko. Our Michael.

I'm not going out. I'm glad to see him — I came here looking for him — but I won't make myself known until I have an idea what's happening.

I see a lot of villagers sitting on the ground around the coffins and the grave and the dirt piles. Michael argues — battles — with a large woman. He and this screamer are the only ones standing, stalking one another in a circle ten meters wide, keeping the people and the coffins and the double grave between them.

I'm able to count twenty-nine sitting on the ground. Women wearing long skirts and tops with bold patterns and colors, men in sweaters or large T-shirts with washed-out logos, all of them looking as if they'd rolled in the mud and didn't care. Two women with children laid across their laps. Both kids naked and bony and sick, eyes open and staring at another world. One woman in a brilliant but filthy wrap and headscarf sits on top of a dirt pile, her legs out straight.

Michael holds a machete two-handed. Sometimes he raises it above his head as if he means to chop the sun out of the sky. He and the woman scream in some kind of Creole or Lugbara unintelligible to me.

★ ★ ★

My guess: the woman is the village queen, La Dolce, down from her tree — I recognize her tennis shoes — and these people have gathered for the funeral of the two dead children, and Michael must have stopped it with his screams and his machete. He and La Dolce howl at each other to the point of strangling on their hatred, but not both at once — it's back and forth — that is, it seems to proceed as a debate while they orbit around the others.

★ ★ ★

She wears a long black skirt and a man's sleeveless undershirt torn off just below her breasts, which, by their outlines, are narrow and pendulous.

She's got a buzz-cut Afro on her hippopotamus head, eyes leaping from the sockets and eyelids like birds' beaks closing over them — her mouth is tiny and round,

but it opens to shocking hugeness, displaying many square white teeth. A broad nose like a triangle biscuit smashed onto her face. She's fat and laughing, hips banging as she struts around, keeping the people and the coffins and the grave between her and Michael.

The hair on Michael's head is growing back. He tromps around in rubber sandals, blue jeans, a gray hooded sweatshirt, waving the machete with his left hand, slapping his right hand against his chest, where it says HARVARD.

Mainly throughout all this I feel thirsty. I've had nothing to drink since yesterday afternoon, and all this drama — and the whole sky, and the earth — and the oceans — seem tiny beside my thirst.

★ ★ ★

One minute ago Michael started chopping away with his machete at the woman's chair, which rests on the ground beside her tree, and she shimmied toward him majestically and plopped herself right down in it, daring him to keep up the destruction and split her in pieces as well.

He's speaking English — 'I'll destroy this place!'

Now she doesn't howl, but rather sings of

252

her power, I think, sitting on her throne, and cries out I think Bring me food! Bring me food! until a woman delivers something on a plastic plate and backs away apologizing. La Dolce flings grain into her mouth, it spills all over her bare belly, which even from here I can see is covered with stretch marks. Water now! Bring me water! They hurry to bring her a liter of bottled water — bottled Goddamn water. She anoints her own head from it and sprinkles her face. The drops remain while she says to Michael in English:

'I am El Olam — the Everlasting God!'

They've stopped everything. He's catching his breath. Listen, Davidia — his face frightens me. The blade is twitching in his hands.

She laughs at him.

I need water and I'm going out now before Michael kills her.

[OCT 27 ca. 5:30 PM]

The sun is low and very red and mean. I can't look west.

Down to double digits: 94 hours to go. Plus 30 minutes. Still 5000 KM to cover.

I've drunk my fill at the creek. No matter. The toxins work slowly. Thirst would have

253

killed me by tomorrow. I'm resting beside the creek among some new associates, that is, four skeletal sad-eyed Brahma cattle and the three herdsmen who tend them. Later I'll tell you all about these guys. I don't intend to move from this haven, I'm at my leisure to write and also to drink, and not just water, and I'll tell you all about that too, but first — as to this morning's romp —

When I came out of my hiding-hut, Michael was declaring again:

'I'll destroy this place!' With a sweep of his machete he said, 'You people are crazy!'

I stood by my doorway till Michael noticed. At first he didn't, but the villagers watched me. Without the usual smiling and laughing, their mouths took up no room in their faces and their eyes seemed abnormally huge.

The sight of me slapped Michael awake. His recognition of me seemed to travel up from his feet and when it got to his face I came closer, but not in reach of the machete.

He looked around himself: a dozen or so huts; the one tree — deceased; two piles of red dirt; two purple coffins, and a hole; also his clansmen huddling together on the ground like survivors of a shipwreck.

He said: 'Where is she?' He meant you, Davidia.

'The Americans had us,' I said. 'Your outfit, the Tenth.'

'Where is she, Nair?'

'She's gone. She got on a chopper and didn't look back.'

His spine withered. The weapon dangled at his side. 'Sometime during Arua, she took her heart away from me. I felt it. In Arua, something happened.'

I wanted to take him away from this scene and talk about that other scene, about you, Davidia, and the colonel and the prop-wash and the noisy cloud that ate you up.

However: the Dolce woman strode up to my face and gave out a hearty, phony laugh and cried, 'God knocked backwards!'

Michael said, 'This woman is insane.'

I said, 'You must be La Dolce.'

She yelped, 'You've got an English for us!!??' (I punctuate excessively because her manner came straight out of comic books. She communicated in yelps, whoops — what else — guffaws, huzzahs, preachments, manifestos — and I had to agree instantly with Michael that she was insane.) 'You are right, because I am!!! — I AM LA DOLCE!!!'

'What a stupid name to call yourself,' Michael said.

She raised her face to Heaven and sang ha-hah.

'I understand she's the village queen or something.'

'More than that. She's a priestess of genocide.'

La Dolce addressed her brethren, pointing at Michael's head. 'Do you hear the Devil talking in his mouth?'

'She calls me her prisoner,' Michael said. 'She tells them I'm being kept here by her power.'

'She speaks good English.'

'She's from Uganda. She's the cousin of my uncle.'

La Dolce pointed at me now, almost touching my nose: 'This one's clan is called Bong-ko. Their lies make you laugh!!!'

Michael said, 'They know the truth about you.' I said What? — he said, 'Aren't you a liar? Why are you here without Davidia? If the Tenth got hold of you, how did you get away? Did you sell me for your freedom? How long before they come for me?' He raised high the machete. 'I feel like cutting the lies right out of you!'

The blade didn't scare me so much — only the look of him. His beard was growing out in streaks and whorls. Nappy head, red eyes, fat parched lips. He'd plastered the laceration on his forearm with red mud. His greasy black face, his mangled sweatshirt, his mistreated

jeans — all dabbed and smeared with it. His sandals and feet were tainted with the same African muck.

'Michael. Lower your weapon. I need water.'

'I can't help you. Do you see her crazy eyes?' La Dolce sat in her wooden chair like an enormous toddler, broadcasting happy rage. 'This woman is calling for a sacrifice. She wants to bury someone alive. If I don't keep an eye on her, she'll throw one of these people into the grave.'

'Has she got more bottled water?'

'She's got a whole commissary.'

'Where? — Please.'

'Die of thirst, Nair. You sold me to the machine.'

'I've got no time for your accusations.'

'You should be the one to go in the grave with those children.'

'Lower your weapon and help your friend.'

'Sacrifice for sacrifice.'

'Two things,' I said, backing away. 'First, water. And then we get out of here.' I guess I looked stupid, stumbling off. And he looked stupid with his cutlass in the air, as if it was stuck there and he couldn't get it down.

I poked my head into several huts and found one stacked with half a dozen cases of bottled water and boxes of cereal and canned

goods, its entrance guarded by a man leaning on a hoe. He took it up like a cudgel when I got near. I tried to bribe him with all my Ugandan shillings, then with US dollars — twenty, a hundred, two hundred — but he wouldn't share.

I experienced a sort of dislocation here. The next several minutes have gotten away from me, and I'm not sure I remember things in their actual order.

I saw the villagers all standing around the grave, shuffling their feet in place as they moaned and trembled. They were dancing. Singing.

La Dolce and Michael had resumed their own dance, circling the scene.

I didn't notice that the purple coffins had gone until they reappeared on the shoulders of four men coming two-by-two from behind me. The dead children, I assumed, traveled inside them. The crowd made way, still chanting and moving in a zombie trance.

The diggers waited in their hole and each coffin was just shoved over into their double embrace and let down to the floor with a little sploosh, and then helping hands raised one of the men from his work, while the other simply stepped onto one of the coffins and clambered out on his own, leaving behind the smeary impression of his bare foot.

La Dolce screamed at some length, and Michael spoke briefly in a much lower tone, both in Lugbara, I supposed.

The mob circled the grave on their knees, shoving dirt into it with their hands. They tossed the piles back into the holes and then bowed their heads while their queen made a speech that included much repetition of 'La Dolce, La Dolce.' When she got near me, she took up her theme in English: 'What is that name? I am La Dolce Vita!! You know it means that life is sweet. That's me. I bring life. Life is sweet. But first we must sacrifice. First God will take what he wants. He takes the babies into his jaws. Can we stop him?' She went among the crowd, looking into face after face, bending close: 'Can you stop God? — Can you stop God? What about you? — Can you stop God? No!! You cannot!!! And now God is angry that you have not sacrificed. I know this because I am God!' I doubt they comprehended.

Michael said to her, 'The Newada people are not animists and sacrificers like that. This village used to be Christian' — he pronounced it Chrishen. Then he shouted, still in English:

'Go home! The grave is full enough! Go home!'

Many of the mob stood up and wandered

away. Some of them wept, nobody talked. A dozen or so stayed with their queen.

La Dolce watched the others go, and I got the sense that Michael had triumphed here.

The queen performed a kind of slow elephantine dance, singing ha-hah, ha-hah. She pointed at Michael's crotch and said, 'I'm going to my sleep now. When I dream, your parts will turn into a white stone!'

Michael laughed. It was false, but loud, from deep in his lungs. He said, 'Woman! If I had diesel, I would soak you and burn you alive.'

'La Dolce is going up!' The queen lowered her butt into her throne with an ostentatious lot of wiggling. The two diggers hurried to help her.

Next to the tree stood a rough-hewn table with some items on it — a few liters of bottled water — empty — a whole cassava, some mangoes, and some of the green oranges they eat in this region. From nails hammered into the trunk hung plastic shopping bags by their knots, full of what I don't know. Clothes, probably, food. A pole jutted from the earth nearby, and between it and the tree some bright things flapped on a length of twine — a scarf, a skirt, a T-shirt. A pair of white athletic socks. Stair treads had been hacked in a zigzag up the trunk, but La

Dolce didn't use them.

La Dolce raised one finger and made a winding motion with it and two stout women and a man took hold of her rope. She laughed and laughed while, by a system of pulleys anchored out of sight above, they hoisted her chair off the ground, and she ascended into the boughs.

We tilted back our heads to watch — the chair swaying, the rope rasping against the tree's rough hide, the crowd's murmurs and exclamations — ayeee ayeee — the wind coming across the expanse.

She pointed down at Michael. 'Hees name shall rot!'

I remembered a spider I'd seen swinging in just such a manner from Michael Adriko's toothbrush. I thought: Yes, everything's coming together now.

I wouldn't have thought that anything could distract me from my thirst, but now I heard the sound of an engine, and a burst of hope lifted me. 'Is that a car?'

It was a cow. Another one also moaned.

I said, 'Shit. We can't ride out of here on cattle.'

Michael took a couple of strokes at the tree with his machete. He gave it up and seemed about to walk off somewhere.

'Michael — I need you to focus now. I

talked to some missionaries. Tomorrow they can take us out of here to Bunia.'

'Good for them.'

'Don't do this. Jesus, man — not now. I need to get to Freetown, and I'm out of ideas.'

'Leave me alone.'

'I need your help.'

'Leave me alone.'

When he's like that, he's like that. I left him alone.

I followed the path down the hill.

While a humpbacked Brahma cow was loosing a stream of piss two meters away, I sponged up creek water in a dirty sock and squeezed it into my mouth. No liquid so sweet has ever touched my lips, until perhaps five minutes later — because gathered around a stump quite near to where I'd fallen on my knees, three remnant herdsmen had convened. One of them offered me a gourd. I thought he meant it for a water glass, but in fact it was already swimming with a filmy yellow liquid, pungently alcoholic, and I knew I'd come among my tribe.

★　★　★

Three fine men: one younger, two older. I forget their names. They have the puffy look

of corpses floating in formalin. And three stunted, starving cows and one bull who drags his chin across the ground because he can't hold up his own horns.

As far as I make out through the language barrier, they've been trading off the last of their cattle for plantain and sugar cane, which they bury together in a formula that ferments and emerges as a remarkable beverage they call Mawa. I don't think it's good for the teeth — they've got none. But these dregs in the gourd, I'll bet you, give strength to the bones.

I can't say whether they're from Michael's clan or some neighboring society. They wear rope sandals. Long-sleeved shifts of coarse cloth, brown or gray, depending on the light.

I fell asleep by the creek, I woke from a long nap, and I've been sitting here writing away with no intention of leaving this spot because, if I take their meaning, a new batch of Mawa comes up from the earth around sundown, and I plan to be here for the resurrection. Prior to my nap, I only got a few swallows.

I'm not going back up that hill to deal with Michael. I'd sooner take my chances on the Tenth Spec Forces than hang my hopes on Michael Adriko, the lunatic comedian.

I should stay sober and alert for the sound of a blue-and-white Isuzu.

Really? Kiss off. What difference does it make? It's been two weeks since we left Arua and I've come altogether about fifty kilometers.

[SAME-SAME, 6:30PM?]

Oh, Davidia! Or maybe I mean
   Oh, Tina!
Whichever is your name, I call to you, oh woman of my heart.
The Mawa decants out of 2 five-liter jugs.
The gourd bowl goes round and round.
My flat black silhouette comrades. Right now they stand against the sunset. Behind them it looks like Dresden's burning. I forget their names. I'll ask again.
   — Oudry
   — Geslin
   — Armand
Priests of the nectar, ministers to the flock, of whom I am one.
If I can't buy or think my way out of this by tomorrow, I'll go back to the Americans and say, Prison? Fine.

★　★　★

264

My handwriting may be illegible — let's blame the dark.

Also my pencil must be dull, but come on, enough — it worries the mind and body to have to sharpen a utensil every half page.

Oudry, Geslin, and Armand have kindled a fire from dried dung on a bed of former thatch, and our laughter flies up into the blackness with its sparks.

Incidentally, Davidia, that's why they're tearing the huts apart around here. For firewood.

Davidia, I wish you could meet Tina.

Tina, I'm not sure I'd like you to meet Davidia.

Do I contradict myself? Not to worry. I'll soon be transcribing these notes in a prison cell, with plenty of time to get my thoughts in order.

Let's face it. I've got to go back to the Yanks.

I've improved the plan a bit: take the last of my cash to Bunia, lavish it on a finale of booze and prostitutes, then advise the UN to arrest me.

★ ★ ★

Fifty kilometers in 14 days. Per my calculations, a circus clown walking on his

hands would have made better progress.

Tina.

You're sexy, Tina. And smart. But not glamorous in the Michael's-woman way. Still. You might have had dealings with Michael. I think you might have dealt with him. You know what I mean? I mean, did you fuck him, Tina? I always suspected you did but I never asked, so I'm asking. Did you fuck Michael?

[OCT 28 ca. 8AM]

When next I encountered Michael Adriko, I found him continuing in a wretched state. He looked like he'd been beaten about the face with a bat, but it was just sadness, only misery, it was nothing physical, it was all from the inside. That was last night.

A few words about remorse.

This remorse twists in me like seasickness.

If you've been seasick lately you know what I mean. This remorse is physically intolerable.

I climbed the hill last night after drinking with my fellow herdsmen. What are their names? God. I've lost their names — and the herdsmen as well, and their cattle. Where are they? I'm alone by the creek.

There's a reason they call them spirits. They enter in, they take control, they speak

and walk around. Wicked, wicked spirits.

Last night I thought I heard Michael chopping with his machete atop this hill. Striking at La Dolce's tree and calling, Nair! with every stroke, Nair! Nair!

It must have been well past midnight, because the moon rode high and gave plenty of light to see by. I floated zigzag up the hill and now report I was hallucinating. Nobody was bothering the tree.

Michael sat against its base with his legs splayed before him and his machete sticking upright at the midpoint between his feet, his arms limp beside him, his chin on his chest — in Kandahar I once saw a man sitting exactly like that, and he was dead.

I said, 'I don't care if you're awake, or dead, or what.'

'I'm defeated, that's all.'

'We need to go, man. What's keeping you here?'

'Something has to happen that hasn't happened.'

'What could possibly happen?'

'Davidia might come.'

'Davidia's not coming. She was disgusted right down through. She didn't look back, Michael. Not one glance.'

'I put her to too harsh a test.'

'Did you think you'd be the king here, and

Davidia would reign beside you as queen?'

'You're making my experience sound shallow. You're wrong. This is cutting me very deep. I never meant to keep her here. No, I only meant to bring my wedding to these people as a great gift, and then leave. I always meant for us to leave.'

'Leave how?'

'There's always a plan for extraction. How many times have I told you that?'

'What plan? Who extracts us?'

'In this case, we extract ourselves.'

'Then let's do it. For God's sake, Michael.'

'What are you made of, Nair? Why did you betray us?'

'Will you leave it for another time? Let's get out of here, if you know a way.'

'I'm not leaving.'

'Come and have some Mawa with these folks down the hill. Let's relax, and talk this over.'

He wouldn't respond. I walked away in the hope he'd hop up and follow me, as a dog might.

The truth was that we'd finished the Mawa to the last molecule and sopped up all the dregs. For this reason, if I had an errand in walking away, I forgot it.

My feet turned me around, and I stood over Michael once again. 'Very good, sir.

What's happening?'

'You're drunk.'

'Let's talk a little bit about betrayal.'

'You're an expert.'

'There's betrayal, and there's betrayal.'

'So far I can't argue with you.'

'I need your help.'

'Go away.'

'Gladly.'

I repeated the same business — I had no control over my words or my deeds. The spirits possessed me. Down the hill became up the hill, and I'm back at him.

'Before I go, I just want to say goodbye to the biggest idiot I've ever known.'

'Goodbye then. You won't get far.'

'I'm resigned to that. Let the Yanks play with me awhile. I'm headed for prison.'

'What do they care about you, really?'

'Do you think you're the only idiot with criminal secrets and idiotic criminal scenarios, who does idiotic things?'

'You're raving. If I had some rope, I'd tie you.'

'I'm going to the bottom of the hill and start waiting for these missionaries. They've got a car.'

'Excellent. Maybe you'll pass out, and they'll run you over.'

The spirits carried me down the hill once

more. Demons. Vandals. Fiends. This time a sense of calm overcame me, a desperate counterfeit sobriety in which I realized I'd better talk clearly and persuasively to this stupid asshole.

Michael was actually on his feet when I returned.

'Hey. Where are you going?'

'Don't follow me.'

'I forgot what I wanted to say before. It's just this: there's some business in Freetown I need to conclude in something of a hurry.'

'In a hurry? Where do you think you are?'

'I've negotiated the sale of some material,' I said, 'and the handoff's in Freetown with no fallback, and I'm afraid the deadline has gotten very tight. Thursday afternoon.'

'What's got you so mad for it? Is there money in this?'

'Until the window closes. Can we get to Freetown?'

'There are UN flights out of Bunia.'

'How can we get on a flight?'

'Money and luck.'

'I think we'd better try. Otherwise I'm in a lot of trouble. Yesterday a fellow promised me hell.'

'The promise was true.'

'He meant I couldn't last on the run, I'll end up turning myself in, and you're right

about that much — the promise is true. What else can I do but give myself up? Help me.'

'Not now. Go sleep it off.'

'Goddamn it! You said you had a plan. Oh, well. I'd be a liar if I said I ever actually believed you — I'd be a liar.'

'That's exactly what you are. A liar.'

'Wait. I'm sorry. Wait.'

'I said don't follow me.'

I called him a cowardly little wog, and a black-ass nigger.

'Shall I knock you down?'

'I'll get up, you nigger. I'll get up, and I'll keep coming.'

'You're trying to hurt me. And that hurts me.'

And me. He was, after all, the only man in whose embrace I'd spent the night, more than once, on the cold desert ground outside Jalalabad one November, and in the strength of his arms I grew warm, I rested, I slept . . . I said, 'Goddamn you for a fucking coon.'

'Fine. Go ahead. That's fine.'

'I know every word for you. My mother's people live in Georgia. They still fly the rebel flag over there.'

'Fine, fine. You forget I spent time in North Carolina.'

'Fort Bragg, that's right. Fort Carson. Every American fort there ever was.'

'I've seen those Confederate flags.'

In the orange moonlight he looked down at his feet, really examined them, lifting one and then the other, and it occurred to me I could get in a couple of good blows while he let this pointless business distract him, I could pretty well box his ears. I must have tried it, because I found myself with the breath knocked out of me and white streaks rocketing around the corners of my head. Sucking at a vacuum, it felt like.

'Aren't you going to get up? I heard you say you'd keep coming.'

My mouth and nose were in the mud. The demons made no reply.

He knelt beside me and stuck his blade in the ground one millimeter from my ear. I thought he might finish me off quietly with a chokehold.

'This is why you never got promoted beyond your captain rank. Your childish temper.'

[OCT 30 NOON]

Davidia, and Tina —

If this communication has come to you raw, before I've had a chance to transcribe these notes properly — or blend them with

my someday semi-honest account — then you see the ink. No more pencils. You see my hand is sturdy. You're looking at a fresh page.

You guess my fortunes have turned. In which direction, I'll tell you in a minute. This much for now: I've had a meal or two, and a wash at a sink, and I'm wearing new clothes. Let me finish the story.

After the fight with Michael, I slept facedown on the ground.

In the morning, Michael woke me gently. He said, 'How was the night?'

He seemed very different. He had a liter of delicious bottled water for me to drink. As soon as its mouth touched mine, I drained it away.

The sky was gray through and through. The air seemed soft. Nothing stirred. I wondered if the clan had all died in the night, all of them at once.

When I was able to stand, Michael led me to a part of the creek where I could bathe in it up to my chest with my clothes on, African style. It looked like a genuine creek — a rapids and small falls — a place where folks might come to cool off and to draw good water; but the water was bad, and nobody came.

The clouds blew off and the morning sky turned blue. I came back to life and noticed

some gaunt cows and even a couple of young goats pushing their noses around on the earth nearby. I lay out on a warm flat rock in the sunshine. Michael sat beside me, smoking — how, I'd like to know, does he produce cigarettes out of thin air?

At this point I noticed that my head ached and that I felt, all around, unhappy. Here's a confession: I'd puked while unconscious, and I'd lain all night facedown in my own sick. If I'd passed out while lying on my back I'd have drowned in it, and my labors would be done, but no such luck. Meanwhile Michael was saying:

'Life is short. But the time is long. I look back, I see so much, my childhood . . . '

While I lay in a woozy stew of crapulence — that is an actual word — Michael told me what he'd been doing since his escape from the Congolese Army: traveling without money, stumbling by the roadside, crawling through the fields like the Frankenstein beast. He spent two days camped near the US garrison, but couldn't form a plan. I couldn't help you, Michael said, I couldn't help Davidia, I couldn't help myself. There was nothing I could do. So I just came here — where again, there's nothing I can do. My people are sick, insane, they're burning their own huts, they don't have any food. Not one

of them can remember me. They know the names of my mother and father, my mother's brother, my father's two cousins who owned a business selling cloth and rope — but they don't remember the children, not me, or my brother who died, or my two sisters who also died in the disturbances back then, when I left the clan. And poof, our existence is erased. And this woman, La Dolce. I'd like to kill her . . .

Michael went on to say:

'I believe I was nine years old the first time I killed someone. I'm not sure how old I was — I don't know how old I am now, really.'

'Tell me it was a woman, or a child.'

'What's the point of saying that?'

'I don't know. I think you're trying to be poignant, and I'm trying to undercut you.'

'There were two of them, and I don't know who they were. It was during the reprisals. Our clan did nicely, you know, during the time of Idi Amin Dada, because he was Kakwa too. But when he ran away, the machetes came out against the Kakwa, and this creek ran with our blood. I returned here after the village was taken over . . . This is where it happened. I heard two people talking in a hut, only their voices, not the words, not even the kind of voice — man or woman or

child — and I threw in a stick of dynamite. The hut was right over there. You walked through my first murders with your feet ... Now I return once again, and everything is dead. Have I brought down a curse on my own clan? What have I done? Have I done something?'

I'd never known Michael to be afraid, not really. Certainly not terrified like this.

I lay there on my back, hanging on to my mind, or the equilibrium, let's say, of my essence — then no longer hanging on, realizing there's no point.

Michael said:

'And I was never with Tina. Even if I was with her before you came along, I would have told you.'

'I believe you. I was crazy. And there's something I want to say as well. Are you listening?'

'I hear you.'

I sat up and looked straight at him and tried hard to make him believe this — because it's true — 'I'd never grass a friend. I might try and steal his girl and leave him to drown in shit while — well, while running off with his girl. But I'm not a snitch. Never.'

Michael tossed his machete into the pool and it sank.

'Holy shit, man. We might need that.'

'As God is my witness, and as long as I live, I shall never take another life. I shall never kill even one more person. I will die instead, if I have to.'

He'd stubbed out his cigarette half-smoked and rested it on the rock beside him. Now he straightened it out, took a matchbox from his pants pocket, and spent a couple of minutes lighting it and smoking it down to the filter and looking satisfied with himself. He tossed the butt at the water and stood up, offering me a hand. 'Now it's time to go. Where do we meet the missionaries?'

'At the road down the hill — the east side, where you come in.'

'When do we meet them?'

'I don't even know if they're actually coming. But the lady said sometime today.'

'Let's go and wait for them. We need to get to Bunia.'

'Michael,' I said, 'you can make it here, but I can't. I'm no African. I'm like Davidia that way.'

'So where do you think you're going?'

'I suppose it's prison.'

'Do you think I'd let them put you in prison?'

'Is there any other way?'

'Haven't I told you from the beginning?

There's always a plan for extraction.' He made a sound like a pig at a trough — sucking back tears. His pride in himself, at this moment, had brought on a seizure of sentiment. 'After everything, it's still the two of us.'

★ ★ ★

Davidia: As we walked out of the village, the hippopotamus-woman La Dolce roused her clan and harried them after us partway down the hill. She cried, 'Laugh at them, laugh at them!' and then 'Riez! Riez!'

She said: 'Don't touch them, don't talk to them, do you see the Devil in their eyes? Riez! Riez!'

I didn't think them capable of it, but one or two coughed up shreds of laughter and spit them at us. Soon the whole mob was yammering like dogs. Michael bowed his back. His head hung low. 'Riez! Riez!' Like hens, like terrified geese. I followed behind him as he was driven from his family.

[NOV 16PM]

Dear Tina, Dear Davidia —
Again I'm writing to you by candlelight,

but only because the power's blinked out in our corner of Freetown.

We're staying, now, at the National Pride Suites, which have nothing to be proud of. Out the window, West Africa: a lane like a sewer. Cockeyed shanties. Inexplicable laughter.

Downstairs there's a bar, intermittently air-conditioned, fragrant with liquor and lime and the cologne of prostitutes, but I'm not a patron — I'm on an indefinite drinks moratorium, thanks to a bargain I've made with Michael. And without the drinks, the women seem stripped of their appeal.

In any case, I'm not one hundred percent. Nursing a bit of a belly — that Goddamn Newada creek. Apparently certain microbes thrive on heavy metals.

However, the small percent of me that feels all right feels absolutely wonderful.

I don't need booze, or sex. I've spent the last two hours napping with my head on a sack full of cash. One hundred thousand US dollars. Minus recent expenses. Not a substantial cushion, just one thousand pieces of paper zipped up in a plastic carrier pouch, but oh how comfortable, and how sweet my dreams.

★   ★   ★

Tina, I hope you got out of Amsterdam. Hope you got away. Hope you didn't sit there waiting for the poisonous fallout from my ruin.

Hah. 'Fallout.'

But Tina, I'm serious: someday I'll put it all down in words and send it to you, and I'll enclose this last note on top. I don't know what a thorough confession might do for you, or what it might do to ease this combination of dread and anger working at my insides . . . For whatever it's worth, someday — the story from beginning to end.

And the end will be spectacular: Michael and I riding to Bunia in an Isuzu Trooper all heavenly blue and purified white packed with Seventh-day Adventists, and our intrepid machine rockets us through storms, crashes, earthquakes, I don't know what, really — I slept the entire two hundred kilometers, except for a couple of times when the man on my left, a Congolese youth named Max, woke me to complain I was drooling on his shoulder. The trip ended at the mission's church in Bunia, where those of us with religion went inside, and the two lost souls, Michael and I, stood under the awning of a cycle shop, trying to carve a plan out of the rain.

You have to remember, Tina, that the end

wasn't yet, that all I had was Michael Adriko, meaning all I had was bitterness and doubt — and 68 hours to make the next 4800 kilometers.

Michael said, 'Let's wear collars, you and I.'

'Dog collars? Do I look like a dog?'

'Clerical collars.'

'Do I look like a clerk?'

'I think it would help with questions.'

'It's a lousy cover. Everyone wants to approach you.'

'Who approached those Adventist people? We moved right through the checkpoints.'

'I wouldn't know,' I admitted. 'I was asleep. But are you serious?'

'It's a joke. Come on, smile.'

'I hate it when people tell me to smile. People like that disgust me.'

'Nair, I have a bit of news: tomorrow afternoon we'll board a plane for Accra. We'll land in Kotoka International by next day's dawning.'

'I don't believe you. Is that a surprise?'

'You'll believe me before too much longer. And then when I tell you to smile, you'll smile.'

We passed the night at Le Citizen Hôtel, mostly in the café, where we sent out for fresh clothes, and where Michael got me drunk

enough to promise I'd drink no more if we reached Freetown in time to make my rendezvous — still about sixty hours distant, and still no closer on the map. Therefore, I gave him my promise . . . The room we took came with its own sink. I vomited in it.

The next morning I lay in bed resting, or dying, while Michael went out to trip a lever, or touch a magic eye — in retrospect it looks that simple, the work of a finger — to set going his plan for extraction.

Even now, as I write this, with everything, or a good bit of everything, having turned out all right, I feel irritated with Michael's coy dramatics. I'm forced to give him credit, I admit that gratefully. We've crawled from the wreck, we've walked away, and all of that is Michael's doing. I'd just sort of rather it weren't.

At noon on Oct 29, with 52 hours to go, we hired a car with one of my twenty-dollar bills, and in thirty minutes we reached the checkpoint outside Bunia's airfield.

A guard in khaki peered inside the car, had us step out a minute, waved his wand at us, ignored its squeaks, then prodded aside a couple of goats with his boot and unhooked a rope to let us through.

Three flagpoles, two drooping flags, a red dirt runway. A concrete kiosk. In front of it

some men in uniform loitered, laughing. Nothing else but a sort of restaurant with a wooden porch. I said, 'I don't see any planes.'

'Do you see those Ghanaian uniforms?'

'I see uniforms.'

'Ghanaian. Wait here. But first give me money.'

'How much?'

'Everything. If we want to get out of here, we have to pay.'

He left me in the café. I found nobody inside. There were some tables and a cold-box full of drinks — unplugged — but nothing zestier than Coke. I guzzled a warm one. Michael joined me after ten minutes. He sat down without a drink and said, 'When we get to Accra, I'll leave you at the airport terminal while I get the Ghanaian passports.'

'Wonderful.'

'You want diplomatic, or private?'

'One of each. And while you're about it, get me a medical diploma.'

'I'm glad you don't believe me. It heightens the enjoyment later.'

'Care to reveal how we get there?'

'Where?'

'Accra, Goddamn it.'

'Ghanaian Air Force, flying for the UN.'

'The UN? Their planes are never on time.'

'You're very negative. Here's one hundred

eighty dollars back. The pilots were reasonable in their requirements.'

At Kotoka International in Accra, he handed me a cube of Big G Original Gum in a red wrapper and said, 'Here, keep yourself busy,' and next he went into the city and accomplished the unthinkable — although by then I was allowing myself to think it, because he'd gotten us this far, and because two Ghanaian thugs wearing dark business suits came in a Mercedes to collect him at the terminal.

That's where I sat for the next many hours — fifteen, I believe — until Michael returned around 11 that night.

He found me at the Teatime Kiosk at Kotoka, where I happened to be writing my last communication to you, Davidia, or to you, Tina, or to both of you . . . He laid out on the tabletop four Ghanaian documents, a pair of them for each of us — one a civilian passport, and the other a diplomatic, both stamped with visas for Sierra Leone, Uganda, and Liberia. 'I started to come for you, to get your photo snapped — but there was a fellow there, an English, who looked just like you. A perfect double. He agreed to substitute.'

'This doesn't look at all like me.'

'It looks like you exactly,' Michael insisted.

'Of course it does. To an African.'

284

I can't tell you my name, Tina. But don't ask for Roland Nair.

'I'm born in Kumasi, and you in Accra. Both of us on the same day, because we're brothers.'

'But I didn't give you any money.'

Apparently he'd paid none. 'I told you — I saved the president's life. I've told you many times.'

'I don't remember any such lie. President who? Mahama? Is that his name?'

'No. It was in 2005. President John Kufuor. When we have privacy, I'll open my pants for you.'

'What-what?'

'I took a bullet for him. I'll show you the scar.'

* * *

At six the following morning, October 31st, we boarded a Kenya Airlines flight to Lungi International in Freetown.

The whole trip, from the sorrows of Newada Mountain to the comfort of the National Pride Suites, took 71 hours.

On the plane I said something which, though it came from my own mouth, I could scarcely believe: 'Michael, if we don't crash, I'll make it on time. We'll get to Freetown

285

with five hours to spare.'

It didn't matter that a swarm of unforesee-ables waited ahead, that anything could sink us. To be back in the running felt like triumph.

'How much for your enterprise?'

'What?'

'How much will you profit, Nair, how much money?'

'One hundred K US. That's the price for betraying absolutely everyone.'

'But, Nair — you didn't betray me.'

'Not quite. Not yet.'

'The slate is clean between us.'

'I tried to steal your girl.'

'I take it as a compliment.'

★   ★   ★

When we landed here in Freetown, Michael took a car to the National and I took another, first to the Paradi Restaurant for the briefest and happiest of errands — retrieving a bit of computer equipment — and then to the Bawarchi, where I waited until my friend Hamid arrived with one hundred thousand dollars in a blue plastic pouch with a zipper. I held the money in my lap while he used his own computer to examine the goods, and then we parted ways. No handshake. But if

the chance comes again, I think we'll do business.

Late last night Michael and I met with some men in the bar downstairs and arranged to hire a boat, a big one. Experienced captain, plenty of fuel, and next stop — anywhere. Abidjan, perhaps. Though neither of us has much French.

Meanwhile we'll confine ourselves to this building, because too many people know Michael by sight. We share a suite of two rooms. The air conditioner and TV seldom work — no generator at the National — so it's hot, and it's boring. This afternoon for entertainment I watched Michael cut the stitches in his arm with barber scissors and pull them out with his teeth.

We'll wait till after midnight to break camp.

Maybe Liberia. Much is possible there. We'll claim a patch of jungle and a strip of beach, and I'll start my semi-honest account while Michael maps out a scheme or two for international conquest.

We don't have to put down roots. Maybe we'll keep moving. Michael and I both liked Uganda. Why not? The climate's pleasant.

When I left him two hours ago, Michael was downstairs in the bar, bent over a bulky very out-of-date video game machine, saying

to it, 'Pchew! Pchew! Pchew! In yo face, outa space!'

For him, Davidia, you were simply Fiancée Number Five. But for me. Good Lord. For me.

* * *

Tina, you more than once predicted that the coldness of my heart would someday make you a bitter woman. I think you chose me for exactly that reason. You must have wanted it. If you're bitter, you devised to become that way, and I think you chose me as your instrument. So stop it. Stop going on and on about it in my mind.

* * *

Maybe back to Ghana. Maybe Senegal. There's always Cameroon.

Or we might leave this continent behind us and fly to Kuwait, where Michael counts on a most enthusiastic welcome, having once, he revealed to me this morning, spent several months reorganizing and polishing every aspect of personal security for that country's emir, Sheikh Sabah IV Al-Ahmad Al-Jaber Al-Sabah, 'thus prolonging his joy for many years.'

I'm inclined to believe it.

We do hope that you have enjoyed reading this large print book.

Did you know that all of our titles are available for purchase?

We publish a wide range of high quality large print books including:
Romances, Mysteries, Classics
General Fiction
Non Fiction and Westerns

Special interest titles available in large print are:
The Little Oxford Dictionary
Music Book
Song Book
Hymn Book
Service Book

Also available from us courtesy of Oxford University Press:
Young Readers' Dictionary
(large print edition)
Young Readers' Thesaurus
(large print edition)

For further information or a free brochure, please contact us at:
Ulverscroft Large Print Books Ltd.,
The Green, Bradgate Road, Anstey,
Leicester, LE7 7FU, England.
Tel: (00 44) 0116 236 4325
Fax: (00 44) 0116 234 0205

Other titles published by Ulverscroft:

THINGS WE HAVE IN COMMON

Tasha Kavanagh

The first time I saw you, you were standing at the edge of the playing field. You were looking down at your little brown straggly dog — but then you looked up, your mouth going slack as your eyes clocked her. Alice Taylor. I was no different. I used to catch myself gazing at the back of her head in class, at her silky fair hair swaying beneath her shoulder blades. If you'd glanced just once across the field, you'd have seen me standing in the middle on my own, looking straight at you. But you didn't. You only had eyes for Alice . . .

9 780982 598313

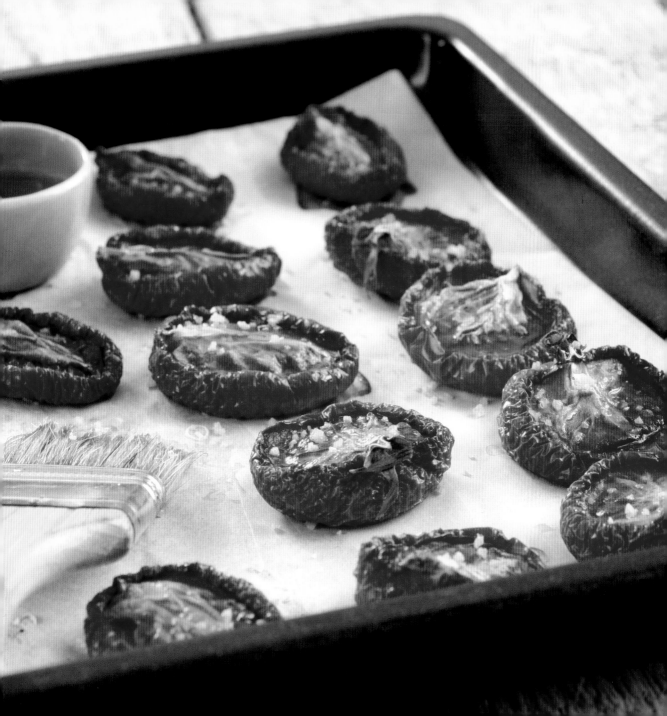

FRESH HERB-TOMATO CONFIT

This recipe, inspired by a French method of preserving food, involves slow-cooking tomatoes with herbs and olive oil.

INGREDIENTS

Makes 3 cups

2 pounds plum tomatoes, peeled, cored, and seeded (page 9)

4 sprigs fresh basil

4 sprigs fresh parsley

2 sprigs fresh thyme

2 cloves garlic

1 teaspoon salt

1 cup extra-virgin olive oil

PREPARATION

1. Preheat oven to 250°F.

2. In a deep baking dish, arrange tomatoes cut-side down and close together. Distribute basil, parsley, thyme, garlic, and salt evenly over top. Pour over oil and cook until tomatoes are wrinkled and deep red, about 2½ to 3 hours.

3. Cool to room temperature, then transfer tomatoes and oil to an airtight container and refrigerate for up to 1 week.

Opposite: Fresh Herb-Tomato Confit

PICKLED GREEN TOMATOES

Use green or partially green tomatoes for this recipe. If possible, use green cherry tomatoes, as they make lovely bite-size pickles!

INGREDIENTS

Makes about 4 pounds

2 quarts cold water

¼ cup coarse salt

1 red chile, cut lengthwise and seeded

2 cloves garlic

½ cup fresh parsley sprigs

4 stalks celery

4 pounds firm green or partially green tomatoes

PREPARATION

1. In a 1-gallon glass jar with a tight-fitting lid, place water, salt, and chile. Shake vigorously.

2. Mix in garlic, parsley, and celery. Add tomatoes, making sure every tomato is completely immersed in liquid.

3. Close jar securely and place on a windowsill, preferably one that gets plenty of direct sunlight. Let sit for 2 days.

4. After 2 days, shake jar gently and return to windowsill. Let sit for another 2 days, then shake jar gently again. Return to windowsill for another 2 days.

5. If windowsill is exposed to plenty of sunlight, the pickles will be ready after 5 or 6 days. If windowsill is shaded, the pickling process may take up to 8 days. Taste pickles to check for readiness. The flavor should be delicately salty and sour. Immersed in brine, pickles may be refrigerated for up to 3 months.

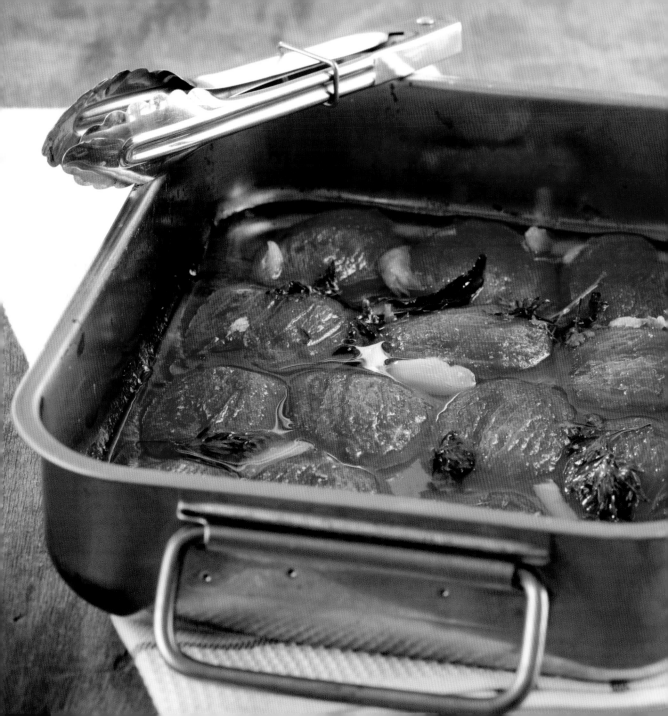

HOT SMOKED CHILE AND TOMATO SPREAD

Spicy and fresh, this spread is a perfect complement to Mexican or Caribbean dishes.

INGREDIENTS

Makes about 5 cups

3 pounds very ripe tomatoes, peeled, cored, and seeded (page 9)

2 tablespoons corn oil

¼ cup finely ground smoked Mexican chile

1 tablespoon salt

1 tablespoon sugar

2 teaspoons garlic powder

PREPARATION

1. Place tomatoes in a food processor and process until smooth.

2. In a large pot over very low heat, heat oil, chile, salt, and sugar. Make sure heat is as low as possible, so the ingredients at the bottom of your pan don't burn.

3. Transfer puréed tomatoes to pot and mix well. Continue heating over low heat, stirring occasionally, so that mixture bubbles gently but does not boil. Cook until thick and smooth, from 2 to 2½ hours, depending upon water content of tomatoes.

4. Cool to room temperature, then transfer to an airtight container. Refrigerate for up to 4 days, or freeze for up to 1 month.

FRESH KETCHUP

Here's a homemade version of the condiment most beloved by children. Prepare for a party when you have burgers and French fries on the menu!

INGREDIENTS

Makes about 3 cups

4 to 6 medium tomatoes, peeled, cored, and seeded (page 9)

½ cup extra-virgin olive oil

1 tablespoon honey

1 small onion, finely chopped

1 clove garlic, minced

1 tablespoon red wine vinegar

2 tablespoons salt

1 tablespoon chili powder or Tabasco sauce (optional)

PREPARATION

1. Place tomatoes, oil, honey, onion, garlic, vinegar, and salt in a blender. Blend until smooth. To make spicy ketchup, mix in chili powder.

2. Transfer to an airtight container and refrigerate for up to 2 days.

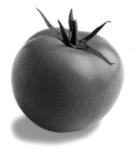

ROASTED GARLIC AND TOMATO SPREAD

I discovered this spread while working in Mediterranean restaurants. Add it to sauces or diverse dishes, or spread it on crisp toast. Replace black pepper with chili powder for a Mexican touch.

INGREDIENTS

Makes about 2 cups

2 heads of garlic, peeled

½ cup extra-virgin olive oil

½ pound plum tomatoes, halved lengthwise

2 teaspoons salt

1 teaspoon freshly ground black pepper or chili powder

PREPARATION

1. Preheat oven to 250°F.

2. In a small baking dish or ovenproof pot, place garlic and oil. Cover with aluminum foil and bake for 1 hour.

3. Heat a heavy skillet over high heat until skillet is very hot. Do not add oil.

4. Working in batches, place tomatoes skin-side down on hot skillet, roasting until black lines appear. Set aside.

5. Remove roasted garlic from oven and cool slightly. Using a slotted spoon, transfer garlic to a food processor. Reserve oil.

6. Add tomatoes, salt, and pepper to garlic, and process until smooth. Slowly pour in reserved oil, and continue processing until mixture is smooth and light.

7. Cool to room temperature, transfer to an airtight container, and refrigerate for up to 3 days.

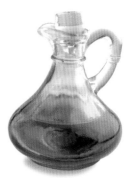

CHERRY TOMATO JAM

This sweet concoction is delicious on creamy vanilla ice cream.

INGREDIENTS

Makes about 3 cups

1½ cups sugar

2 tablespoons water

1 pound cherry tomatoes, sliced

PREPARATION

1. In a medium saucepan, heat sugar and water over low heat until syrupy.

2. Add tomatoes and continue heating until mixture comes to a gentle boil.

3. Mix well and continue to cook over low heat, mixing occasionally, until mixture thickens, about 45 minutes.

4. Remove from heat and cool to room temperature. Transfer to sterilized jars and seal with airtight lids. Refrigerate for up to 1 week.

HOMEMADE TOMATO PASTE

This is the real stuff—thick, creamy, and flavorful.

INGREDIENTS

Makes 7 to 8 cups

6 pounds very ripe tomatoes, peeled, cored, and seeded (page 9)

2 tablespoons extra-virgin olive oil

2 tablespoons salt

3 tablespoons sugar

PREPARATION

1. Place tomatoes in a food processor and process until smooth.

2. In a large pot, heat oil, salt, and sugar over very low heat. Make sure heat is as low as possible, so the ingredients at the bottom of your pot don't burn.

3. Transfer puréed tomatoes to pot and mix well. Continue heating over low heat, stirring occasionally, so that mixture bubbles gently but does not boil. Cook until thick and smooth, from 3 to 5 hours, depending upon water content of tomatoes.

4. Cool to room temperature, then transfer to an airtight container. Refrigerate for up to 4 days, or freeze for up to 1 month.

Opposite: Cherry Tomato Jam

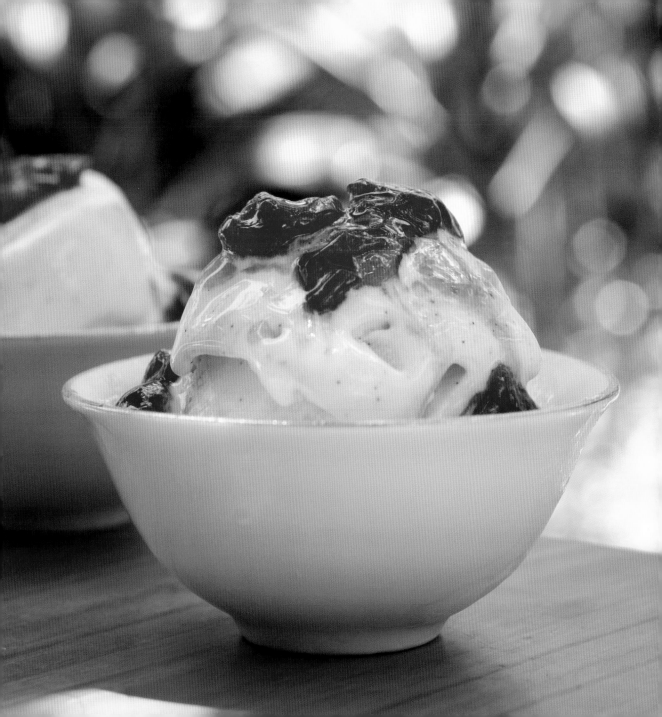

CILANTRO AND TOMATO SALSA

This salsa is excellent with crispy nacho chips. It's best fresh, so prepare just before serving if possible.

INGREDIENTS

Makes about 2 cups

½ pound very ripe tomatoes, roughly chopped

3 cloves garlic, peeled

¼ cup chopped fresh cilantro

1 tablespoon chopped fresh parsley

1 teaspoon red wine vinegar

1 tablespoon extra-virgin olive oil

2 teaspoons salt

1 red chile, seeded and chopped

PREPARATION

1. In a food processor, place tomatoes, garlic, cilantro, parsley, vinegar, oil, salt, and chile, and process until smooth.

2. Serve immediately, or transfer to an airtight container and refrigerate for up to 24 hours.

TOMATO CHUTNEY

This refreshing condiment is perfect for garnishing roasted meats and for spicing up sauces.

INGREDIENTS

Makes about 4 cups

2 tablespoons canola oil

2 medium white onions, finely chopped

3 cloves garlic, minced

2 tablespoons honey

1 teaspoon freshly ground black pepper

1 teaspoon cayenne pepper

1 tablespoon salt

2 teaspoons sweet paprika

2 tablespoons red wine vinegar

2 pounds crushed tomatoes

PREPARATION

1. Heat a deep, heavy skillet over medium heat. Add oil and onions, and cook until onions are translucent, about 5 minutes.

2. Add garlic and cook for another 2 minutes.

3. Mix in honey, black pepper, cayenne pepper, salt, and paprika. Pour in vinegar and cook for another 2 minutes.

4. Mix in tomatoes, reduce heat to low, and simmer until mixture is thick, about 30 to 40 minutes.

5. Cool to room temperature, transfer to an airtight container, and refrigerate for up to 1 week. Best served at room temperature.

Opposite: Cilantro and Tomato Salsa

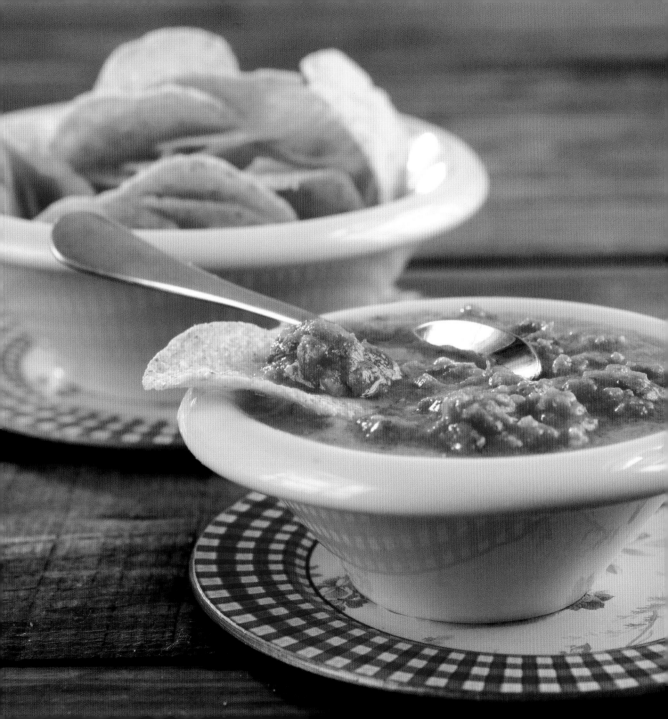

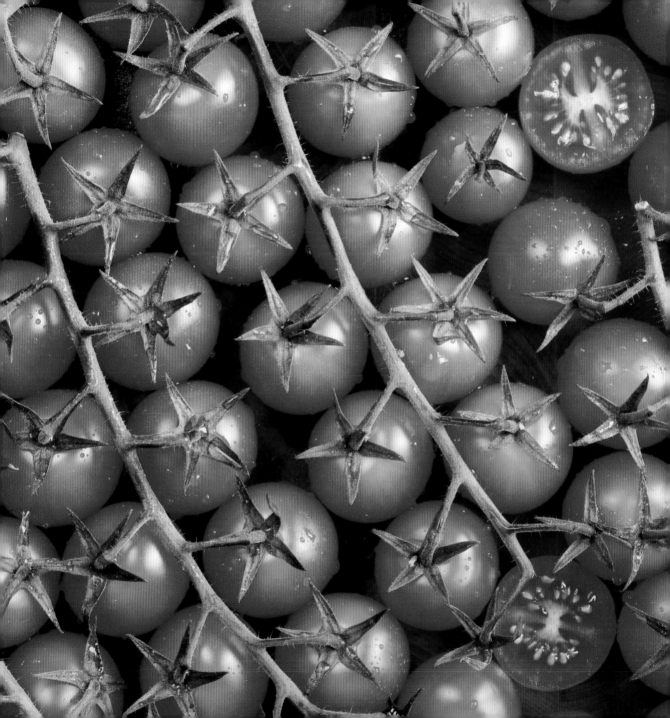

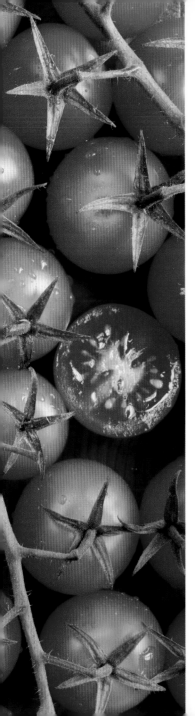

SOUPS

TOMATO AND BREAD SOUP

I first tried this soup on a cold wintry day, while wandering through a colorful market in Florence. A friendly restaurateur was happy to share the recipe with me, and I'm delighted to pass it on to you.

INGREDIENTS

Serves 4

3 tablespoons extra-virgin olive oil

1 medium red onion, finely diced

2 stalks celery, cut into ½-inch dice

2 cloves garlic, minced

2 carrots, cut into ½-inch dice

Two 16-ounce cans diced tomatoes

1 tablespoon salt

1 teaspoon freshly ground black pepper

1 tablespoon chicken soup powder

½ cup white wine

2 cups water

½ pound crusty white bread, ripped into large chunks

2 tablespoons coarsely chopped fresh basil

2 tablespoons grated Parmesan cheese, for garnish

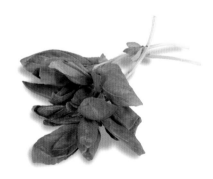

PREPARATION

1. In a large pot over medium heat, cook oil, onion, celery, garlic, and carrots for 3 minutes.

2. Mix in canned tomatoes with their juices, salt, pepper, and soup powder. Increase heat and bring to a boil.

3. Pour in wine and cook for 5 minutes. Add water and return to a boil. Reduce heat, cover, and simmer for 30 minutes. At this stage, soup may be cooled to room temperature, transferred to an airtight container, and refrigerated for up to 2 days. Reheat gently before serving.

4. Just before serving, mix bread and basil into hot soup. Transfer to serving dishes, sprinkle with cheese, and serve immediately.

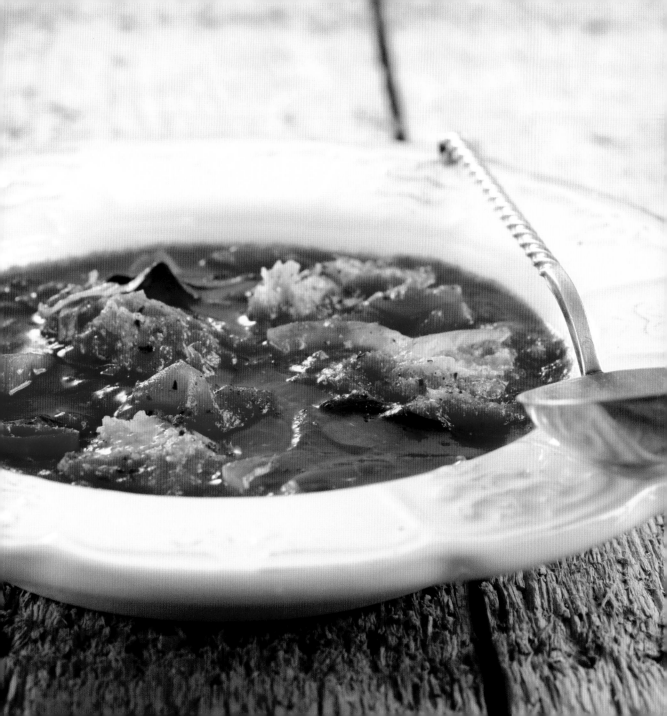

GAZPACHO

Cool and refreshing. This summertime soup originates in the Spanish Mediterranean islands.

INGREDIENTS

Serves 4

4 large tomatoes, quartered

1 red bell pepper, seeded and cut into large chunks

1 small red onion, finely chopped

3 cloves garlic, minced

¼ cup extra-virgin olive oil, plus more for garnish

1 tablespoon tomato paste

1 tablespoon freshly squeezed lemon juice

1 tablespoon red wine vinegar

2 teaspoons salt

1 red chile, seeded and finely diced

1 tablespoon chopped fresh parsley

1 English cucumber, finely chopped

1 small white onion, finely diced, for garnish

½ red chile, seeded and finely diced, for garnish

½ green chile, seeded and finely diced, for garnish

PREPARATION

1. Place tomatoes, red pepper, red onion, garlic, oil, tomato paste, lemon juice, vinegar, salt, chile, and parsley in a blender and blend until smooth.

2. Refrigerate for at least 30 minutes, to chill and allow flavors to blend. At this stage, soup may be stored in an airtight container in the refrigerator for up to 24 hours.

3. To serve, transfer chilled soup to bowls, add cucumber, and drizzle with a little olive oil. Serve with white onion, red chile, and green chile for garnish.

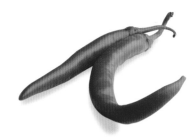

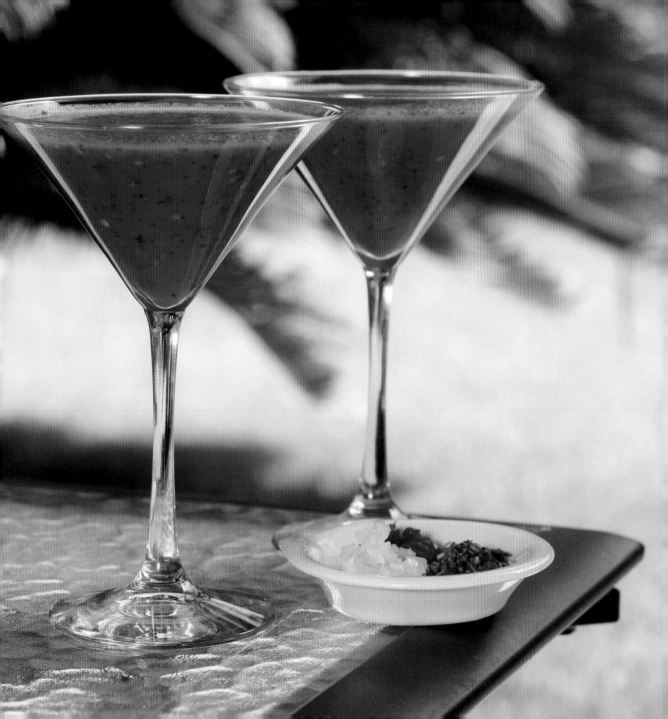

FRESH HERB AND TOMATO SOUP

This soup makes a lovely light meal, any time of day, any season.

INGREDIENTS

Serves 4

2 tablespoons extra-virgin olive oil

1 medium white onion, finely diced

3 cloves garlic, minced

1 tablespoon finely chopped oil-packed sun-dried tomatoes

½ pound cherry tomatoes, finely chopped

One 16-ounce can diced tomatoes

3 cups water

1 tablespoon chicken soup powder

1 tablespoon chopped fresh thyme

1 tablespoon chopped fresh oregano

1 tablespoon salt

2 teaspoons white pepper

2 tablespoons chopped fresh parsley, for garnish

1 tablespoon chopped fresh basil, for garnish

PREPARATION

1. In a large pot over medium heat, cook oil, onion, garlic, and sun-dried tomatoes for 3 minutes.

2. Mix in cherry tomatoes and cook for 5 minutes, stirring occasionally.

3. Mix in canned tomatoes with their juices, increase heat, and bring to a boil.

4. Add water and return to a boil. Add soup powder, thyme, oregano, salt, and pepper. Reduce heat, cover, and simmer for 30 minutes. At this stage, soup may be cooled to room temperature, transferred to an airtight container, and refrigerated for up to 2 days. Reheat gently before serving.

5. To serve, transfer to serving dishes and garnish with parsley and basil.

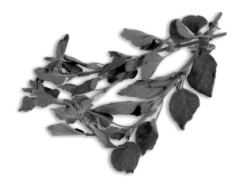

28

TOMATO SOUP WITH BEEF AND MARROW

I first tried this hearty soup on a wintry day in Paris. Years later, the scent of it cooking in my own kitchen always reminds me of that first taste.

INGREDIENTS

Serves 4

2 tablespoons extra-virgin olive oil

1 medium red onion, finely diced

1 stalk celery, cut into ½-inch dice

3 cloves garlic, minced

2 carrots, cut into ½-inch dice

One 16-ounce can whole tomatoes, coarsely chopped

1 tablespoon tomato paste

½ tablespoon chopped fresh rosemary

1 tablespoon salt

2 teaspoons freshly ground black pepper

2 tablespoons chicken soup powder

1 cup red wine

3 cups water

Four 3-inch beef marrow bones, split lengthwise

½ pound beef tenderloin, cut into ¼-inch strips

PREPARATION

1. In a large pot over medium heat, cook oil, onion, celery, garlic, and carrots for 3 minutes.

2. Mix in canned tomatoes and their juices, tomato paste, rosemary, salt, pepper, and soup powder. Increase heat and bring to a boil.

3. Pour in wine and cook for 5 minutes. Add water, bones, and beef, and return to a boil. Reduce heat, cover, and simmer for 1½ hours.

4. Serve immediately or cool to room temperature, transfer to an airtight container, and refrigerate for up to 3 days. Reheat gently before serving.

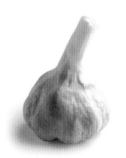

TUSCANY BEAN AND TOMATO SOUP

This Italian soup is warm, filling, and satisfying.

INGREDIENTS

Serves 4

1 cup white beans, soaked overnight in 1½ quarts water

2 tablespoons extra-virgin olive oil

1 medium red onion, finely diced

3 cloves garlic, minced

2 carrots, cut into ½-inch dice

½ pound beef tenderloin, cut into ½-inch cubes

1 tablespoon chopped fresh thyme

1 tablespoon salt

1 teaspoon freshly ground black pepper

2 tablespoons chicken soup powder

Two 16-ounce cans diced tomatoes

1 cup red wine

1 quart water

PREPARATION

1. Rinse and drain beans. Set aside.

2. In a large pot over medium heat, cook oil, onion, garlic, and carrots for 3 minutes.

3. Mix in beef, thyme, salt, pepper, and soup powder, and cook while stirring for 3 minutes, until beef browns.

4. Mix in canned tomatoes and their juices and cook for 5 minutes, stirring occasionally. Add wine and drained beans, and cook for 5 minutes.

5. Add water and bring to a boil. Reduce heat, cover, and simmer for 1½ to 2 hours, until beans are soft.

6. Serve immediately or cool to room temperature, transfer to an airtight container, and refrigerate for up to 3 days. Reheat gently before serving.

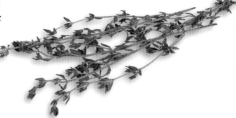

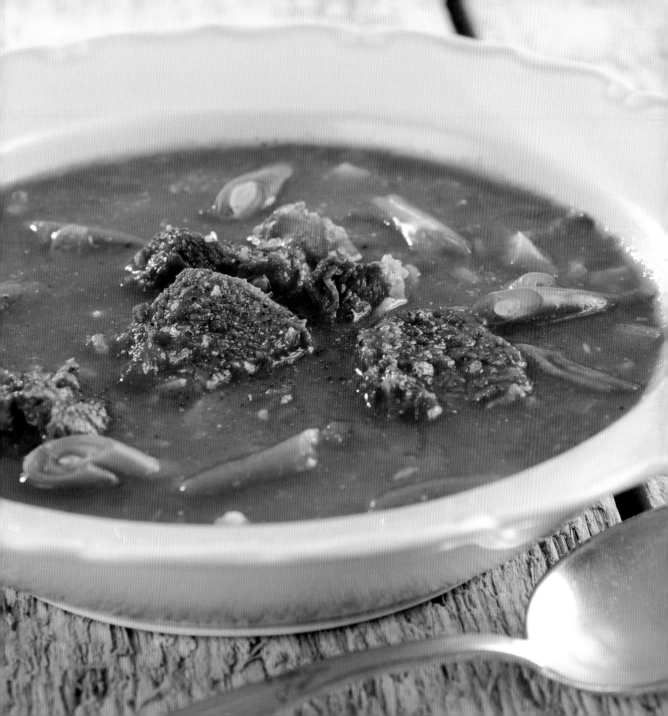

TOMATO AND SEAFOOD SOUP

The French may be famous for their fish soup, but this Italian version is no less delicious.

INGREDIENTS

Serves 4

¼ cup extra-virgin olive oil

1 small red onion, finely diced

3 cloves garlic, minced

½ pound fresh mussels, scrubbed well

½ pound clams, scrubbed well

2 cups white wine

Two 16-ounce cans diced tomatoes

2 tablespoons chopped fresh basil

1 tablespoon salt

2 teaspoons white pepper

3 cups water

½ pound small calamari, cleaned and cut into strips

½ pound fresh crabmeat (or frozen and thawed at room temperature)

½ pound shrimp, cleaned and peeled

PREPARATION

1. In a large pot over medium heat, cook oil, onion, garlic, mussels, and clams for 3 minutes.

2. Pour in wine, cover, and cook for 15 minutes.

3. Add canned tomatoes and their juices, basil, salt, and pepper, and cook for 10 minutes. Add water and bring to a boil.

4. Add calamari and crabmeat, reduce heat, cover, and simmer for 15 minutes. At this stage, soup may be cooled to room temperature, transferred to an airtight container, and refrigerated for up to 2 days. Reheat to boiling before serving.

5. Just before serving, add shrimp to hot soup and cook on low heat for 3 minutes. Transfer to serving dishes and serve immediately.

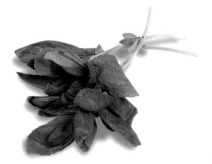

SPANISH TOMATO AND BEEF SOUP

I first tasted this soup while traveling near Madrid. It is colorful, distinct, and flavorful—much like the city itself.

INGREDIENTS

Serves 4

2 tablespoons extra-virgin olive oil

2 medium white onions, finely diced

3 cloves garlic, minced

1 red bell pepper, seeded and finely diced

½ pound beef tenderloin, cut into ½-inch cubes

1 tablespoon salt

1 tablespoon Spanish paprika

2 tablespoons chicken soup powder

2 tablespoons tomato paste

1 teaspoon white pepper

1 cup white wine

1 pound tomatoes, finely diced

2 cups water

1 tablespoon red wine vinegar

PREPARATION

1. In a large pot over medium heat, cook oil, onions, garlic, and bell pepper for 5 minutes.

2. Mix in beef, ½ tablespoon salt, and paprika, and cook for 10 minutes, stirring occasionally.

3. Add soup powder, tomato paste, remaining ½ tablespoon salt, pepper, and wine, and bring to a boil.

4. Add tomatoes, water, and vinegar, and return to a boil. Reduce heat, cover, and simmer for 1½ hours.

5. Serve immediately or cool to room temperature, transfer to an airtight container, and refrigerate for up to 2 days. Reheat gently before serving.

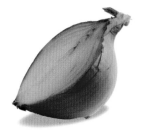

SHRIMP CREOLE SOUP

Whenever I find myself longing for the smells, tastes, and colors of New Orleans,
I prepare a batch of this soup.

INGREDIENTS

Serves 4

1 pound beefsteak tomatoes, peeled, cored, and seeded (page 9)

½ cup butter

2 medium white onions, finely diced

3 cloves garlic, minced

1 tablespoon Old Bay Seasoning

1 tablespoon salt

1 tablespoon chicken soup powder

½ cup heavy cream

1 cup water

½ pound shrimp, cleaned and peeled

PREPARATION

1. Place tomatoes in a food processor and process until smooth.

2. Heat a large pot over medium heat. Add butter, onions, and garlic, and cook for 3 minutes. Add Old Bay Seasoning, salt, soup powder, and cream, and heat until boiling.

3. Mix in puréed tomatoes and bring to a boil. Pour in water, reduce heat to low, cover, and simmer for 1 hour. At this stage, soup may be cooled to room temperature, transferred to an airtight container, and refrigerated for up to 2 days. Reheat to boiling before serving.

4. Just before serving, add shrimp to hot soup and cook over low heat for 3 minutes. Transfer to serving dishes and serve immediately.

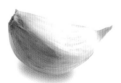

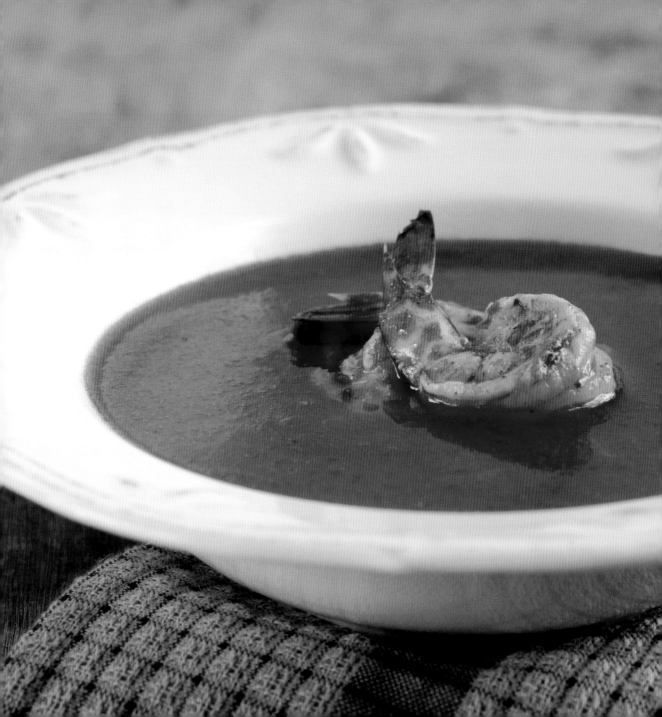

PASTA SOUP

My wife and I discovered this dish while traveling in Greece and it quickly worked its way into our kitchen.

INGREDIENTS

Serves 4

2 tablespoons extra-virgin olive oil

2 medium red onions, finely diced

1 stalk celery, finely diced

3 cloves garlic, minced

1 tablespoon chopped fresh oregano

1 tablespoon salt

1 teaspoon freshly ground black pepper

2 tablespoons chicken soup powder

Two 16-ounce cans diced tomatoes

1 cup red wine

2 tablespoons tomato paste

1 quart water

1 cup shell pasta

PREPARATION

1. In a large pot over medium heat, cook oil, onions, celery, and garlic for 3 minutes.

2. Add oregano, salt, pepper, and soup powder, and cook while stirring for 3 minutes.

3. Mix in canned tomatoes with their juices and cook, stirring occasionally, for 5 minutes.

4. Add wine and tomato paste and cook for 5 minutes. Add water and bring to a boil. Reduce heat, cover, and simmer for 40 minutes. At this stage, soup may be cooled to room temperature, transferred to an airtight container, and refrigerated for up to 2 days. Reheat to boiling before serving.

5. Just before serving, add pasta to boiling soup and continue to boil for 10 minutes. Transfer to serving dishes and serve immediately.

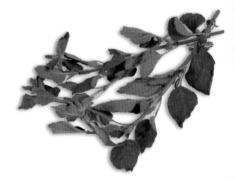

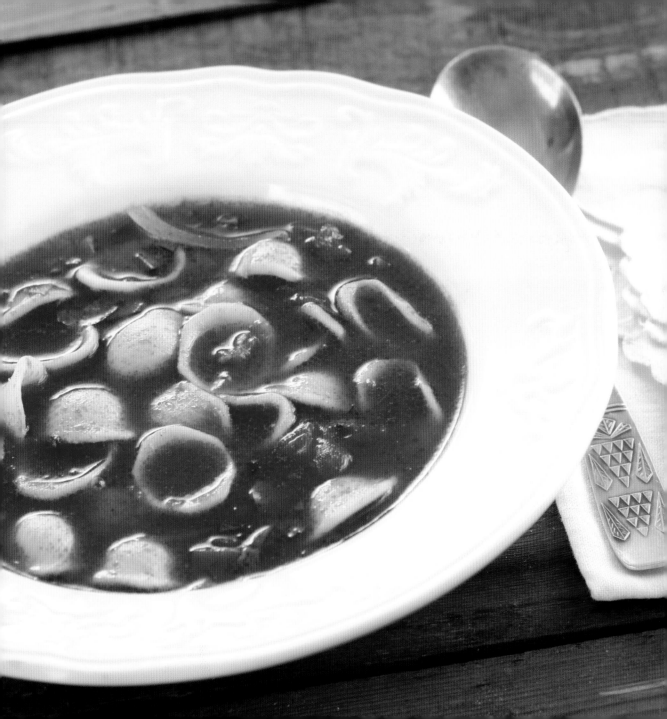

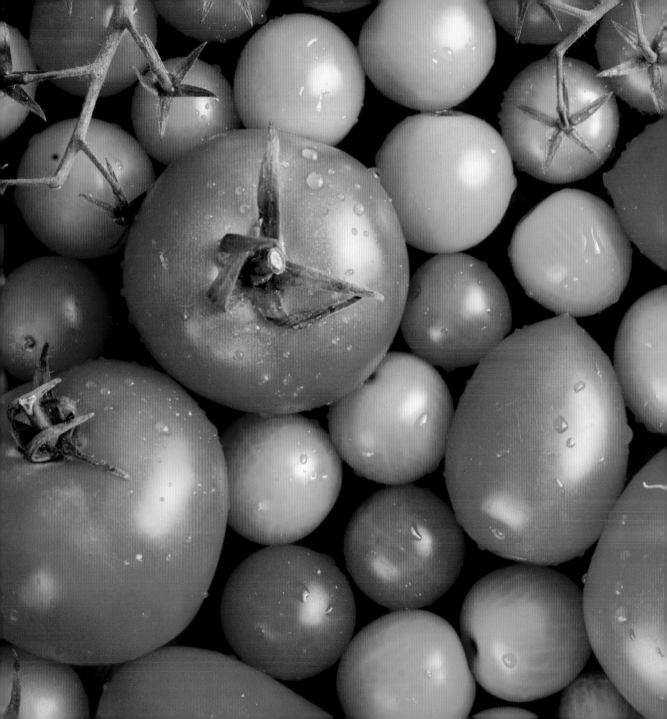

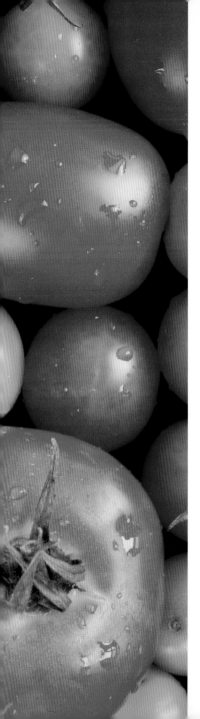

STARTERS,
SALADS,
AND
LIGHT
MEALS

CATALONIAN CROSTINI

In this delicious appetizer, the flavor of the garlic and tomato are rubbed into the grilled bread. The process is simple but flavorful.

INGREDIENTS

Serves 4

8 slices crusty white bread (preferably San Francisco sourdough)

4 cloves garlic, peeled and halved

4 large tomatoes, halved

1 tablespoon extra-virgin olive oil

2 teaspoons salt

PREPARATION

1. Heat a grill pan over high heat until very hot. Grill bread slices on both sides until dark lines are visible.

2. Immediately after grilling, rub each slice with ½ garlic clove, and discard garlic. Do this while bread is still hot to ensure that the flavor of the garlic is absorbed.

3. Immediately after rubbing with garlic, rub each slice with a tomato half. Discard tomato.

4. Arrange bread on a serving platter and drizzle with oil. Sprinkle with salt and serve immediately.

TOMATO AND FETA SALAD

No meal in Greece is complete without this signature salad.

INGREDIENTS

Serves 4

4 medium tomatoes, quartered

1 green bell pepper, seeded and cut into ½-inch dice

1 English cucumber, cut into ½-inch dice

1 medium red onion, cut into ⅛-inch slices

2 tablespoons extra-virgin olive oil

1 tablespoon red wine vinegar

2 teaspoons salt

1 teaspoon freshly ground black pepper

½ pound feta cheese, cut into ½-inch cubes

1 tablespoon coarsely chopped fresh oregano

PREPARATION

1. In a large bowl, mix together tomatoes, bell pepper, cucumber, onion, 1 tablespoon oil, vinegar, salt, and black pepper. Cover with plastic wrap and refrigerate for at least 15 minutes.

2. Immediately before serving, transfer salad to serving dishes, distribute cheese over top, sprinkle with oregano, and drizzle with remaining tablespoon oil.

Opposite: Catalonian Crostini

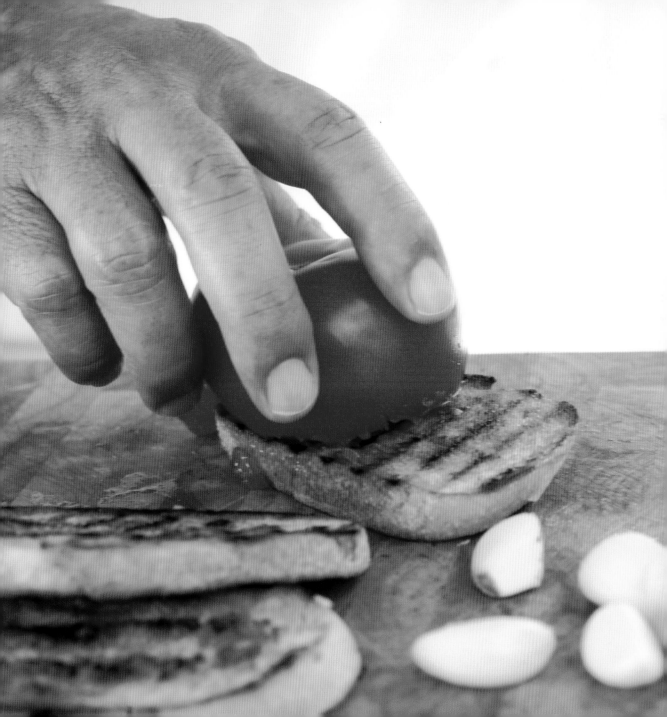

LEBANESE TABBOULEH

When I studied baking in Paris, I often traded freshly baked pastries with a Lebanese friend who made a delicious tabbouleh salad. The secret to her recipe: drain the bulgur thoroughly and use only fresh ingredients.

INGREDIENTS

Serves 4

½ pound bulgur

1 quart water

2 medium tomatoes, finely diced

1 cup finely chopped fresh parsley

3 tablespoons extra-virgin olive oil

2 tablespoons freshly squeezed lemon juice

2 teaspoons salt

1 teaspoon white pepper

PREPARATION

1. Place bulgur and water in a medium bowl and set aside for at least 2 hours. When bulgur is soft (test by pressing between your fingers), transfer to a fine sieve to drain. Be sure to drain as thoroughly as possible.

2. In a separate bowl, mix together tomatoes, parsley, oil, lemon juice, salt, and pepper.

3. Add drained bulgur to tomato mixture and mix until well combined.

4. Cover, transfer to refrigerator, and chill for at least 1 hour to allow flavors to blend, or for up to 24 hours.

5. Remove from refrigerator at least 30 minutes before serving to allow to come to room temperature.

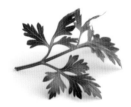

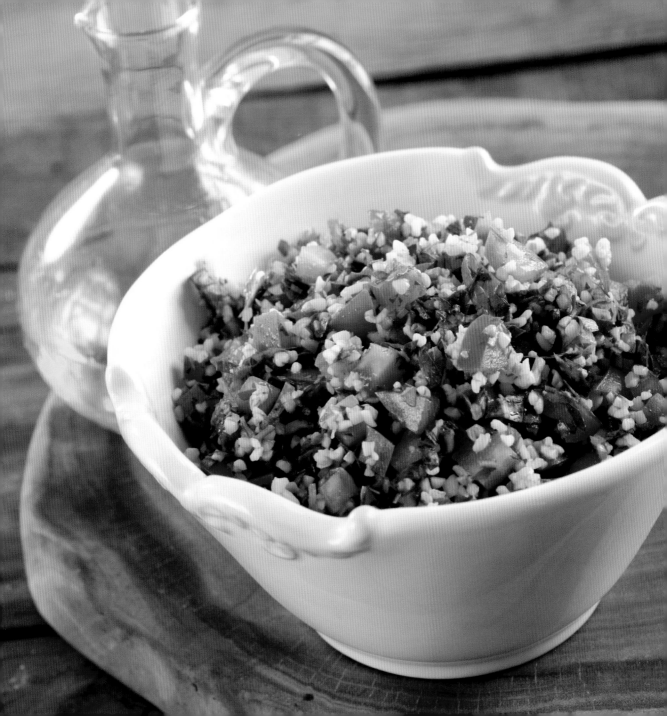

MOZZARELLA AND TOMATO SALAD

This simple salad is known as insalata caprese *in its native Italy, but it is simply delicious by any name!*

INGREDIENTS

Serves 4

3 large very ripe tomatoes, sliced into ¼-inch rounds

2 mozzarella balls, sliced into ¼-inch rounds

1 teaspoon salt

1 teaspoon freshly ground black pepper

2 tablespoons extra-virgin olive oil

½ tablespoon red wine vinegar

1 tablespoon fresh basil leaves

PREPARATION

1. Arrange tomato slices in an overlapping ring on a large serving platter.

2. Tuck a slice of mozzarella between each tomato slice, ensuring that some of the tomato is visible behind each slice of mozzarella.

3. Sprinkle salt and pepper over top, drizzle with oil and vinegar, sprinkle with basil, and serve immediately.

TOMATOES IN PARSLEY AND GARLIC SAUCE

This salad has a distinct Mediterranean flavor. Use the freshest ingredients possible for best flavor.

INGREDIENTS

Serves 4

4 large tomatoes, cut into ½-inch slices

¼ cup extra-virgin olive oil, plus more for garnish

½ cup chopped fresh parsley

2 tablespoons red wine vinegar

2 teaspoons salt

1 teaspoon freshly ground black pepper

3 cloves garlic, minced

1 teaspoon freshly squeezed lemon juice

PREPARATION

1. Arrange tomato slices on a large serving platter and set aside.

2. Mix together oil, parsley, vinegar, salt, pepper, garlic, and lemon juice in a small bowl.

3. Pour mixture evenly over tomato slices, making sure every slice is covered. Cover with plastic wrap and refrigerate for 30 minutes.

4. Garnish with a little olive oil just before serving.

Opposite: Mozzarella and Tomato Salad

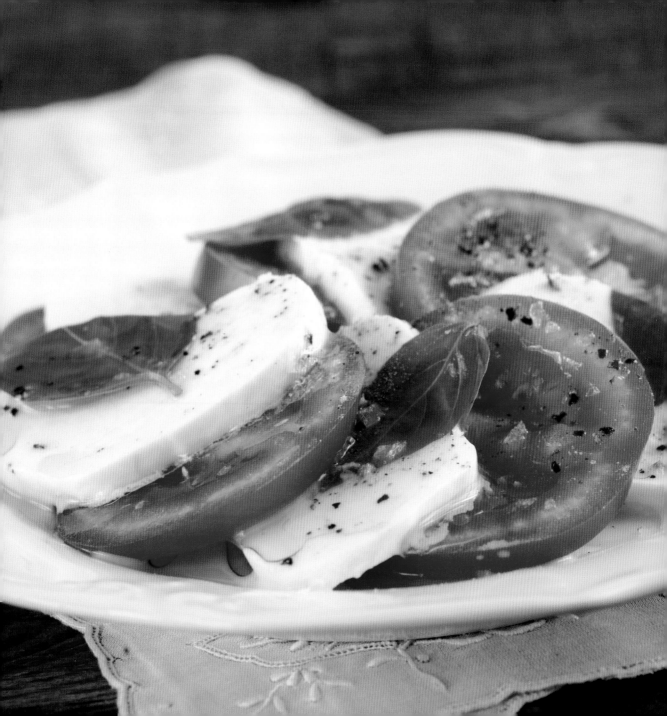

BRUSCHETTA WITH GOAT CHEESE

Conjure up the atmosphere of a holiday in Italy with the goat cheese, fresh tomatoes, and olive oil in this dish.

INGREDIENTS

Serves 4

½ pound cherry tomatoes, quartered

2 cloves garlic, minced

2 tablespoons extra-virgin olive oil

1 tablespoon red wine vinegar

2 teaspoons salt

1 teaspoon freshly ground black pepper

1 tablespoon coarsely chopped fresh basil

8 slices crusty white bread (preferably San Francisco sourdough)

¼ cup crumbled goat cheese

PREPARATION

1. In a medium bowl, mix together tomatoes, garlic, oil, vinegar, salt, pepper, and basil. Set aside.

2. Heat a grill pan over high heat until very hot. Grill bread slices on both sides until dark lines are visible, then arrange on a serving dish.

3. Place a generous tablespoon of tomato mixture on each bread slice, sprinkle cheese over top, and serve immediately.

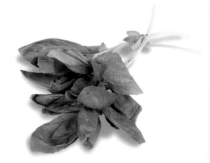

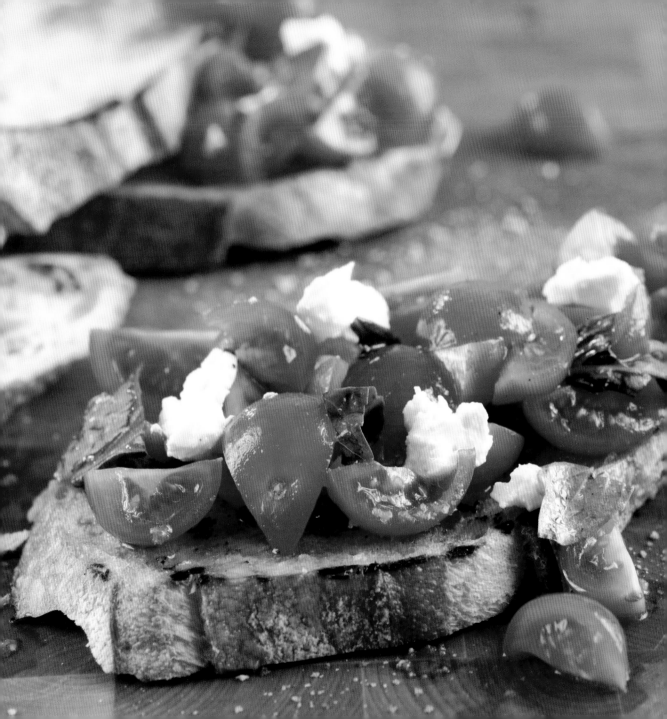

ROASTED CHERRY TOMATOES WITH QUINOA

Quinoa is a nutritious, high-protein grain that is a lovely complement for diverse ingredients. Use white, brown, or black quinoa in this dish.

INGREDIENTS

Serves 4

½ pound quinoa

1½ quarts water

1 tablespoon plus 3 teaspoons salt

¾ pound cherry tomatoes, halved

4 tablespoons extra-virgin olive oil

2 teaspoons white pepper

1 tablespoon chopped fresh thyme

2 tablespoons red wine vinegar

PREPARATION

1. Preheat oven to 450°F.

2. In a large pot over medium heat, bring quinoa, water, and 1 tablespoon salt to a boil.

3. Reduce heat to low and cook for 15 minutes, until quinoa softens. Transfer cooked quinoa to a fine sieve to drain. Be sure to drain as thoroughly as possible.

4. Arrange tomatoes on a baking sheet. Drizzle with 2 tablespoons oil, sprinkle 1 teaspoon salt over top, and roast for 10 minutes. Remove from oven and transfer to a large bowl.

5. Transfer drained quinoa to bowl with tomatoes. Add remaining 2 tablespoons oil, 2 teaspoons salt, pepper, thyme, and vinegar. Mix well.

6. Let cool to room temperature and serve immediately, or transfer to an airtight container and refrigerate for up to 2 days. Remove from refrigerator at least 30 minutes before serving to allow to come to room temperature.

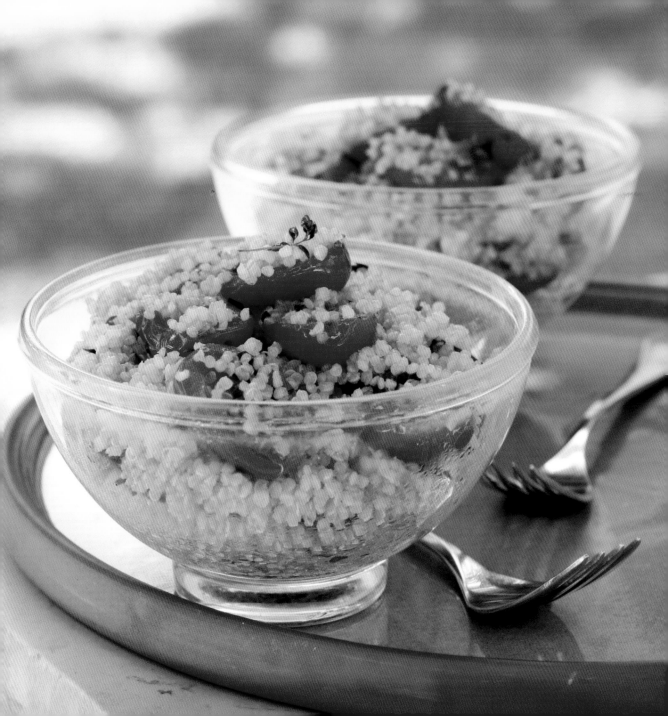

TOMATO AND FRESH GOAT CHEESE TART

These attractive tarts are perfect for serving at Sunday brunch. Fresh, flavorful, and sure to impress.

INGREDIENTS

Serves 6

All-purpose flour, for dusting

1 pound frozen puff pastry, thawed

¾ pound fresh goat cheese, cut into ¼-inch slices

1½ cups Fresh Herb-Tomato Confit (page 14)

1 teaspoon coarse salt

2 tablespoons extra-virgin olive oil

PREPARATION

1. Preheat oven to 425°F.

2. On a lightly floured surface, roll out pastry to ⅛ inch thick and cut out a 12 × 16-inch rectangle. Transfer to a baking sheet and bake for 10 minutes.

3. Place a second baking sheet directly on top of pastry and bake for 15 minutes, or until pastry is brown and very flaky. (The weight of the second baking sheet will flatten the pastry as it bakes.) Transfer pastry to a wire rack to cool for 20 minutes.

4. Cut cooled pastry into twelve 4-inch squares. Place a square on a serving dish and arrange 4 cheese slices on top. Spread tomato confit on cheese, then lay a square of pastry on top. Arrange 4 more cheese slices, and spread another layer of confit. Repeat to assemble 5 more tarts.

5. Sprinkle coarse salt over each tart, drizzle with a little oil, and serve immediately.

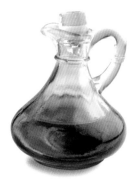

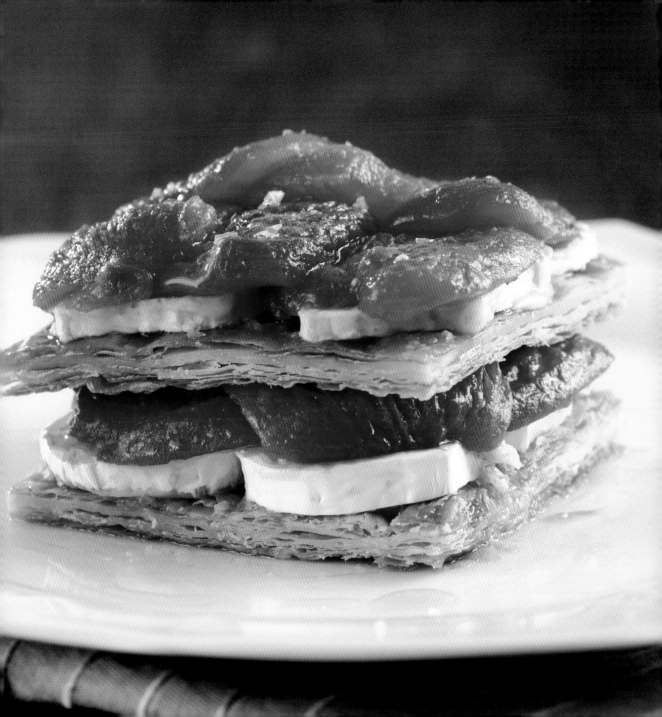

PANZANELLA SALAD

The first time I tried this salad was at a market in Florence, and every time I have it, I am transported back. The key to its success is using the freshest vegetables available.

INGREDIENTS

Serves 4

½ pound day-old white bread (preferably San Francisco sourdough), ripped into large chunks

6 medium ripe tomatoes, quartered

2 medium red onions, cut into ⅛-inch slices

2 tablespoons extra-virgin olive oil

1 tablespoon freshly squeezed lemon juice

2 teaspoons salt

1 teaspoon white pepper

2 tablespoons coarsely chopped fresh parsley

PREPARATION

1. Preheat oven to 450°F.

2. Arrange bread chunks on a large baking sheet and bake until toasted.

3. In a large bowl, mix together tomatoes, onions, oil, lemon juice, salt, and pepper. Cover with plastic wrap and refrigerate for at least 10 minutes.

4. Immediately before serving, mix in toasted bread chunks and parsley.

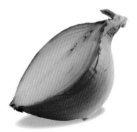

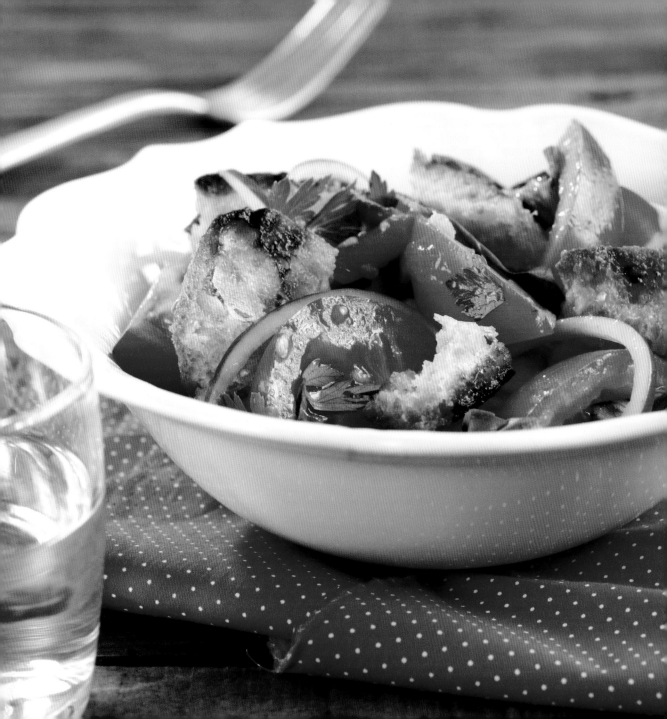

ARUGULA AND TOMATO SALAD

This lovely salad is a regular lunchtime feature in my home kitchen.

INGREDIENTS

Serves 4

4 medium tomatoes, quartered

1 cup cherry tomatoes, halved

2 tablespoons extra-virgin olive oil

1 tablespoon red wine vinegar

2 teaspoons salt

1 teaspoon freshly ground black pepper

½ pound fresh arugula

½ pound mixed baby greens

PREPARATION

1. In a medium bowl, mix together tomatoes, cherry tomatoes, oil, vinegar, salt, and pepper. Cover with plastic wrap and refrigerate for at least 10 minutes.

2. Immediately before serving, mix in arugula and baby greens.

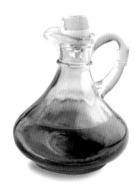

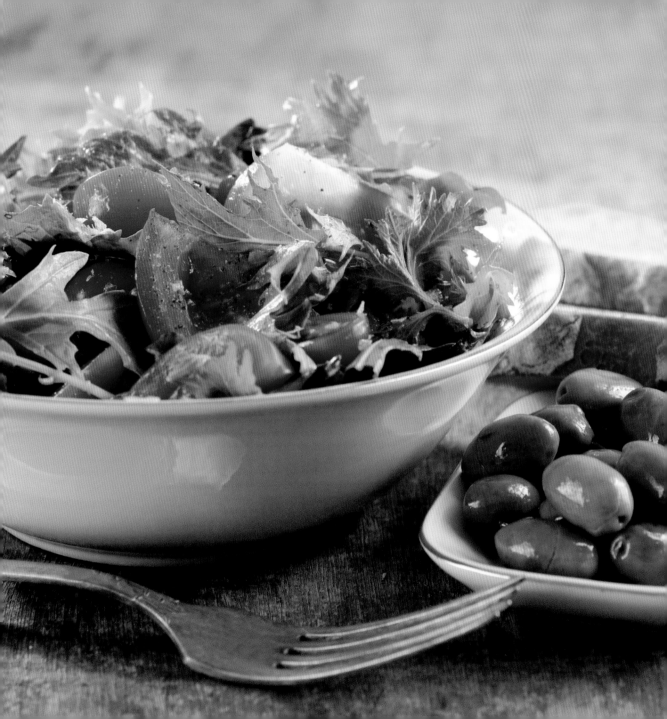

FENNEL, TOMATO, AND RED ONION SALAD

The flavors in this dish are subtle. Even people who generally shy away from fennel will enjoy this salad.

INGREDIENTS

Serves 4

4 medium tomatoes, quartered

2 medium fennel bulbs, thinly sliced lengthwise

1 medium red onion, thinly sliced lengthwise

2 tablespoons coarsely chopped parsley

2 tablespoons extra-virgin olive oil

1 tablespoon balsamic vinegar

1 tablespoon freshly squeezed lemon juice

2 teaspoons salt

1 teaspoon white pepper

PREPARATION

1. In a large bowl, mix together tomatoes, fennel, onion, parsley, oil, vinegar, lemon juice, salt, and pepper.

2. Cover with plastic wrap and refrigerate for at least 15 minutes. Serve directly from refrigerator.

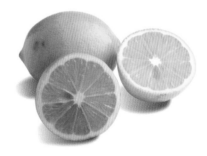

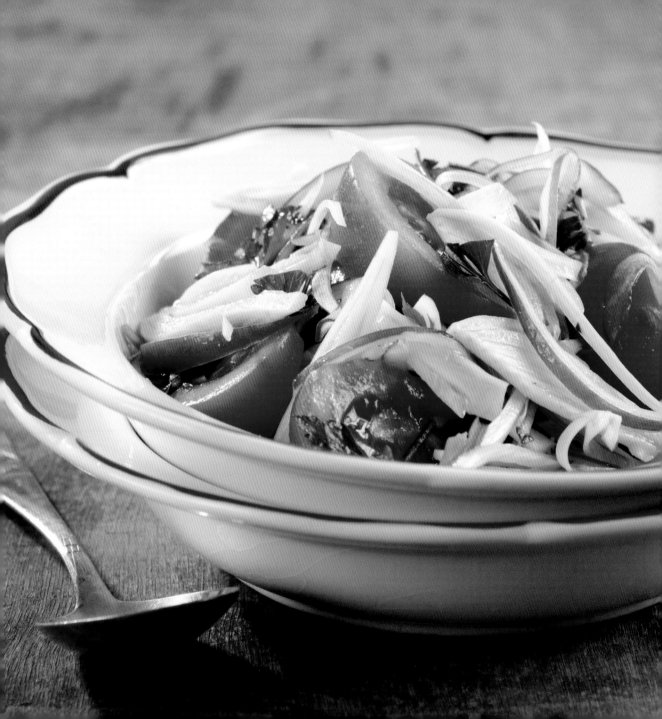

STUFFED TOMATOES

*The inspiration for this dish came during the photo shoot for this recipe book.
Since then, it has become a favorite in our kitchen.*

INGREDIENTS

Serves 6

¾ pound fresh saltwater
whitefish fillet (such as sea
bass, halibut, or snapper),
finely diced

3 tablespoons extra-virgin
olive oil

2 tablespoons freshly squeezed
lemon juice

1 tablespoon finely chopped
fresh cilantro

1 tablespoon finely chopped
fresh chives

2 tablespoons salt

1 teaspoon white pepper

1 teaspoon Tabasco sauce

6 large plum tomatoes

PREPARATION

1. In a medium bowl, place fish,
oil, lemon juice, cilantro, chives,
salt, pepper, and Tabasco sauce,
and mix until well combined.
Cover with plastic wrap and
refrigerate for 15 minutes.

2. In the meantime, cut tomatoes
in half lengthwise. Remove seeds
with a teaspoon, leaving a thick,
even shell.

3. Carefully fill each tomato
half with chilled fish mixture.
Arrange on a platter and
serve immediately.

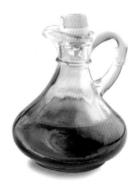

58

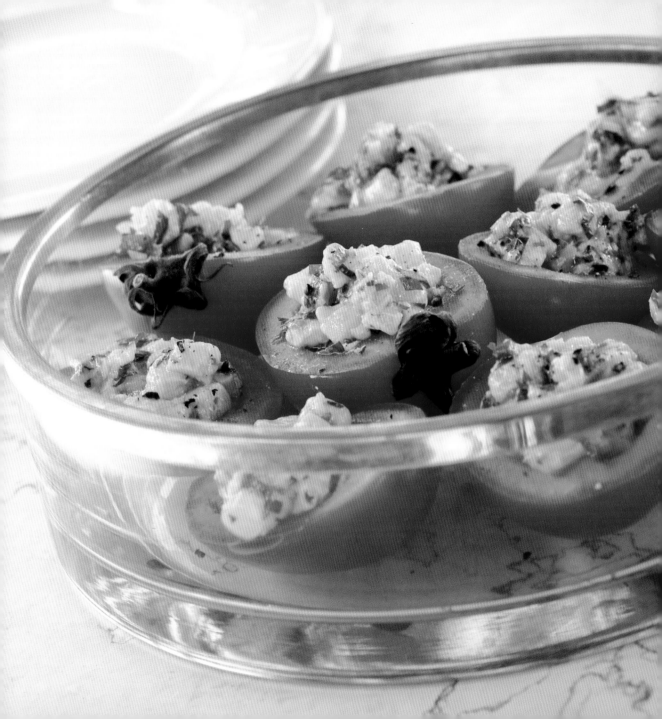

TORTILLA TOMATO AND CHICKEN WRAP

This dish is easy to prepare and fun to eat.

INGREDIENTS

Serves 2

1 tablespoon extra-virgin olive oil

2 cloves garlic, minced

1 red chile, seeded and finely diced

½ pound cherry tomatoes, halved

1 teaspoon salt

1 teaspoon Spanish paprika

½ pound fresh chicken breast, cut into ½-inch strips

2 large tortillas

¼ cup coarsely chopped fresh cilantro

PREPARATION

1. Heat a large skillet over medium heat. Add oil, garlic, and chile, and cook for 3 minutes, stirring occasionally.

2. Add tomatoes, salt, and paprika, and cook for 5 minutes, stirring occasionally.

3. Add chicken strips and cook for 6 minutes, stirring occasionally.

4. At the same time, heat a large cast-iron skillet over high heat until very hot. Toast one tortilla at a time until golden brown, about 3 or 4 minutes for each side.

5. To serve, place chicken mixture in a strip along the middle of each tortilla. Sprinkle with cilantro, roll up tortilla, and serve immediately.

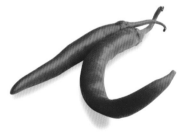

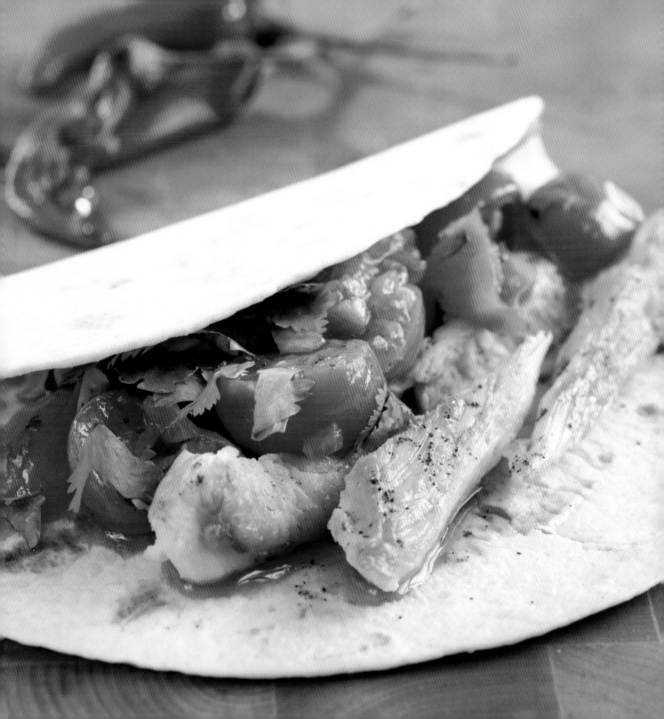

CHERRY TOMATO TART

This impressive starter dresses up any affair. It may take a little effort to prepare, but it's worth it.

INGREDIENTS

Serves 6

1 pound cherry tomatoes, with stems

¼ cup extra-virgin olive oil

1 teaspoon coarse salt

1 teaspoon freshly ground black pepper

All-purpose flour, for dusting

1 pound frozen puff pastry, thawed

1 large egg, beaten

½ pound salted ricotta cheese

PREPARATION

1. Preheat oven to 425°F.

2. Place cherry tomatoes in a deep baking sheet. Add oil, salt, and pepper, and bake for 10 minutes. Set aside.

3. Line a baking sheet with parchment paper. On a lightly floured surface, roll out half of the pastry into an 8 x 12-inch rectangle and cut into six 4-inch squares. Arrange squares on baking sheet.

4. Roll and cut remaining pastry in the same way. From the middle of each of these squares, cut out a smaller, 3-inch square, leaving a 1-inch pastry frame.

5. Brush pastry squares on baking sheet with half the beaten egg. Lay a pastry frame on top of each square and brush with remaining beaten egg. Bake for 15 to 20 minutes, until pastry is high, flaky, and golden brown.

6. Transfer baked pastry squares to a wire rack and cool for 10 minutes. Use a sharp knife to cut along the inside edge of the frame, making a space for the filling.

7. Arrange several baked cherry tomatoes inside each square, crumble cheese over top, drizzle with juice from baked tomatoes, and serve immediately.

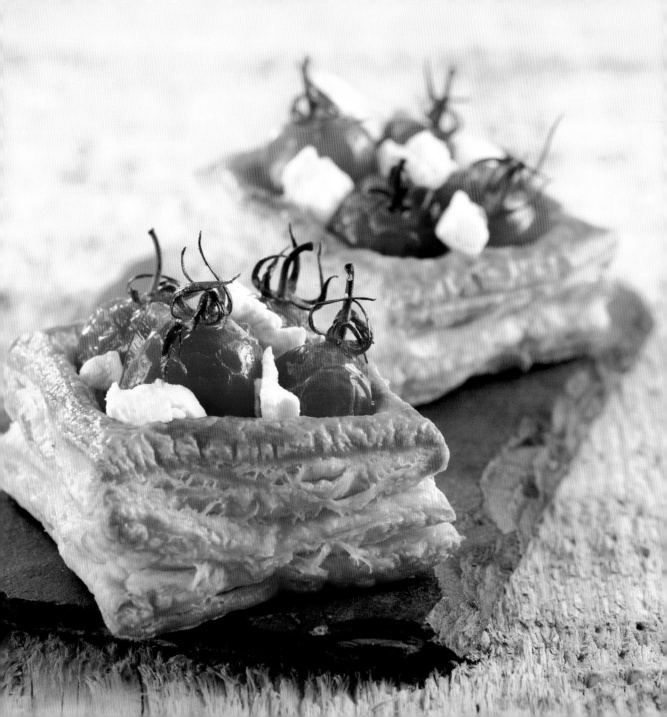

BEEF AND TOMATO SANDWICH

This dish makes a hearty, filling lunch when you don't have too much time for preparation.

INGREDIENTS

Serves 2

3 large tomatoes, cut into ⅓-inch slices

2 tablespoons extra-virgin olive oil

1 teaspoon salt

1 teaspoon freshly ground black pepper

¾ pound beef sirloin, very thinly sliced

2 fresh ciabatta

1 handful mixed salad greens

PREPARATION

1. Heat a cast-iron skillet over high heat until skillet is very hot. Roast tomato slices for 2 minutes on each side, then transfer to a large bowl. Add oil, salt, and pepper, and mix well.

2. Clean skillet and return to heat, once again heating until very hot. Add beef slices and roast for 3 minutes on each side.

3. To serve, cut ciabatta in half widthwise and layer one half with beef slices, tomato slices, and salad greens. Pour over sauce from tomatoes and close sandwich. Serve immediately.

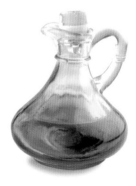

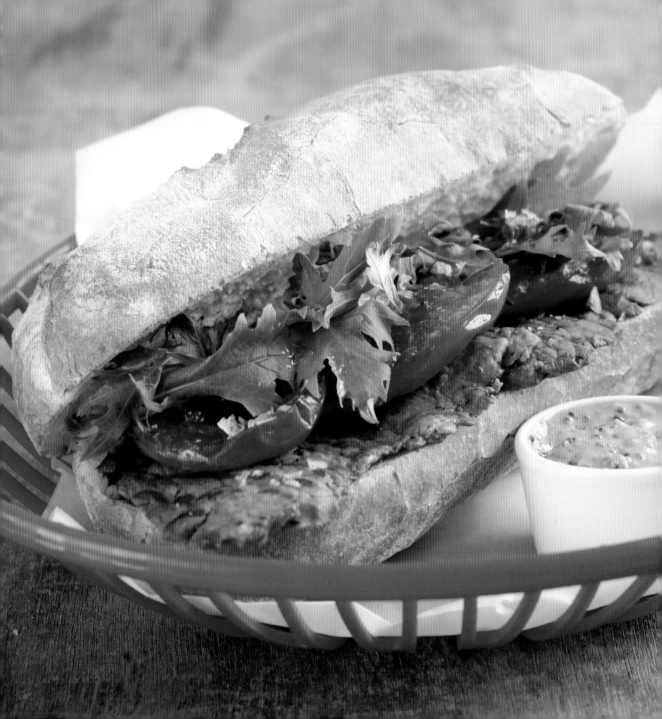

TOMATO BREAD

Use this bread for sandwiches, or serve with creamy butter alongside salads, cheeses, and meats. Day-old bread is ideal for making bruschetta or pizza wheels.

INGREDIENTS

Serves 6

½ cup cold water

2 tablespoons extra-virgin olive oil

1 teaspoon dry yeast

½ cup crushed tomatoes, canned or fresh

3 cups bread flour, plus more for dusting

¼ cup coarsely chopped fresh basil

2 teaspoons salt

PREPARATION

1. In the bowl of an electric mixer fitted with the dough hook, place water, oil, yeast, crushed tomatoes, flour, and basil. Mix on low speed for 3 minutes.

2. Continue mixing, add salt, and increase speed to medium. Mix for another 8 minutes. Dough will be a light red color, with specks of green from the basil.

3. Remove dough from bowl and shape into a ball. Dust mixing bowl lightly with flour, then return dough, cover with a kitchen towel, and let rise in a warm place for 1 hour, or until doubled in size.

4. Line a baking sheet with parchment paper. Turn out dough onto a lightly floured surface and roll into a 12-inch cylinder with tapered ends. Transfer to baking sheet and let rise in a warm place for 1 hour, or until doubled in size.

5. Preheat oven to 450°F. Make sure that oven is thoroughly and evenly heated before baking. Bake bread for 10 minutes at 450°F, then reduce heat to 400°F and bake for another 30 minutes. Bread is ready when a tap on the bottom sounds clear and hollow.

6. Transfer to a wire rack and cool completely before slicing. Store in a breadbox for up to 2 days.

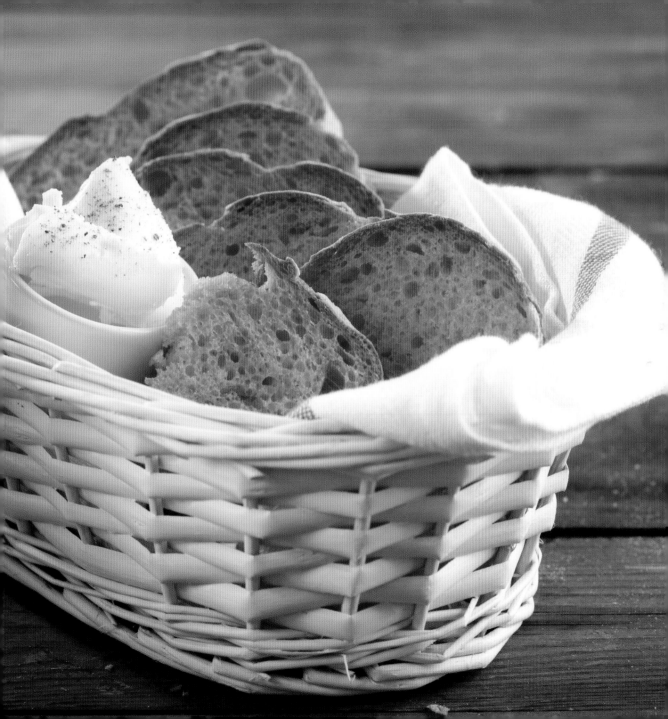

POLENTA WITH TOMATO SAUCE

Polenta, a staple in Italy and many other parts of Europe, is filling and warm. The exact cooking time varies according to its texture, so keep an eye on the polenta as it cooks.

INGREDIENTS

Serves 6

3 tablespoons extra-virgin olive oil

3 cloves garlic, minced

One 16-ounce can diced tomatoes

½ cup red wine

1 teaspoon white pepper

1 tablespoon plus 2 teaspoons salt

4 cups water

1 cup coarse Italian polenta

¼ cup butter

¼ cup grated Parmesan cheese, plus more for topping

PREPARATION

1. Heat a deep, heavy skillet over medium heat. Add oil and garlic and cook, stirring occasionally, for 3 minutes.

2. Increase heat and add canned tomatoes and their juices. Cook, stirring occasionally, for 5 minutes.

3. Add wine, pepper, and 2 teaspoons salt. Cook, stirring occasionally, for 3 minutes. Remove from heat, cover, and set aside until ready to serve.

4. In a medium pot over medium heat, bring 2 cups water to a boil and add remaining tablespoon salt and polenta. Cook, stirring constantly, until mixture thickens, about 10 to 15 minutes.

5. In the meantime, bring the remaining 2 cups water to a boil in a separate, small pot. Add 1 cup boiling water to the thickened polenta and continue to cook, stirring constantly, until thickened again.

6. Reduce heat and add remaining cup boiling water. Cook, stirring constantly, until thickened, then remove from heat. Mix in butter and cheese.

7. To serve, spoon polenta onto serving dishes and flatten into a mound with the back of a spoon. Top with a generous spoonful of tomato sauce and extra cheese.

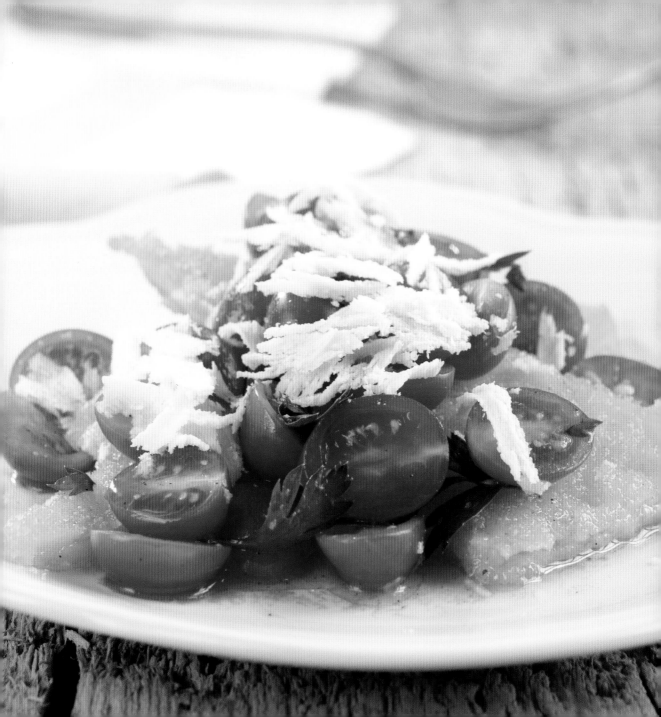

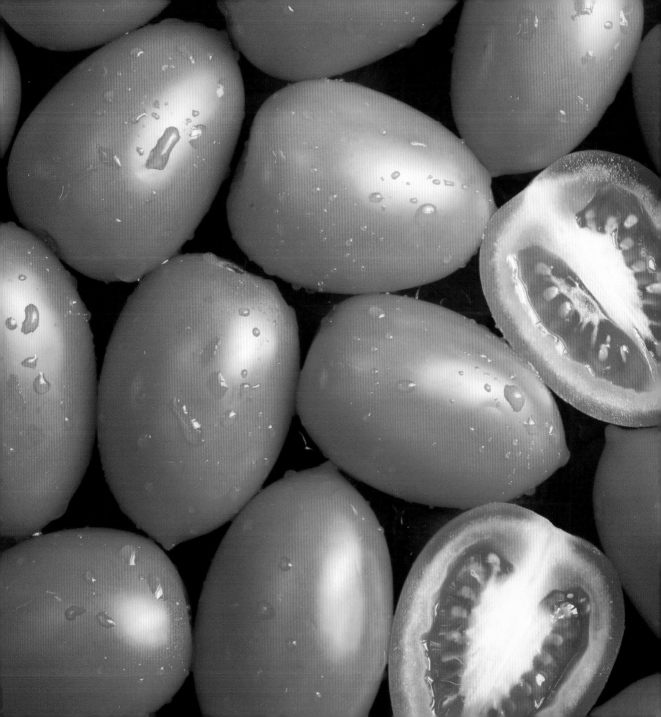

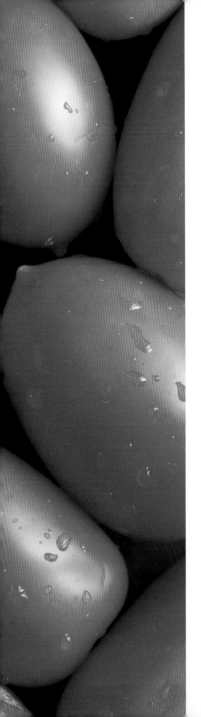

FISH AND SEAFOOD

MOROCCAN FISH AND TOMATO BAKE

This traditional Moroccan dish has a rich, spicy flavor. Serve with steamed couscous and plenty of crusty bread for soaking up the sauce.

INGREDIENTS

Serves 4

¼ cup extra-virgin olive oil

2 cloves garlic, minced

1 tablespoon Spanish paprika

2 tablespoons tomato paste

One 16-ounce can crushed tomatoes

1 red chile, seeded and finely diced

1 lemon, cut into ¼-inch slices

1 teaspoon ground cumin

2 teaspoons salt

4 tomatoes, cut into ½-inch dice

2 pounds whitefish fillets

1 tablespoon chopped fresh cilantro

1 tablespoon chopped fresh parsley

PREPARATION

1. In a wide saucepan with a lid, cook oil, garlic, and paprika over medium heat while stirring for 3 minutes.

2. Reduce heat and mix in tomato paste, canned tomatoes, chile, lemon slices, cumin, and salt. Simmer over low heat for 20 minutes.

3. Mix in diced tomatoes. Arrange fish fillets on top, cover, and cook over low heat for 30 minutes.

4. Remove pan from heat. Sprinkle cilantro and parsley over fish, cover, and let sit for 10 minutes.

5. Serve immediately or cool to room temperature, transfer to an airtight container, and refrigerate for up to 2 days. Reheat gently before serving.

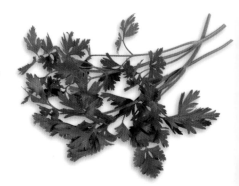

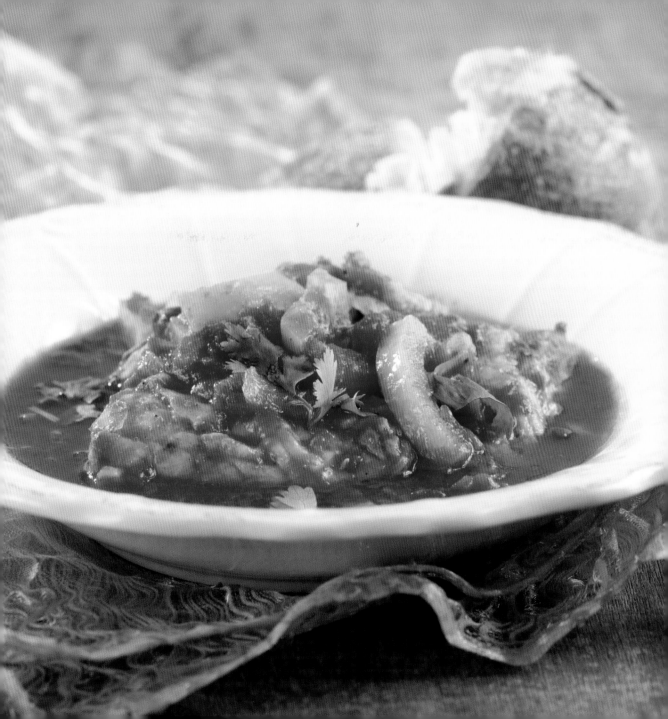

MULLET IN TOMATO SAUCE

For me, this dish conjures the sounds, smells, and memories of summer evenings in Greece, sitting with friends in a local tavern.

INGREDIENTS

Serves 4

2 tablespoons extra-virgin olive oil

1 small white onion, finely diced

2 teaspoons salt

3 cloves garlic, thinly sliced

One 16-ounce can diced tomatoes

1 teaspoon Spanish paprika

1 teaspoon freshly ground black pepper

12 fresh whole mullets, cleaned

PREPARATION

1. Preheat oven to 425°F.

2. In a medium ovenproof saucepan over medium heat, cook oil, onion, and 1 teaspoon salt until onion is translucent, about 5 minutes.

3. Mix in garlic, canned tomatoes and their juices, paprika, pepper, and remaining teaspoon salt, and bring to a boil.

4. Reduce heat and simmer for 15 minutes.

5. Arrange fish on top of sauce, transfer pan to oven, and bake for 6 minutes. Gently turn over fish and bake for another 10 minutes. The fish is ready when it flakes easily with a fork.

6. To serve, arrange fish on a serving dish and top generously with sauce.

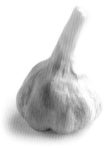

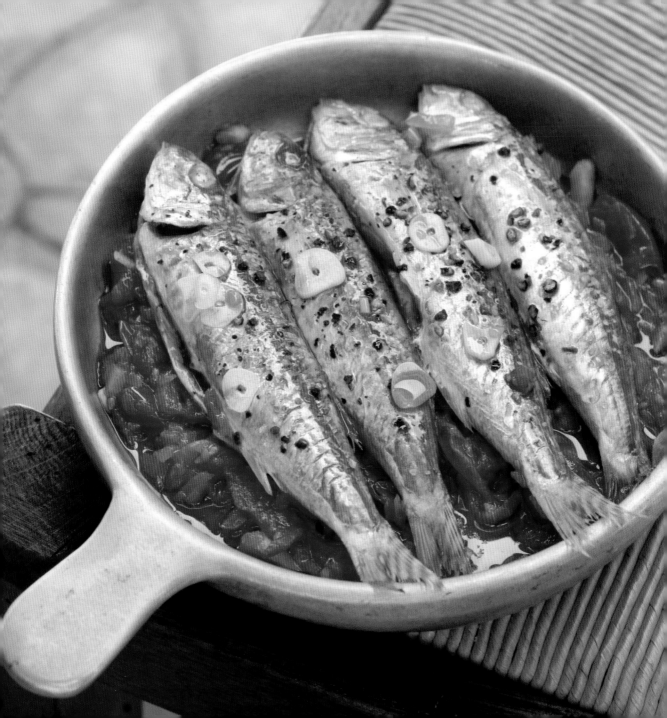

WHITEFISH CARPACCIO WITH TOMATO MARINADE

For all carpaccio dishes, make sure the fish is very thinly sliced. I recommend asking your fishmonger to slice it for you. The sauce in this recipe has a rich, interesting flavor.

INGREDIENTS

Serves 4

¾ pound fresh whitefish fillet, skinless and very thinly sliced

¼ cup finely chopped oil-packed sun-dried tomatoes

1 cup finely diced cherry tomatoes

1 tablespoon aged balsamic vinegar

2 teaspoons extra-virgin olive oil

1 tablespoon freshly squeezed lemon juice

2 teaspoons salt

1 teaspoon white pepper

½ teaspoon Tabasco sauce

1 tablespoon chopped fresh chives, for garnish

PREPARATION

1. In a large bowl, place fish slices, sun-dried tomatoes, cherry tomatoes, vinegar, oil, lemon juice, salt, pepper, and Tabasco sauce. Carefully mix with a large spoon, taking care not to rip fish slices. Cover with plastic wrap and refrigerate for 30 minutes.

2. Arrange fish slices in a single layer on a large serving dish. Slices should be close together, but not overlapping.

3. Pour sauce from bowl over top and sprinkle with chives. Serve immediately.

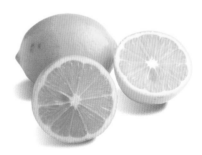

SHRIMP IN SUN-DRIED TOMATO BUTTER

Elegant yet easy to prepare. Serve this dish as a light summer supper with a bottle of chilled white wine.

INGREDIENTS

Serves 4

¼ cup oil-packed sun-dried tomatoes

1 tablespoon extra-virgin olive oil

2 cloves garlic, minced

2 tablespoons white wine

⅓ cup butter

2 teaspoons salt

1 teaspoon freshly ground black pepper

1 teaspoon freshly squeezed lemon juice

2 pounds large shrimp, cleaned and peeled

PREPARATION

1. Place sun-dried tomatoes and their oil in a blender and blend until smooth.

2. Heat a large skillet over medium heat. Add oil, garlic, and puréed sun-dried tomatoes, and cook for 4 minutes. Pour in wine and cook for another 4 minutes.

3. Add butter and continue to cook while stirring. When butter is melted, add salt, pepper, lemon juice, and shrimp.

4. Cook while stirring for about 4 minutes, until shrimp turn pink and shrink a little. Serve immediately.

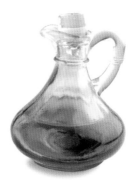

GROUPER CARPACCIO WITH TOMATO VINAIGRETTE

For all carpaccio dishes, make sure the fish is very thinly sliced. I recommend asking your fishmonger to slice it for you. The dressing in this dish is quite delicate, really bringing out the flavor of the fish.

INGREDIENTS

Serves 4

¾ pound fresh grouper fillet, skinless and very thinly sliced

2 teaspoons salt

½ cup cherry tomatoes, halved lengthwise

3 tablespoons extra-virgin olive oil

1 tablespoon freshly squeezed lemon juice

½ teaspoon freshly ground black pepper

1 teaspoon chopped fresh thyme, for garnish

PREPARATION

1. On a large serving dish, arrange fish slices so that they are close together, but not overlapping.

2. Sprinkle with 1 teaspoon salt, cover with plastic wrap, and refrigerate for 10 minutes.

3. In the meantime, squeeze juice and seeds from cherry tomatoes into a small bowl. Discard peels. Add oil, lemon juice, remaining teaspoon salt, and pepper to bowl, and whisk together.

4. Pour mixture evenly over fish, taking care that every piece is covered. Garnish with thyme and serve immediately.

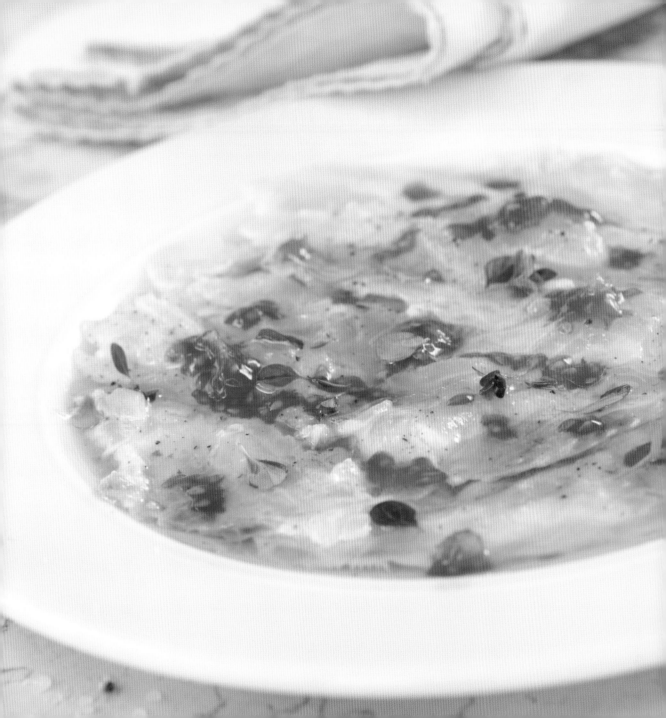

ROASTED SNAPPER
WITH TOMATOES

*This elegant dish makes an impressive main course
for dinner with really good friends.*

INGREDIENTS

Serves 4

Four 8-ounce fresh snapper
fillets

3 tablespoons extra-virgin olive
oil, plus more for rubbing

1 teaspoon freshly ground
black pepper

2 teaspoons salt

2 cloves garlic, minced

3 large tomatoes, cut into
½-inch dice

1 tablespoon white wine

1 teaspoon Spanish paprika

1 teaspoon white pepper

1 tablespoon chopped fresh
parsley

1 tablespoon chopped fresh
cilantro

PREPARATION

1. Preheat oven to 450°F.

2. Lay fish fillets on a large
baking sheet and rub with a little
olive oil. Sprinkle with black
pepper and 1 teaspoon salt, and
cook for 12 minutes, until fish
flakes easily with a fork.

3. In the meantime, heat a heavy
skillet over high heat until very
hot. Add oil, garlic, and
tomatoes, and cook while stirring
for 2 minutes. Add wine,
remaining teaspoon salt, paprika,
and white pepper, and cook for
another 3 minutes. Remove from
heat and mix in parsley and
cilantro. Set aside until fish
is ready.

4. To serve, divide tomato
mixture among 4 plates using a
slotted spoon. Top each with a
fish fillet, then pour tomato sauce
over top. Serve immediately.

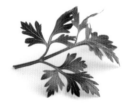

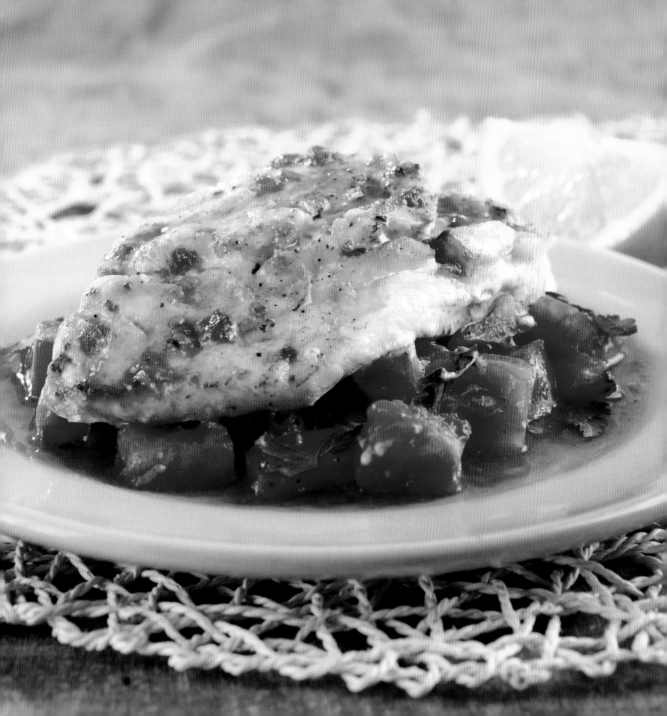

SEAFOOD AND TOMATO STEW

This satisfying dish makes a lovely winter meal. Serve with a full-bodied red wine.

INGREDIENTS

Serves 6

3 tablespoons extra-virgin olive oil

3 cloves garlic, finely minced

1 red chile, seeded and finely diced

2 teaspoons salt

1 tablespoon finely diced oil-packed sun-dried tomatoes

¾ pound cherry tomatoes, coarsely chopped

½ pound fresh mussels, scrubbed well

½ pound clams, scrubbed well

1 tablespoon chopped fresh oregano

½ pound small calamari, cleaned and cut into rings

½ pound shrimp, cleaned and peeled

PREPARATION

1. Heat a medium pot over medium heat. Add oil, garlic, chile, and 1 teaspoon salt, and cook for 2 minutes.

2. Add sun-dried tomatoes, cherry tomatoes, mussels, clams, and oregano. Cover and cook for about 8 minutes, until mussels and clams open. If many shells remain closed, cover and cook for another 5 minutes. Discard any shells that have not opened.

3. Mix in calamari and cook uncovered for 3 minutes, stirring occasionally.

4. Add shrimp and remaining teaspoon salt. Cook, stirring constantly, for 4 minutes, until shrimp turn pink and shrink a little. Serve immediately.

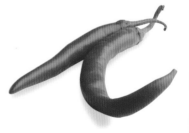

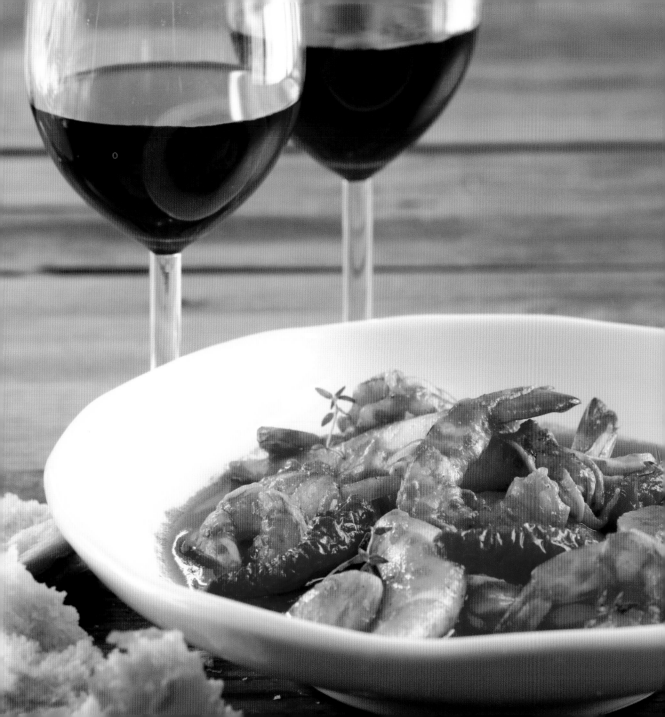

FRESH SARDINES IN SPICY TOMATO SAUCE

This is my rendition of a favorite Moroccan dish.

INGREDIENTS

Serves 4

¼ cup extra-virgin olive oil

3 cloves garlic, minced

2 red chiles, seeded and finely diced

2 tablespoons finely diced oil-packed sun-dried tomatoes

One 16-ounce can puréed tomatoes

2 teaspoons salt

1 teaspoon Old Bay Seasoning

8 fresh Portuguese sardines, cleaned and filleted

PREPARATION

1. Heat a large skillet over medium heat. Add oil, garlic, and chiles, and cook for 2 minutes.

2. Add sun-dried tomatoes, canned tomatoes, salt, and Old Bay Seasoning, and heat until boiling. Reduce heat to low and simmer for 20 minutes.

3. Add sardines, cover, and cook for another 10 minutes.

4. Serve immediately or cool to room temperature, transfer to an airtight container, and refrigerate for up to 2 days. Reheat before serving.

5. To serve, spoon a little sauce into 4 serving dishes. Carefully lay 2 sardines into each dish, then pour a little sauce over top. Serve extra sauce in a small bowl on the side.

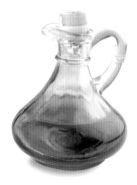

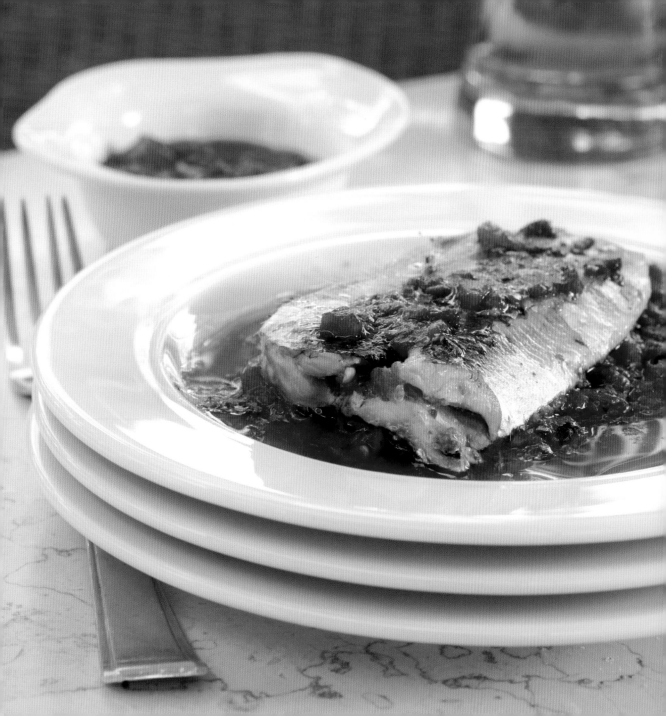

BOUILLABAISSE

Make this soup for a really special occasion, since it requires many ingredients and quite a bit of preparation. When ordering fish for this dish, be sure to ask the fishmonger to package the bones and heads as well. Serve with fresh San Francisco sourdough bread.

INGREDIENTS

Serves 6

2 tablespoons extra-virgin olive oil

1 medium white onion, thinly sliced

3 cloves garlic, minced

2 stalks celery, cut into ½-inch slices

1 carrot, cut into ½-inch dice

1 tablespoon chopped fresh thyme

1 tablespoon chopped fresh oregano

½ tablespoon chopped fresh rosemary

2 bay leaves

1 teaspoon fennel seeds

1 teaspoon saffron

2 teaspoons freshly ground black pepper

1 pound fish heads and bones (such as grouper, snapper, or sea bass)

4 fresh blue crabs, cleaned and halved

6 large tomatoes, cut into ½-inch cubes

3 potatoes, cut into 1-inch cubes

Water

1 tablespoon salt, plus more to taste

1 teaspoon cayenne pepper

2½ pounds fresh fish fillets (such as grouper, snapper, or bass), cut into 2-inch pieces

½ pound small calamari, cleaned and cut into rings

½ pound fresh mussels, scrubbed well

½ pound shrimp, cleaned and peeled

2 tablespoons anise liqueur (such as Pastis or Ricard)

PREPARATION

1. In a large pot over medium heat, cook oil, onion, garlic, celery, and carrot until vegetables are golden, about 6 minutes. Add thyme, oregano, rosemary, bay leaves, fennel, saffron, and black pepper, and cook for another 3 minutes.

2. Add fish heads and bones, crabs, tomatoes, and potatoes. Add enough water to triple the volume in the pot, and bring soup to a boil. Do not cover.

3. Add salt and cayenne pepper, reduce heat, and gently boil for 40 minutes. Skim off foam as it rises.

4. Remove stock from heat. Using a slotted spoon, remove bones and shells from the stock and discard.

LOBSTER IN TOMATO SAUCE

When choosing the lobsters for this dish, be sure to select ones with their tails curled under. That's a sure sign that the lobsters were fresh when cooked.

5. Blend stock with an immersion blender and pour through a sieve into a large bowl.

6. Return strained stock to pot, and discard strained bones and shells. Bring stock to a boil over medium heat. Add salt to taste.

7. Just before serving, add fish, calamari, mussels, and shrimp to hot soup and cook for 2 minutes. Pour in anise liqueur, transfer to deep serving dishes, and serve immediately.

8. At this point, the soup may also be cooled to room temperature, transferred to an airtight container, and refrigerated for up to 2 days. Reheat gently before serving.

INGREDIENTS

Serves 4

3 tablespoons extra-virgin olive oil

1 medium red onion, coarsely chopped

2 teaspoons salt

3 cloves garlic, minced

½ pound cherry tomatoes, halved

1 tablespoon chopped fresh oregano

One 16-ounce can diced tomatoes

1 teaspoon freshly ground black pepper

Two 1¼-pound fresh lobsters, steamed, chilled, and cut in half lengthwise

PREPARATION

1. Heat a large pot over medium heat. Add oil, onion, and 1 teaspoon salt, and cook until onion is translucent, about 5 minutes.

2. Add garlic and cook for 2 minutes.

3. Mix in cherry tomatoes and oregano, and cook for 10 minutes, until tomatoes soften and mixture thickens to a sauce.

4. Mix in canned tomatoes with their juices, pepper, and remaining teaspoon salt. Reduce heat and simmer for 20 minutes.

5. Add lobsters, cover, and cook for 15 minutes.

6. To serve, place half a lobster on each serving dish and cover with sauce. Serve immediately.

SPICY MOROCCAN FISH

*My wife's grandmother prepared this spicy North African dish every weekend.
My take on the traditional recipe can be used to spice up grouper, sole, or any
other whitefish. Serve with fresh bread for soaking up extra sauce.*

INGREDIENTS

Serves 4

½ cup vegetable oil (such as
canola, corn, or sunflower)

6 cloves garlic

½ cup tomato paste

2 tablespoons finely chopped
oil-packed sun-dried tomatoes

1 tablespoon Spanish paprika

2 teaspoons ground cumin

1 teaspoon ground caraway
seeds

2 teaspoons salt

1 teaspoon cayenne pepper

Four 8-ounce whitefish fillets
(such as sea bass, sole, or cod)

1 cup water

PREPARATION

1. In a medium pot over very
low heat, heat oil and garlic for
20 minutes, until garlic is very
soft. Make sure heat is very low,
so garlic doesn't burn.

2. Add tomato paste, sun-dried
tomatoes, paprika, cumin,
caraway seeds, salt, and cayenne
pepper, and mix well. Continue
to cook over very low heat for
10 minutes.

3. Add fish and water, increase
heat to medium, and cook until
mixture comes to a boil.

4. Turn heat down to low, cover,
and cook for 15 minutes. Serve
immediately or cool to room
temperature, transfer to an
airtight container, and refrigerate
for up to 2 days. Reheat gently
before serving.

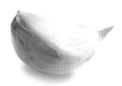

PRAWNS IN TOMATO SAUCE

The combination of almonds and tomatoes in this dish evokes the fine aromas of the Catalonian kitchen.

INGREDIENTS

Serves 4

2 tablespoons extra-virgin olive oil

¼ cup coarsely chopped blanched almonds

3 cloves garlic, coarsely chopped

1 teaspoon chopped fresh thyme

One 16-ounce can diced tomatoes

2 tablespoons dry sherry

1 tablespoon Spanish paprika

2 teaspoons salt

2 pounds fresh prawns, peeled and cleaned

1 tablespoon chopped fresh parsley, for garnish

PREPARATION

1. Heat a large deep pan over medium heat. Add oil, almonds, and garlic, and cook for 3 minutes.

2. Add thyme, canned tomatoes with their juices, sherry, paprika, and salt. Cook for 10 minutes, stirring occasionally.

3. Mix in prawns, cover, and cook for 5 minutes.

4. Transfer to serving dishes, garnish with parsley, and serve immediately.

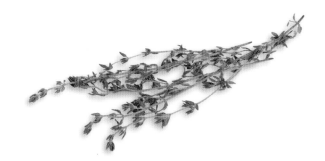

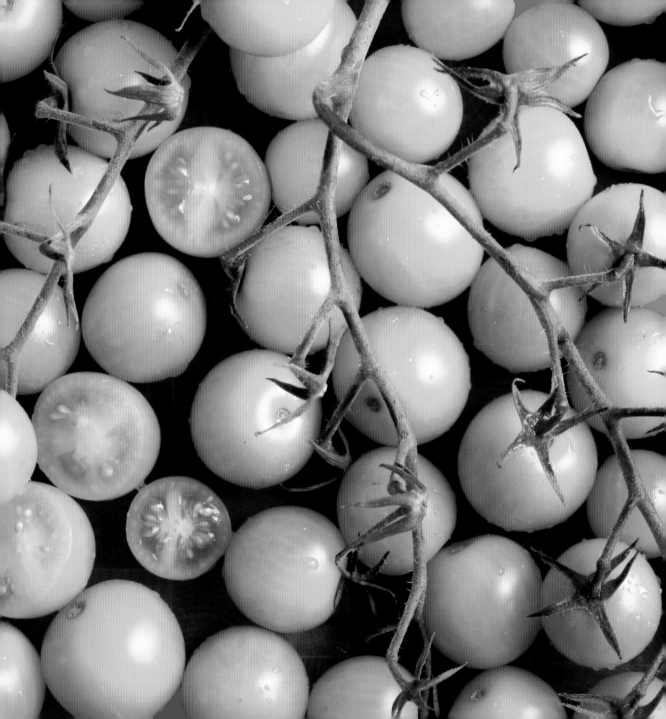

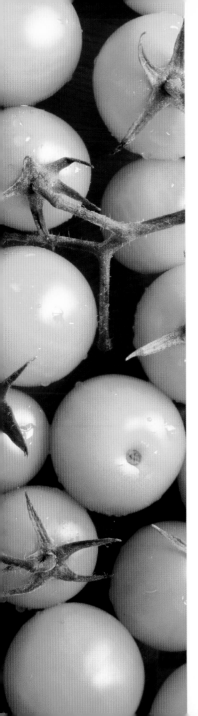

PASTA
AND
RISOTTO

TOMATO AND PORCINI MUSHROOM RISOTTO

This dish hails from northern Italy. It's perfect for warming (and filling) the stomach on a brisk autumn afternoon.

INGREDIENTS

Serves 6

2 teaspoons extra-virgin olive oil

1 medium white onion, finely diced

2 cloves garlic, minced

¾ cup dried porcini mushrooms

1½ pounds cherry tomatoes, quartered

1½ cups risotto rice

½ cup white wine

1 tablespoon chicken soup powder

1 tablespoon salt

1 teaspoon white pepper

2 cups boiling water

⅓ cup grated Parmesan cheese

2 tablespoons butter

PREPARATION

1. In a wide saucepan over medium heat, heat oil, onion, garlic, and mushrooms until onion is translucent, about 5 minutes.

2. Add cherry tomatoes and cook for 5 minutes, stirring occasionally. Mix in rice, then add wine and soup powder. Cook while stirring for 5 minutes.

3. Add salt, pepper, and boiling water and cook while stirring for 17 to 20 minutes, until all liquid evaporates.

4. Add cheese and butter, remove from heat, and stir until well blended.

5. Transfer to serving dishes and serve immediately.

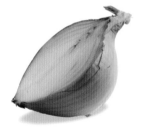

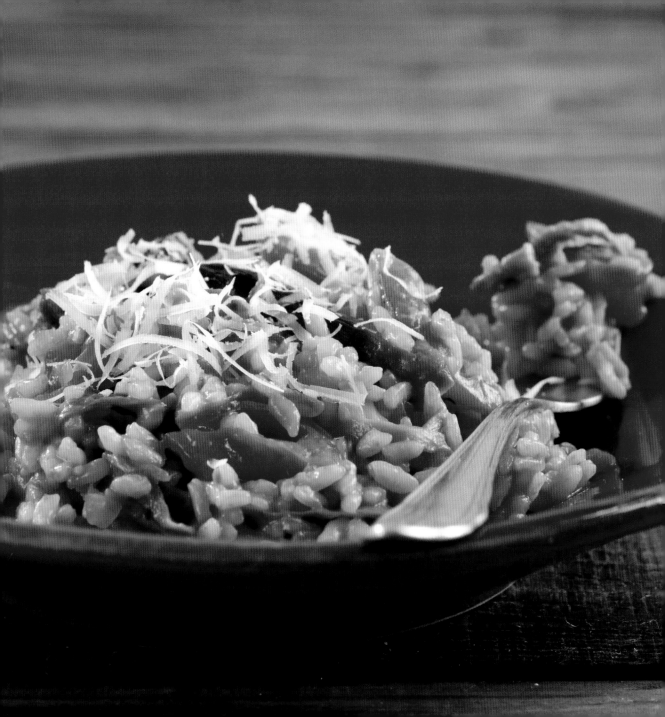

NEW YORK–STYLE SPAGHETTI AND MEATBALLS

This is the version of this world-famous dish that we make in our kitchen. It's a guaranteed crowd-pleaser.

INGREDIENTS

Serves 6

½ pound ground beef

2 medium onions, finely diced

3 teaspoons salt

2 teaspoons freshly ground black pepper

2 tablespoons extra-virgin olive oil

1 carrot, cut into ¼-inch dice

3 cloves garlic, minced

⅓ cup red wine

1 tablespoon finely chopped fresh thyme

One 16-ounce can diced tomatoes

⅔ cup frozen peas

4 quarts water

3 tablespoons coarse salt

One 16-ounce package thin spaghetti

PREPARATION

1. In a large bowl, place beef, half the onion, 1½ teaspoons salt, and 1 teaspoon pepper. Mix together with a fork until well combined, then refrigerate for 30 minutes.

2. Heat a large, deep skillet over medium heat. Add oil, remaining onion, carrot, and garlic, and cook for 3 minutes while stirring.

3. Add wine, thyme, and remaining 1½ teaspoons salt and 1 teaspoon pepper, and cook for 5 minutes.

4. Add canned tomatoes with their juices and bring to a boil. Reduce heat and simmer while you prepare the meatballs.

5. With wet hands, shape chilled beef mixture into 1-inch balls and place in simmering tomato sauce. Cover and cook over low heat for 30 minutes.

6. Remove from heat and mix in peas. Cover and set aside while you prepare pasta. At this stage, meatballs may be may be cooled to room temperature, transferred to an airtight container, and refrigerated for up to 2 days. Or freeze for up to 1 month, then defrost at room temperature and reheat before serving.

7. In a large pot, bring water and coarse salt to a boil. Add spaghetti and cook until al dente, according to instructions on package. Drain in a colander.

8. To serve, arrange pasta on serving dishes. Top each serving with meatballs and pour sauce over top.

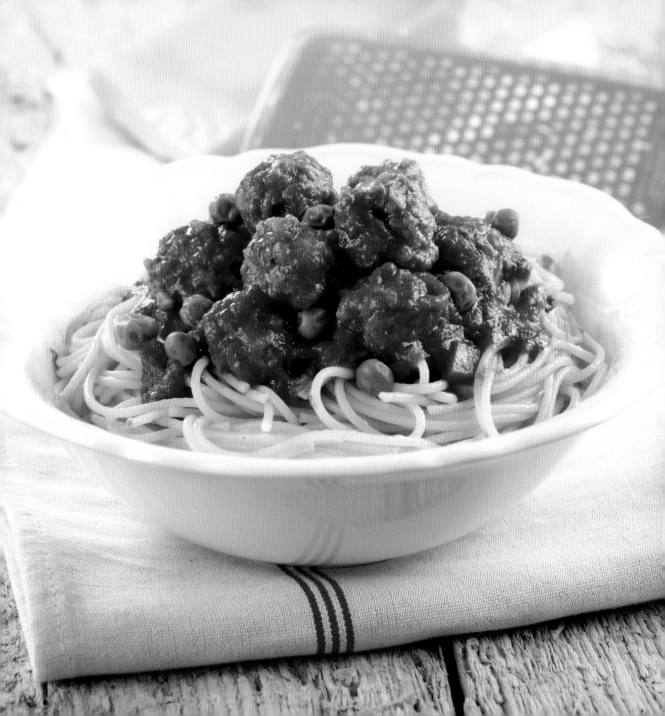

SPAGHETTI BOLOGNESE

This recipe is a traditional favorite. Make a double batch of the sauce and use it to prepare lasagna (page 100) or cannelloni (page 110).

INGREDIENTS

Serves 6

Sauce:

2 tablespoons extra-virgin olive oil

½ pound ground beef

3 garlic cloves, minced

1 carrot, finely diced

1 large onion, finely diced

1 stalk celery, finely diced

1 tablespoon salt

2 teaspoons finely ground black pepper

2 tablespoons finely chopped oil-packed sun-dried tomatoes

1 cup red wine

One 16-ounce can diced tomatoes

Pasta:

4 quarts water

3 tablespoons coarse salt

One 16-ounce package thick spaghetti

½ cup grated Parmesan cheese

PREPARATION

1. Make sauce: Preheat oven to 425°F.

2. Heat a large, deep saucepan or ovenproof pot over medium heat. Add oil and beef, and cook while stirring for 10 minutes, until meat turns gray.

3. Mix in garlic, carrot, onion, celery, salt, pepper, and sun-dried tomatoes. Cook for 5 minutes, stirring occasionally.

4. Add wine and cook until completely evaporated, about 10 to 15 minutes.

5. Stir in canned tomatoes and their juices, and remove from heat. Cover with aluminum foil and bake for 30 minutes. At this stage, sauce may be cooled to room temperature, transferred to an airtight container, and refrigerated for up to 2 days. Or freeze for up to 1 month, then defrost overnight in the refrigerator and reheat before serving.

6. While sauce is baking, prepare pasta: In a large pot, bring water and coarse salt to a boil. Add pasta and cook until al dente, according to instructions on package. Drain in a colander and return to pot.

7. Pour sauce and ¼ cup cheese over drained pasta in pot and mix well. Transfer to serving dishes, top with remaining ¼ cup cheese, and serve immediately.

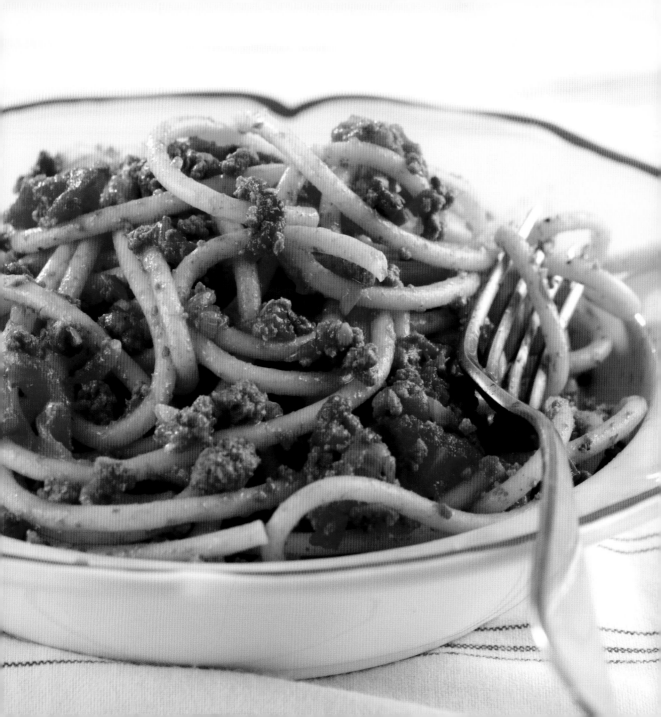

PASTA WITH GORGONZOLA CHEESE AND TOMATOES

This rich dish is perfect for people who love fine cheese.

INGREDIENTS

Serves 6

4 quarts water

3 tablespoons coarse salt

One 16-ounce package short pasta (such as penne, fusilli, or gemelli)

2 tablespoons extra-virgin olive oil

3 cloves garlic, minced

4 large tomatoes, cut into ½-inch cubes

2 teaspoons salt

1 teaspoon white pepper

¼ cup white wine

1 tablespoon coarsely chopped fresh basil

½ pound Gorgonzola cheese

PREPARATION

1. In a large pot, bring water and coarse salt to a boil. Add pasta and cook until al dente, according to instructions on package. Drain in a colander and return to pot.

2. While pasta is cooking, heat a large, deep saucepan over medium heat. Add oil and garlic, and cook for 3 minutes, stirring occasionally.

3. Increase heat to high and add tomatoes. Cook for 5 minutes, stirring occasionally. Add salt, pepper, and wine, and cook for another 3 minutes, stirring occasionally. Remove from heat and stir in basil.

4. Pour sauce over drained pasta in pot and mix well. Transfer to serving dishes, crumble cheese over top, and serve immediately.

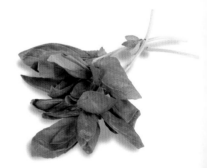

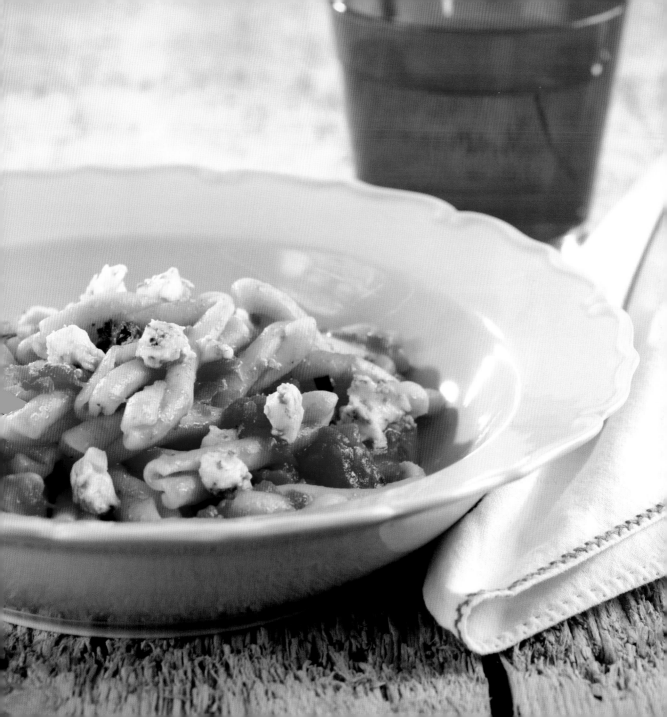

LASAGNA WITH BOLOGNESE SAUCE

Lasagna lovers will clamor for an invitation to supper when they hear you're making this dish.

INGREDIENTS

Serves 8

2 tablespoons butter

2 tablespoons all-purpose flour

2 teaspoons salt

1 teaspoon white pepper

1 teaspoon ground nutmeg

3 cups milk

2 pounds lasagna sheets

1 batch Bolognese sauce (page 96)

Extra-virgin olive oil, for greasing

PREPARATION

1. Preheat oven to 375°F. Grease an 8 × 14 × 3-inch baking pan with olive oil.

2. In a medium saucepan over medium heat, stir together butter and flour until butter is melted and bubbles begin to form.

3. Add salt, pepper, nutmeg, and 1½ cups milk, and continue to cook, stirring constantly, until mixture comes to a boil.

4. Pour in remaining 1½ cups milk and cook, stirring constantly, until mixture thickens and boils again. If mixture boils but isn't thick yet, reduce heat slightly and continue to cook, stirring constantly, until thickened. Remove from heat and set aside.

5. Arrange a layer of lasagna sheets in the bottom of the baking pan, overlapping them slightly. Spoon one-third of the Bolognese sauce on top, then pour over one-third of the white sauce. Arrange another layer of lasagna sheets on top, this time side by side and not overlapping. Spoon on another third of Bolognese sauce, and another third of white sauce. Arrange a final layer of lasagna sheets side by side and top with remaining Bolognese and white sauces.

6. Transfer to oven and bake until top is golden brown, about 30 minutes. Let sit for 15 minutes before serving, or cool to room temperature, cover with aluminum foil, and refrigerate for up to 24 hours. Reheat before serving.

TOMATO AND EGGPLANT PASTA

Looking for an alternative to meat when serving pasta?
This dish is filling and flavorful.

INGREDIENTS

Serves 6

2 large eggplants, cut into
½-inch dice

4 tablespoons extra-virgin
olive oil

4 teaspoons salt

2 teaspoons coarsely ground
black pepper

3 cloves garlic, minced

One 16-ounce can diced
tomatoes

1 tablespoon finely chopped
parsley

1 tablespoon coarsely chopped
fresh basil

4 quarts water

3 tablespoons coarse salt

One 16-ounce package penne
pasta

¼ cup grated Parmesan cheese

PREPARATION

1. Preheat oven to 425°F.

2. In a large bowl, mix together
eggplant, 2 tablespoons oil,
2 teaspoons salt, and 1 teaspoon
pepper. Arrange in a single layer
on a large baking sheet and bake
for 20 minutes.

3. In the meantime, heat a large,
deep saucepan over medium heat.
Cook garlic and remaining
2 tablespoons oil for 3 minutes,
stirring occasionally. Add canned
tomatoes and their juices and
cook, stirring occasionally, for
10 minutes.

4. Stir in remaining 2 teaspoons
salt and 1 teaspoon pepper.
Remove from heat and stir in
cooked eggplant, parsley, and
basil. Cover and set aside while
you prepare pasta.

5. In a large pot, bring water and
coarse salt to a boil. Add pasta
and cook until al dente,
according to instructions on
package. Drain in a colander and
return to pot.

6. Pour sauce over drained
pasta in pot and mix well.
Transfer to serving dishes, top
generously with cheese, and
serve immediately.

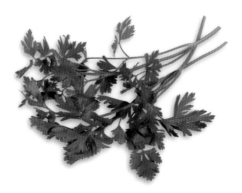

SPAGHETTI WITH FRESH TOMATO AND RICOTTA SAUCE

This is a popular summer dish in our house. Light and fresh, it's perfect for serving when the weather is warm.

INGREDIENTS

Serves 6

4 quarts water

3 tablespoons coarse salt

One 16-ounce package thick spaghetti

3 large tomatoes, peeled, cored, seeded, and grated (page 9)

1 clove garlic, minced

2 tablespoons extra-virgin olive oil

1 tablespoon salt

1 teaspoon white pepper

1 tablespoon finely chopped fresh parsley

1 tablespoon freshly squeezed lemon juice

½ pound fresh ricotta cheese

PREPARATION

1. In a large pot, bring water and coarse salt to a boil. Add pasta and cook until al dente, according to instructions on package. Drain in a colander.

2. While pasta is cooking, add grated tomatoes to a large bowl and mix in garlic, oil, salt, pepper, parsley, and lemon juice. Add drained pasta and mix well.

3. Transfer to serving dishes, crumble cheese over top, and serve immediately.

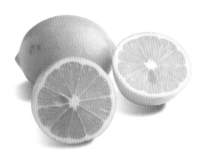

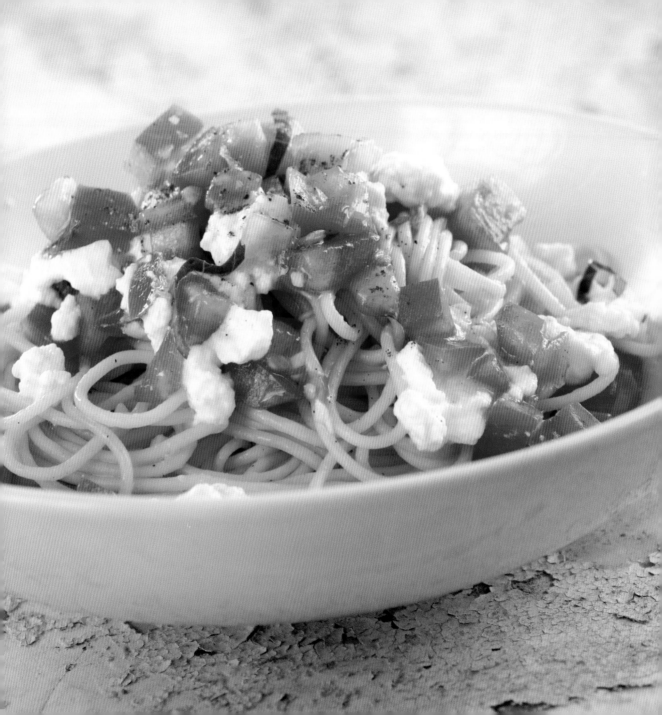

NEAPOLITAN SEAFOOD PASTA

In a small seafood restaurant beside a marina in Italy, this was my favorite dish. The secret to its success—use only fresh seafood.

INGREDIENTS

Serves 6

4 quarts water

3 tablespoons coarse salt

One 16-ounce package pappardelle pasta

3 tablespoons extra-virgin olive oil

3 cloves garlic, minced

½ pound small calamari, cleaned and cut into rings

½ pound fresh mussels, scrubbed well

½ pound fresh clams, scrubbed well

2 fresh crabs, cleaned and halved

½ cup white wine

One 16-ounce can diced tomatoes

2 teaspoons salt

1 teaspoon white pepper

½ pound shrimp, cleaned and peeled

2 tablespoons coarsely chopped fresh basil

PREPARATION

1. In a large pot, bring water and coarse salt to a boil. Add pasta and cook until al dente, according to instructions on package. Drain in a colander and return to pot.

2. While pasta is cooking, heat a large, deep saucepan over medium heat. Cook oil and garlic over medium heat for 3 minutes, stirring occasionally.

3. Increase heat to high and add calamari, mussels, clams, and crabs. Cook for 2 minutes while stirring. Add wine and continue cooking until half the wine evaporates.

4. Mix in canned tomatoes with their juices, salt, and pepper, and continue to cook, stirring occasionally, for 10 minutes.

5. Add shrimp and cook while stirring for 2 minutes. Remove from heat and stir in basil.

6. Pour sauce over drained pasta in pot and mix well. Transfer to serving dishes and serve immediately.

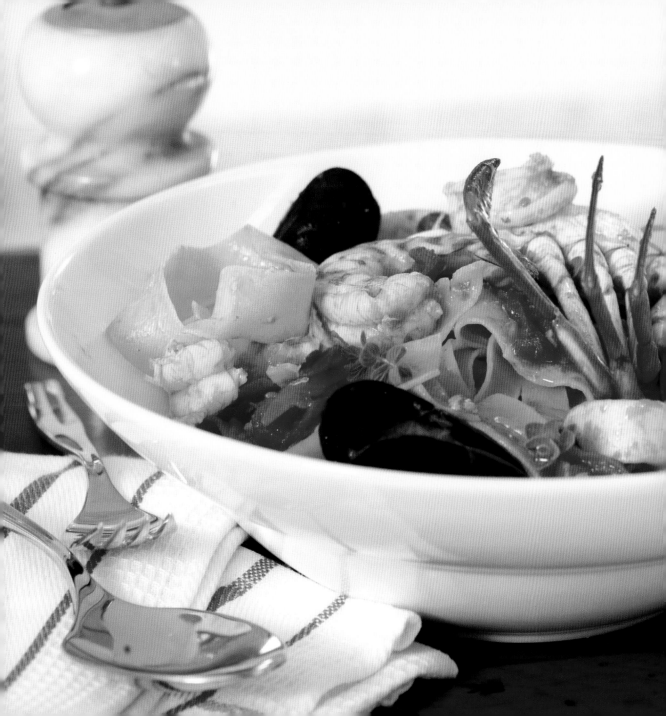

CRAB RAVIOLI IN TOMATO BUTTER SAUCE

This dish takes a bit of time to prepare, but the result is worth it. It's perfect for celebrating a very special occasion.

INGREDIENTS

Serves 4

Pastry:

2 large eggs

2 tablespoons extra-virgin olive oil

2½ cups all-purpose flour, plus more for dusting *591≈>300yp.*

1 teaspoon salt

Filling:

½ pound crab meat *118≈>60y.*

1 teaspoon salt

½ teaspoon ground nutmeg

1 tablespoon butter, softened

1 tablespoon grated Parmesan cheese

Sauce:

1 cup cherry tomatoes *236≈>118y.*

2 tablespoons finely chopped oil-packed sun-dried tomatoes

1 tablespoon chopped fresh thyme

1 teaspoon salt

1 teaspoon freshly ground black pepper

1 clove garlic, minced

½ cup butter, cold

3 quarts water

2 tablespoons coarse salt

¼ cup grated Parmesan cheese

PREPARATION

1. Make pastry: In a food processor, place eggs, oil, flour, and salt, and process until a firm dough forms. Cover with plastic wrap and refrigerate for 30 minutes.

2. Make filling: In a large bowl, mix together crab, salt, nutmeg, butter, and cheese. Refrigerate until ready to use.

3. Turn out chilled pastry onto a lightly floured surface. Roll out using a rolling pin, or run through a pasta machine. Shape into a ball, flatten and roll out again, then shape into a ball again. Repeat this process 3 or 4 times to make pastry smooth and elastic.

4. Roll out pastry as thin as possible. Cut into 2-inch squares using a pastry wheel or ravioli cutter. Place 1 tablespoon filling in middle of each square and fold into triangles by drawing two opposite corners together. Rub a little water along edges to stick. Arrange on a lightly floured plate, taking care that ravioli don't touch each other. Set aside until sauce is ready. Refrigerate for up to 1 day, or freeze for up to 1 month.

(continued on page 108)

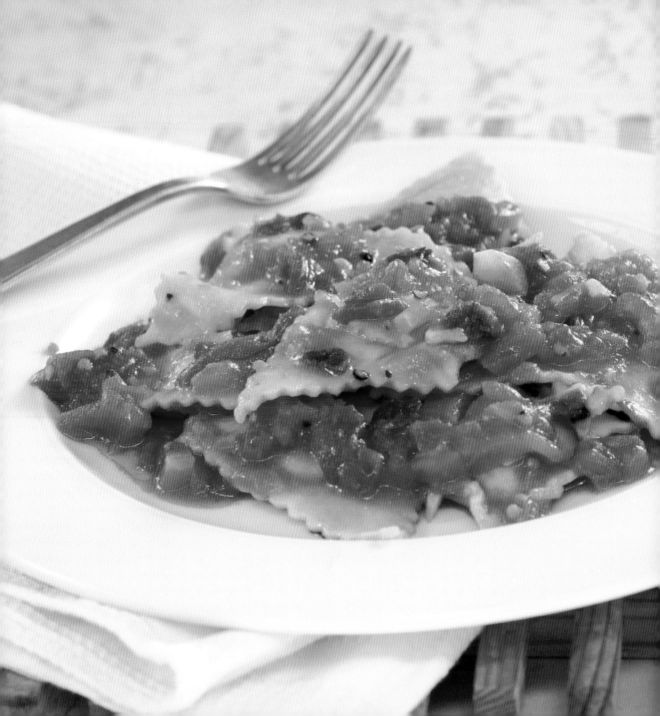

(continued from page 106)

TOMATO AND SEAFOOD RISOTTO

Make this Italian dish with the freshest seafood you can find.

5. Make sauce: In a blender, place cherry tomatoes, sun-dried tomatoes, thyme, salt, pepper, and garlic. Blend until smooth.

6. Heat a large saucepan over medium heat. Add tomato mixture and cook for 5 minutes. Stir in butter until melted. Remove from heat and set aside.

7. In a large pot, bring water and coarse salt to a boil and add ravioli. When ravioli begin to float, cook for another 2 minutes, then transfer to a colander and drain.

8. Add drained ravioli to sauce and mix gently with a large spoon. Transfer to serving dishes, top with cheese, and serve immediately.

INGREDIENTS

Serves 6

3 tablespoons extra-virgin olive oil

1 medium white onion, finely diced

3 cloves garlic, minced

½ pound small calamari, cleaned and cut into rings

½ pound fresh mussels, scrubbed well

½ pound clams, scrubbed well

1 cup white wine

1½ cups risotto rice

1 pound cherry tomatoes, quartered

1 tablespoon chicken soup powder

2 cups boiling water

1 tablespoon salt

1 teaspoon white pepper

½ pound shrimp, cleaned and peeled

PREPARATION

1. In a wide saucepan over medium heat, heat oil, onion, and garlic until onion is translucent, about 5 minutes.

2. Add calamari, mussels, and clams, and cook while stirring for 4 minutes.

3. Pour in wine and cook for 5 minutes, stirring occasionally.

4. Stir in rice. Add cherry tomatoes, soup powder, and 1 cup boiling water, and cook while stirring for 15 minutes.

5. Add salt, pepper, and remaining cup boiling water. Cook while stirring for 7 minutes.

6. Add shrimp and cook while stirring for 3 minutes.

7. Transfer to serving dishes and serve immediately.

TOMATO AND THREE-CHEESE LASAGNA

This vegetarian dish is as filling as a meat-based version.

INGREDIENTS

Serves 8

2 tablespoons extra-virgin olive oil, plus more for greasing

3 cloves garlic, minced

1 tablespoon chopped fresh thyme

1 pound cherry tomatoes, halved

2 tablespoons chopped oil-packed sun-dried tomatoes

4 teaspoons salt

2 teaspoons white pepper

2 tablespoons butter

2 tablespoons all-purpose flour

1 teaspoon ground nutmeg

3 cups milk

1 cup grated Parmesan cheese

½ cup grated blue cheese

½ cup crumbled feta cheese

2 pounds lasagna sheets

PREPARATION

1. Preheat oven to 375°F. Grease an 8 × 14 × 3-inch baking pan with olive oil.

2. In a large saucepan over medium heat, cook oil, garlic, and thyme for 3 minutes, stirring occasionally.

3. Add cherry tomatoes, sun-dried tomatoes, 2 teaspoons salt, and 1 teaspoon pepper, and mix well. Cook for 10 minutes, stirring occasionally. Remove from heat and set aside.

4. Separately, in a medium saucepan over medium heat, stir together butter and flour until butter is melted and bubbles begin to form.

5. Add remaining 2 teaspoons salt and 1 teaspoon pepper, nutmeg, and 1½ cups milk. Cook, stirring constantly, until mixture comes to a boil.

6. Pour in remaining 1½ cups milk and cook, stirring constantly, until mixture thickens and boils again. If mixture boils but isn't thick yet, reduce heat slightly and continue to cook, stirring constantly, until thickened. Remove from heat and set side.

7. In a medium bowl, mix cheeses together.

8. Arrange a layer of lasagna sheets in the bottom of the baking pan, overlapping them slightly. Spoon one-third of the tomato sauce on top, sprinkle over one-third of the cheese mixture, then one-third of the white sauce. Arrange another layer of lasagna sheets on top, this time side by side and not overlapping. Spoon on another third of tomato sauce, a third of cheese mixture, then a third of white sauce. Arrange a final layer of lasagna sheets side by side and top with remaining tomato sauce, cheeses, and white sauce.

9. Bake until top is golden brown, about 30 minutes. Let sit for 15 minutes before serving, or cool to room temperature, cover with aluminum foil, and refrigerate for up to 24 hours. Reheat before serving.

CANNELLONI IN TOMATO BEEF SAUCE

Looking for comfort food? You'll find it here! This recipe is
a pleasure to prepare and serve.

INGREDIENTS

Serves 6

2 tablespoons extra-virgin olive oil, plus more for greasing

1 medium onion, finely diced

3 cloves garlic, minced

¾ pound ground beef

4 teaspoons salt

2 teaspoons white pepper

4 large tomatoes, cut into ½-inch dice

2 tablespoons finely chopped oil-packed sun-dried tomatoes

2 tablespoons butter

2 tablespoons all-purpose flour

1 teaspoon ground nutmeg

3 cups milk

18 dry cannelloni

½ cup grated Parmesan cheese

PREPARATION

1. Preheat oven to 375°F. Grease an 8 × 14 × 3-inch baking pan with olive oil.

2. In a large saucepan over medium heat, cook oil, onion, and garlic for 3 minutes, stirring occasionally.

3. Add beef, 2 teaspoons salt, and 1 teaspoon pepper. Cook, stirring occasionally, for 10 minutes.

4. Add tomatoes and sun-dried tomatoes, and cook for 15 minutes, stirring occasionally. Remove from heat and set aside.

5. Separately, in a medium pan over medium heat, stir together butter and flour until butter is melted and bubbles begin to form.

6. Add remaining 2 teaspoons salt and 1 teaspoon pepper, nutmeg, and 1½ cups milk. Cook, stirring constantly, until mixture comes to a boil.

7. Pour in remaining 1½ cups milk and cook, stirring constantly, until mixture thickens and boils again. If mixture boils but isn't thick yet, reduce heat slightly and continue to cook, stirring constantly, until thickened. Remove from heat and set aside.

8. Using a spoon, carefully fill cannelloni with tomato sauce and arrange in the baking pan. Mix remaining tomato sauce with white sauce and pour over the cannelloni. Bake until golden brown, about 30 minutes.

9. Cooked cannelloni may be cooled to room temperature, covered with aluminum foil, and refrigerated for up to 24 hours. Reheat before serving. To serve, arrange 3 cannelloni on each serving dish and top with cheese.

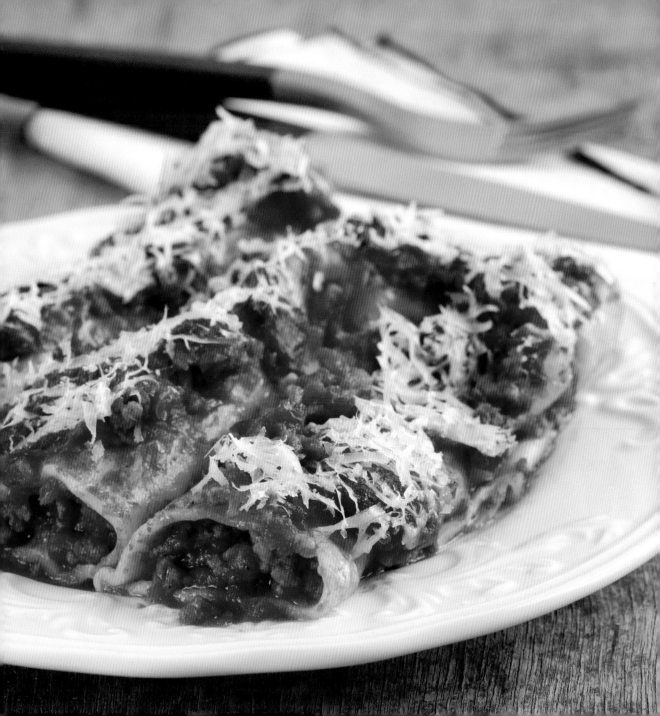

GNOCCHI IN TOMATO SAUCE

I introduced this dish to several friends, and to my delight, they've become fans as well. Select fresh or vacuum-packed gnocchi for best flavor.

INGREDIENTS

Serves 4

2 tablespoons extra-virgin olive oil

3 cloves garlic, minced

½ pound cherry tomatoes, quartered

½ tablespoon chopped fresh thyme

½ tablespoon chopped fresh oregano

2 teaspoons salt

1 teaspoon white pepper

4 quarts water

3 tablespoons coarse salt

One 16-ounce package gnocchi, fresh or vacuum-packed

½ cup grated Parmesan cheese

PREPARATION

1. Heat a large saucepan over medium heat. Add oil and garlic and cook for 3 minutes, stirring occasionally.

2. Add cherry tomatoes, thyme, oregano, salt, and pepper, and cook for 10 minutes, stirring occasionally.

3. In the meantime, bring water and coarse salt to a boil in a large pot. Add gnocchi and cook according to instructions on package.

4. Drain gnocchi in a colander, transfer to pan with sauce, and mix well. Transfer to serving dishes, top with cheese, and serve immediately.

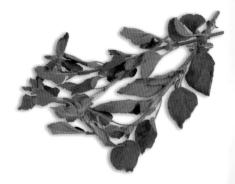

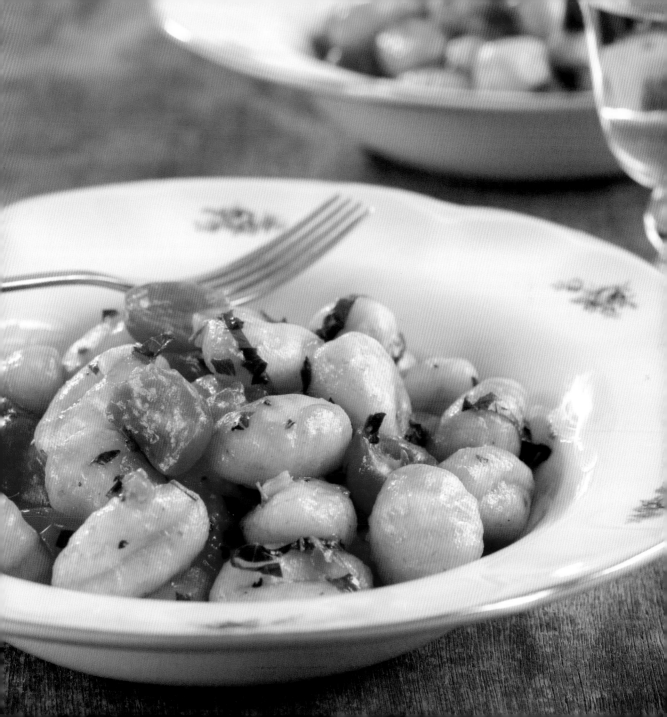

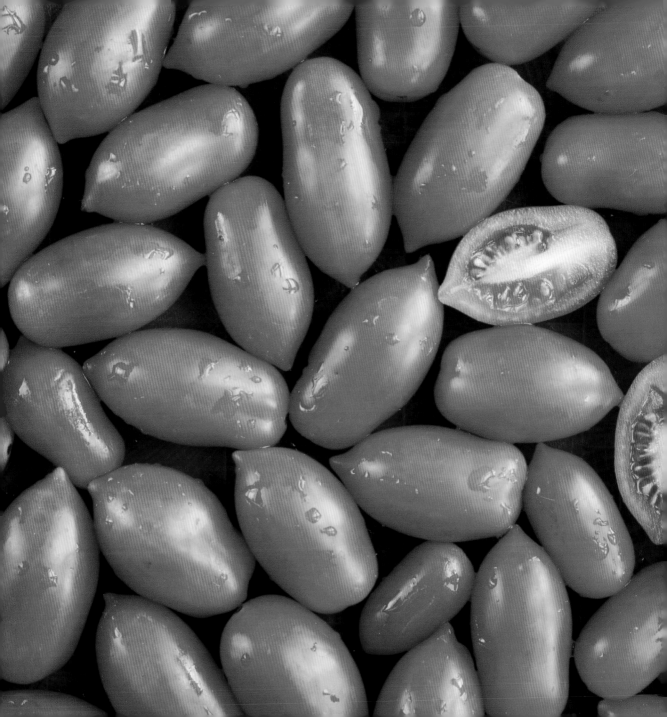

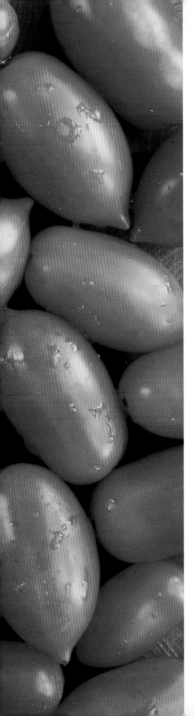

CHICKEN
AND MEAT

ROASTED CHICKEN WITH TOMATOES AND FRESH HERBS

This mouth-watering dish is distinctly Mediterranean. Pouring the pan juices back over the chicken just before serving maximizes the dish's flavor.

INGREDIENTS

Serves 4

Two 14-ounce young chickens

½ pound cherry tomatoes, halved

¼ cup extra-virgin olive oil

2 teaspoons coarse salt

1 teaspoon freshly ground black pepper

1 tablespoon finely chopped fresh thyme

2 cloves garlic, minced

1 teaspoon balsamic vinegar

PREPARATION

1. Preheat oven to 450°F. Place chickens in a deep baking pan.

2. In a bowl, mix together cherry tomatoes, oil, salt, pepper, thyme, garlic, and vinegar. Pour mixture over chicken.

3. Bake chicken at 450°F for 6 minutes, then reduce heat to 400°F and bake for another 20 minutes, or until chickens are brown and tomatoes lighten in color.

4. Transfer chickens to a large serving dish and pour pan juices over top just before serving. The chickens and pan juices may also be cooled to room temperature, transferred to an airtight container, and refrigerated for up to 24 hours. Reheat before serving.

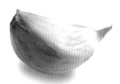

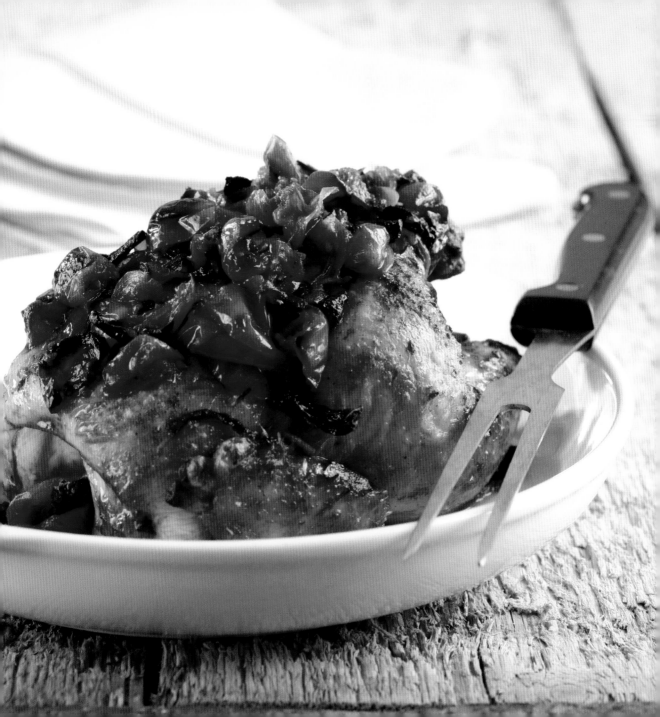

ROASTED BEEF SHOULDER IN TOMATO SAUCE

Serve this satisfying and delicious dish at family gatherings and other special occasions. Perfect with mashed potatoes or steamed rice.

INGREDIENTS

Serves 8

½ cup extra-virgin olive oil

1 medium white onion, finely diced

3 cloves garlic, minced

2 carrots, halved and cut into ½-inch slices

2 stalks celery, finely diced

3 teaspoons salt

One 16-ounce can crushed tomatoes

1 cup red wine

1 cup water

½ cup tomato paste

2 teaspoons freshly ground black pepper

One 5-pound beef shoulder roast

PREPARATION

1. Preheat oven to 375°F.

2. In a large, ovenproof roasting pan over medium heat, cook oil, onion, garlic, carrots, celery, and salt until onion is translucent, about 5 minutes.

3. Add canned tomatoes and wine. Increase heat and cook, stirring occasionally, until mixture comes to a boil.

4. Stir in water, tomato paste, and pepper. Add beef, cover, and transfer to oven. Bake for 2 hours, then turn beef over so that the side that was out of the sauce is now in the sauce. Bake for another hour.

5. Remove lid and bake uncovered for 30 minutes.

6. Remove from oven and let rest for about 15 minutes before slicing. Serve immediately, or cool to room temperature, transfer to an airtight container, and refrigerate for up to 2 days.

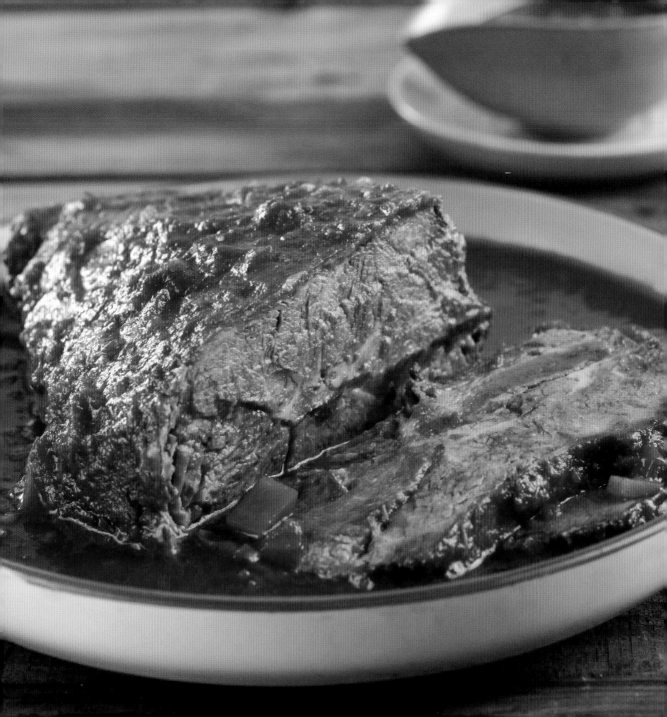

OSSO BUCCO

A classic from the Italian kitchen, this dish is perfect for chasing away wintertime chills. It tastes even better when prepared in advance, as this gives the flavors time to blend.

INGREDIENTS

Serves 6

¼ cup all-purpose flour

2 teaspoons salt

1 teaspoon freshly ground black pepper

6 slices veal shank, with bone

½ cup vegetable oil

1 medium red onion, coarsely chopped

3 stalks celery, cut into ½-inch dice

2 carrots, cut into ½-inch dice

2 cloves garlic, minced

2 cups white wine

Two 16-ounce cans diced tomatoes

2 cups chicken stock

One 19-ounce can chickpeas, drained and rinsed

3 tablespoons extra-virgin olive oil

½ cup chopped fresh parsley

1 tablespoon chopped fresh thyme

PREPARATION

1. In a large bowl, combine flour, 1 teaspoon salt, and 1 teaspoon pepper. Press each veal shank in mixture to coat, shaking excess back into bowl.

2. In a large, heavy, ovenproof saucepan, heat vegetable oil over medium heat. Sear coated veal until golden, about 3 minutes on each side, to seal in juices. Using a slotted spoon, transfer veal to a plate lined with paper towels and set aside.

3. Carefully pour hot oil out of pan and return pan to heat. (Do not rinse.) Add onion, celery, carrots, garlic, and a pinch of salt. Cook over low heat until onion is translucent, about 5 minutes.

4. Preheat oven to 400°F.

5. Add wine to vegetables in pan, increase heat to medium, and cook until liquid is reduced by half.

6. Arrange veal on top of vegetables. Add canned tomatoes and their juices, chicken stock, chickpeas, olive oil, parsley, thyme, and salt and pepper to taste. Increase heat to high and bring to a boil.

7. Remove from heat, cover, and transfer to oven. Bake until veal is very tender, about 1½ hours, then remove cover, increase heat to 450°F, and bake for about 15 minutes, until browned.

8. To serve, transfer a veal shank to each serving dish, place a large scoop of chickpeas alongside, and pour pan sauce generously over top.

SCALLOPINI IN TOMATO SAUCE

Ask your butcher to slice the veal especially thin for this recipe.

INGREDIENTS

Serves 4

3 tablespoons all-purpose flour

2 pounds veal scallopini

3 tablespoons extra-virgin olive oil

1 tablespoon chopped fresh thyme

2 cloves garlic, minced

1 cup white wine

1 pound cherry tomatoes

½ cup butter, cold

1 teaspoon salt

1 teaspoon white pepper

¼ cup grated Parmesan cheese

PREPARATION

1. Place flour in a large bowl or plate and press in each veal slice to coat, shaking off excess.

2. Heat oil in a large pan over medium heat. Fry coated veal slices for about 2 minutes on each side, then transfer to a dish and set aside. Place thyme and garlic in hot pan and fry for 2 minutes.

3. Add wine, increase heat to high, and cook for 3 minutes. Mix in tomatoes, reduce heat to low, and cook for 15 minutes, stirring occasionally.

4. Add butter, salt, and pepper to pan, and stir until butter is melted. Return veal to pan and increase heat to medium. Cook, stirring occasionally, for about 3 minutes, until veal is coated with a thin sauce. Transfer to serving dishes, sprinkle with cheese, and serve immediately.

CHORIZO IN TOMATO SAUCE

Serve these spicy sausages on a heaping serving of buttery mashed potatoes.

INGREDIENTS

Serves 4

8 Spanish chorizo sausages

2 tablespoons extra-virgin olive oil

1 medium white onion, finely diced

3 cloves garlic, minced

One 16-ounce can diced tomatoes

2 teaspoons salt

1 teaspoon white pepper

½ cup chopped fresh parsley

1 tablespoon chopped fresh thyme

PREPARATION

1. Heat a cast-iron skillet or grill pan over high heat until very hot. Grill sausages until golden brown, about 4 minutes each side. Set aside until cool enough to handle, then cut into ½-inch rounds.

2. In a medium pot over medium heat, cook oil, onion, and garlic until onion is translucent, about 5 minutes.

3. Mix in canned tomatoes with their juices, salt, and pepper, and bring to a boil.

4. Reduce heat to low, add sausage rounds, cover, and cook for 30 minutes.

5. Serve immediately, or cool to room temperature, transfer to an airtight container, and refrigerate for up to 2 days. Reheat before serving.

Opposite: Chorizo in Tomato Sauce

CHICKEN LIVERS IN TOMATO SAUCE

This traditional North African dish is excellent with steamed couscous or white rice and fresh crusty white bread.

INGREDIENTS

Serves 4

¼ cup extra-virgin olive oil

1 large white onion, finely diced

2 teaspoons tomato paste

2 teaspoons ground cumin

2 teaspoons Spanish paprika

½ teaspoon ground cinnamon

3 cloves garlic, minced

½ cup water

2 teaspoons salt

1 teaspoon ground black pepper

2 pounds chicken livers

PREPARATION

1. In a large saucepan over medium heat, cook oil and onion until onion is translucent, about 5 minutes.

2. Mix in tomato paste, cumin, paprika, cinnamon, garlic, water, salt, and pepper. Cook, stirring occasionally, until mixture boils.

3. Add livers and stir gently to coat completely with sauce. Reduce heat to low, cover, and cook for 45 minutes.

4. Serve immediately, or cool to room temperature, transfer to an airtight container, and refrigerate for up to 24 hours. Reheat gently before serving.

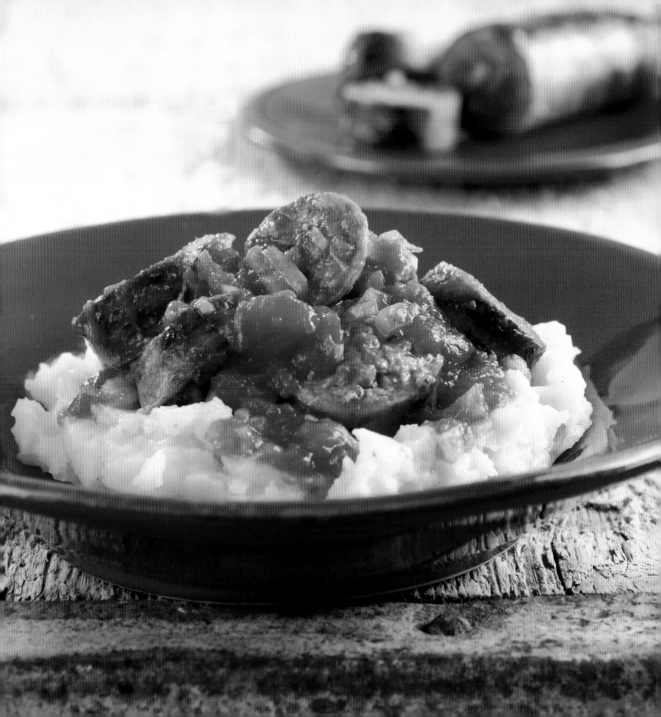

ROASTED LAMB WITH CHERRY TOMATOES

Celebrate a festive occasion with this impressive dish.

INGREDIENTS

Serves 4

2 whole racks of lamb

1 pound cherry tomatoes, halved

3 cloves garlic, minced

¼ cup extra-virgin olive oil

¼ cup white wine

2 teaspoons salt

2 teaspoons freshly ground black pepper

1 tablespoon chopped fresh thyme

PREPARATION

1. Preheat oven to 450°F. Place lamb in a roasting pan.

2. In a large bowl, mix together all remaining ingredients. Pour over lamb and cover with aluminum foil. Bake for 20 minutes.

3. Remove foil, reduce heat to 400°F, and bake for another 20 minutes.

4. Remove from oven and let rest for about 5 minutes. Transfer lamb to a cutting board and slice to separate the ribs. Arrange ribs on serving dishes, pour pan sauce over top, and serve immediately.

Opposite: Roasted Lamb with Cherry Tomatoes

CHICKEN WINGS IN SPICY TOMATO SAUCE

Make this appetizer when you're expecting a group of hungry football fans at your house.

INGREDIENTS

Serves 4

¼ cup tomato paste

2 cloves garlic, minced

1 tablespoon soy sauce

1 tablespoon honey

2 teaspoons salt

1 tablespoon extra-virgin olive oil

2 pounds (about 12) chicken wings

PREPARATION

1. Preheat oven to 400°F. In a large bowl, whisk together tomato paste, garlic, soy sauce, honey, salt, and oil.

2. Rinse chicken wings and pat dry. Add to bowl and mix gently with a large wooden spoon to coat.

3. Transfer to a deep baking dish and bake, turning occasionally and brushing with sauce, for 25 minutes, until wings are a deep brown color.

4. Serve immediately, or cool to room temperature, transfer to an airtight container, and refrigerate for up to 2 days. Reheat before serving.

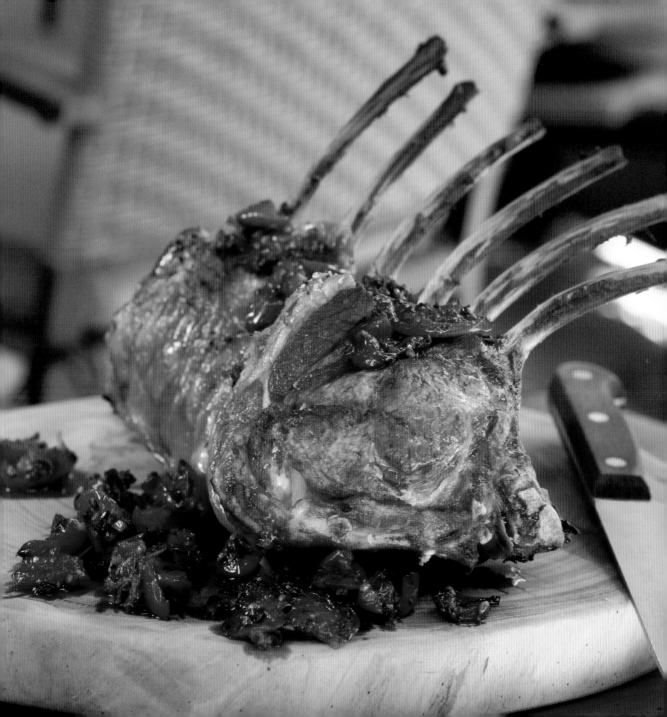

COUSCOUS WITH TOMATOES AND CHICKEN

Couscous is a Middle Eastern staple made from semolina wheat.
Traditional couscous takes hours to prepare, but instant couscous is an excellent
(and easy) alternative.

INGREDIENTS

Serves 4

3 cups water

2 cups instant couscous

3 tablespoons extra-virgin
olive oil

1 tablespoon plus 2 teaspoons
salt

3 cloves garlic, minced

½ pound chicken breast, cut
into strips

3 large tomatoes, cut into
½-inch cubes

2 teaspoons freshly ground
black pepper

1 teaspoon paprika

1 tablespoon chopped fresh
parsley

1 tablespoon finely chopped
scallion

1 tablespoon chopped fresh
cilantro

PREPARATION

1. In a medium pot, bring water
to a boil. Remove from heat and
add couscous, 1 tablespoon oil,
and 1 tablespoon salt. Cover and
set aside for 30 minutes.

2. In a medium pot over
medium heat, heat remaining
2 tablespoons oil. Add garlic and
chicken and cook, stirring
occasionally, for 5 minutes.

3. Add tomatoes, remaining
2 teaspoons salt, pepper, and
paprika. Cook for 10 minutes,
stirring occasionally.

4. Remove from heat and mix in
parsley, scallion, and cilantro.

5. To serve, transfer couscous to
serving dishes, top each dish
with a few strips of chicken, and
pour over a generous spoonful
of sauce.

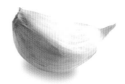

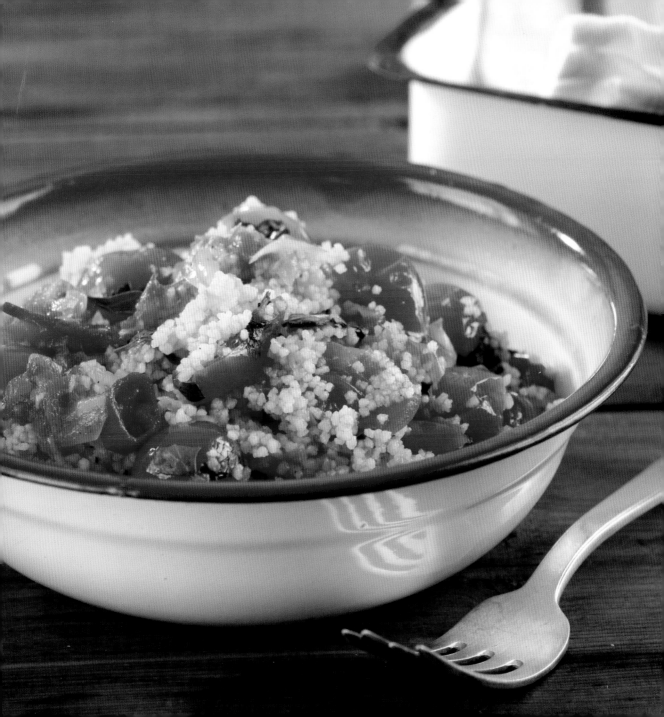

INDEX